500 Health
Questions Answered

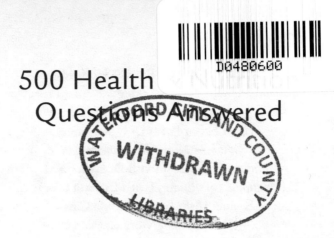

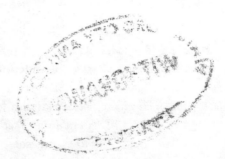

Other books by Patrick Holford

Optimum Nutrition Before, During and After Pregnancy
(with Susannah Lawson)
The H Factor (with Dr James Braly)
Optimum Nutrition for the Mind
Natural Highs Chill (with Dr Hyla Cass)
Natural Highs Energy (with Dr Hyla Cass)
Natural Highs (with Dr Hyla Cass)
The Optimum Nutrition Bible
100% Health
Beat Stress and Fatigue
Say No to Cancer
Say No to Heart Disease
Say No to Arthritis
Improve Your Digestion
Balancing Hormones Naturally (with Kate Neil)
Boost Your Immune System (with Jennifer Meek)
Supplements for Superhealth
The Optimum Nutrition Cookbook (with Judy Ridgway)
The 30-Day Fatburner Diet
Six Weeks to Superhealth
The Little Book of Optimum Nutrition
The Low-GI Diet Bible
The Holford Low-GL Diet
The Holford Diet GL Counter
The Holford Low-GL Diet Made Easy
The 10 Secrets of 100% Healthy People
The Feel Good Factor

500

Top Health & Nutrition Questions Answered

Patrick Holford

piatkus

PIATKUS

First published in Great Britain in 2004 by
Piatkus Books Ltd

Reprinted 2004, 2006, 2007, 2008, 2011

Copyright © 2004 by Patrick Holford

The moral right of the author has been asserted.

A catalogue record for this book is available from
the British Library.

ISBN 978 0 7499 2493 5

Edited by Barbara Kiser
Text design by Jerry Goldie

Papers used by Piatkus are natural, renewable and recyclable
products sourced from well-managed forests and certified
in accordance with the rules of the Forest Stewardship Council.

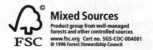 **Mixed Sources**
Product group from well-managed
forests and other controlled sources
www.fsc.org Cert no. SGS-COC-004081
© 1996 Forest Stewardship Council

Typeset by Phoenix Photosetting, Chatham, Kent
Printed and bound in Great Britain by
CPI Mackays, Chatham, ME5 8TD

CONTENTS

Contents

Contents

Contents

This book is dedicated to Joseph Goodman,
a warrior for the truth, for optimum nutrition and for
a healthier, happier future for us all.
Thank you Joe.

Disclaimer

While all the nutrients and dietary changes referred to in this book have been proven safe, those seeking help for specific medical conditions are advised to consult a qualified nutrition therapist, clinical nutritionist, doctor or equivalent health professional. The recommendations given in this book are solely intended as education and information, and should not be taken as medical advice. Neither the authors nor the publisher accept liability for readers who choose to self-prescribe.

All supplements should be kept out of reach of infants and young children.

Guide to Abbreviations and Measurements

Most vitamins are measured in milligrams or micrograms. Vitamins A, D and E used to be measured in International Units (ius) however are now officially measured in mcgs or mgs. I've included both measures to avoid confusion.

1 gram (g) = 1,000 milligrams (mg) = 1,000,000 micrograms (mcg)
1mcg of retinol (1mcg RE) = 3.3ius of vitamin A
1mcg RE of beta-carotene = 6mcg of beta-carotene
100ius of vitamin D = 2.5mcg
100ius of vitamin E = 67mg

The best form of amino acids are the 'l-' form eg l-glutamine, l-lysine. Throughout this book I refer only to the amino acid name eg *glutamine* or *lysine*. When you buy a supplement do, however, check you are getting the l- form.

ACKNOWLEDGEMENTS

I'd like to thank the thousands of people who have sent in their questions, Susannah Lawson and Shane Heaton for helping me research and answer them, Barbara Kiser for organising and editing, and Anna Crago, Gill Bailey and everyone at my publishers Piatkus.

ALLERGIES

An astonishing one in three of us is allergic to some-thing, and approximately half of all allergies are food allergies. So if you have one or suspect you do – whether it's to pollen, peanuts, shellfish, milk or wheat – you're hardly alone.

With an allergy, the immune system produces a protein called an antibody to fight off the allergen that's causing the problem. In a 'classic' allergy, an antibody called IgE is produced, triggering the release of a chemical, histamine, that usually causes a rapid, severe reaction such as swelling of the mucous mem-branes. More common are allergic reactions involv-ing the IgG antibody. This type can cause a delayed reaction – sometimes called a 'food intolerance' – up to 24 hours after exposure to the allergen. While not as obviously dramatic as a classic allergic reaction, a food intolerance can seriously erode your wellbeing. Luckily, it's easy to get to grips with, as you'll find in this section.

General

Q *Why do people get allergies and why do allergies sometimes come on in later life?*

A One man's food is another's poison. This means some of us react to certain foods while others do not. Why this happens is still largely shrouded in mystery, but we do have a pretty good idea of how it happens. First, if foods are introduced too early into a child's diet, their immature immune systems can mistake innocuous foods for harmful invaders and set off an immune response to protect them from the 'attack'. The resulting symptoms are the allergic reaction. It's no coincidence that dairy products and wheat, two of the most common foods fed to infants (as formula and rusks), cause problems in many of them.

Trouble can also hit further along the road. Some adults can eat certain foods for years with no problem, then suddenly start reacting to them. This can happen for a variety of reasons. Perhaps they've eaten too much of a given food – not a rare occurrence these days with wheat, for example. Just think how many people start the day with toast or wheat-based cereal, grab a sandwich for lunch and then settle down to a plate of pasta for dinner! Also, as we age, our stomach acid levels fall and we tend not to chew and digest our food so well. Our digestive system is meant to break food down into molecules, which can be readily used by the body. Poor digestion, however, means fragments of food can enter the bloodstream, where they're treated as hostile invaders by our immune system's scout cells. The same thing can happen if you have a 'leaky' gut, where the intestinal tract lining has become too permeable to do its job properly. Stress, nutrient deficiencies, alcohol and some drugs can all contribute to this condition.

In all these ways, your body can become sensitive to certain foods, and continuing to eat them will mean your body goes on eliciting the same reaction due to its immunological memory.

Q *What do you recommend for someone with lots of allergies?*

A With allergies, it's important to remember that the problem is usually not the food, but how your body is reacting to it – and that means inflammation. This is particularly obvious when you've got a long list of allergies. So controlling inflammation nutritionally is key. It's important to reduce your intake of meat (such as chicken and lamb) and dairy, while upping the amounts of anti-inflammatory foods you eat, including oily fish (sardines, herring, mackerel, organically farmed or wild salmon) and seeds (flax, sunflower and pumpkin). You can also supplement fish oils, ideally 1 gram a day giving 300mg of EPA and 200mg of DHA, and such excellent natural anti-inflammatory herbal remedies as boswellia, from Indian frankincense, and curcumin, from turmeric and ginger. Try avoiding wheat and eat oat or rice cakes instead for 10 days, as wheat can irritate the gut and make you more prone to other sensitivities. Most importantly, get yourself tested with a proper food intolerance blood test.

It's also possible you have a condition called 'leaky gut', where stress, alcohol and other factors make the lining of the intestine increasingly permeable; when this happens, fragments rather than molecules of food can enter the bloodstream, where the immune system treats them as invaders. To treat a leaky gut, you need to strictly avoid foods you are sensitive to, and repair the gut lining with nutrients such as glutamine. It's best to work with a nutritional therapist who can test you for allergies and intolerances, check if you have leaky gut and design a programme to meet your particular needs.

Q **I wake up with a blocked nose and often feel blocked up after a meal. Is this an allergy?**

A It's highly likely. Excessive mucus is an inflammatory – and thus allergic –reaction, probably to something you ate the night before. The top two suspects are wheat and milk, the two foods that trigger the most allergies. Avoid both for 10 days and notice what happens. During this time it's best to avoid alcohol too. A few drinks at night, especially beer and wine, can also leave you feeling blocked up in the morning. If you're still blocked up after the 10-day period, try to locate the real culprit by doing the same avoidance test with the foods you eat most of, one by one.

Q *Every spring I get terrible hay fever. What can I do?*

A Even though allergic reactions to pollen are the cause of hay fever, other factors make one person more likely to sneeze than another. For example, after it was realised that hay fever cases have risen dramatically in cities, compared to rural areas, researchers discovered that pollutants such as exhaust fumes prime the immune system to react.

To combat the itching, sneezing and misery of hay fever, take a good all-round antioxidant supplement containing vitamin A, C, E, beta-carotene, selenium and zinc, plus the amino acids cysteine or glutathione, to increase your resistance. The amino acid methionine in combination with calcium is a very effective antihistamine. You need to supplement 500mg of methionine with 400mg of calcium, twice a day. Vitamin C, 1g a day, also helps to control excessive histamine levels, as does vitamin B5 (pantothenic acid) at 500mg a day.

The three most common allergy-provoking substances are pollen, wheat and milk. Intriguingly, all these substances are either a grass, or a product of grass. It may be that some hay fever sufferers become sensitised to proteins that are common to grains, grasses and possibly milk. Some people report remarkable relief by avoiding wheat and dairy products during hay fever season.

Food allergies

Q *If I eat something I'm allergic to, what does it do to my body?*

A Allergic reactions range from the barely noticeable to the extremely severe, up to and including death. In essence, you body has developed an over-sensitivity to the molecular structure of a certain food, inappropriately identifying it as a foreign invader, that requires a defensive response to protect you from the attack. This immune response sets off various chemical reactions in the body, often causing inflammation that can manifest in different ways in different people.

Common symptoms include headaches, diarrhoea, rashes, fatigue, mental fogginess, constipation, irritable bowel syndrome, sinus problems, acne, abdominal pain, bloating and eczema. Common conditions that are often exacerbated by food allergies include arthritis, ME, migraines and anxiety. The very severe kinds of reaction can induce vomiting, severe rashes, severe digestive problems and anaphylactic shock, and people prone to these will need to exercise great vigilance in avoiding the foods that provoke them. You can get yourself tested for food sensitivities (see Resources, page 483), though the important thing to remember is that it's not the food that's the problem, but how your body reacts to it. So considering ways to reduce your inflammatory response – such as getting sufficient omega-3 essential fats by eating oily fish, seeds and oils – is a good place to start addressing the cause of the allergy, not just the symptoms.

Q *Which type of milk is the most allergenic –*
skimmed or whole, and why?

A I'm not sure that one is more or less allergenic than
the other. I advise someone with a potential dairy
allergy/intolerance to avoid *all* dairy for 10 days and
see if there is any difference and then, when they
start eating or drinking it again, to note any changes.
I wouldn't say, 'switch to skimmed and see if that
helps'. But if you were keen to try it, you could
reintroduce skimmed milk first (and no other dairy
food) and see what happened, then three days later
reintroduce whole.

There is a theoretical reason why full fat *may* be
more allergenic, or at least appear so. It is not typi-
cally the fat that people are allergic to, but the lactose
(sugar) and/or the proteins (casein). But fats are
integral to inflammatory responses such as allergic
reactions, and the kind of fat in dairy, saturated fat, is
pro-inflammatory. If you have too many pro-
inflammatory fats, and not enough anti-inflammatory
fats (omega-3, found in seeds, oily fish and oils), you
will tend to react more to potential allergens. So in
theory, the less saturated fat in milk, the less pro-
inflammatory it is, though upping your anti-
inflammatories is just as, or more, important.

That means getting enough essential fats from oily
fish, seeds and their cold-pressed oils, and also taking
antioxidants such as vitamins A, C and E, B complex
(especially B6) and zinc. A good basic diet is essential,
so drink plenty of water, and curb your sugar intake, too.

Q **My brain seems to scramble after I've eaten bread. I can't even spell correctly! Is this an allergy?**

A This is a common feature of wheat intolerance or allergy. The ubiquitous wheat can literally make you crazy, and sadly does for a large number of people. Studies in psychiatric wards have shown again and again that wheat and other food sensitivities can produce symptoms such as severe depression, nervousness, irritability, loss of motivation and mental blankness. Many people diagnosed with schizophrenia and other mental health problems are found to have sensitivities to wheat, milk, sugar, tobacco and eggs, with wheat being the most common.

The reason for this is fascinating. Certain fragments of wheat protein, called gluten, have a molecular structure that's very similar to that of chemicals naturally occurring in our brain called endorphins and encephalins. The wheat gluten proteins (and dairy proteins too) can actually link with receptors in the frontal lobes and lower limbic regions of our brain in either a stimulatory or suppressive way, and the result is a mild to severe disruption of normal brain activity. If you suspect an allergy to wheat or any other food, avoid it strictly for 10 days and see what happens when you reintroduce it, or better still, see a nutrition consultant and ask for an IgG food intolerance test.

Q **I've read a story about wheat being a 'cereal killer'. Surely this is a myth.**

A Gluten is the substance in wheat that can cause allergic reactions. We used to believe that gluten allergy, known as coeliac disease, was extremely rare, affecting about 1 in 6,000 people. However, according to research from Italy, coeliac's disease may affect almost 1 in 100 people. In other words, it is vastly underdiagnosed. The other myth about gluten is that it only causes digestive problems such as bloating, flatulence and diarrhoea. But there is now compelling evidence that the first diagnosis of coeliac disease is often cancer of the digestive tract! Deaths from such cancers are twice as common within the first year of a coeliac's diagnosis, so perhaps 'cereal killer' is not an exaggeration.

Medical expert Dr James Braly, author of the book *Dangerous Grains*, believes that screening for gluten sensitivity should be routine for high-risk people. This includes anyone with a family member with gluten sensitivity, and people with autoimmune diseases such as insulin-dependent diabetes, rheumatoid arthritis and thyroid problems, as well as women who experience pregnancy problems such as spontaneous abortions.

Sensitivity to gluten, which is also found in rye, barley and oats, but not in rice or corn, can be tested with a simple home test kit that measures IgG antibodies (see Resources, page 483).

DIG DEEPER: Dr Braly's book *Dangerous Grains* (Avery, 2002) is available in bookshops.

Q *I get bloating sometimes – I've heard that this might be a wheat allergy. Is this true in all cases?*

A While wheat *can* be a cause of gas (see 'Why does wheat cause bloating?', page 111), bloating and flatulence can also be the result of poor digestion, dysbiosis (harbouring harmful intestinal bacteria), an overgrowth of the fungus *Candida albicans*, other allergies or parasites. Start by improving your digestion. If food is not completely broken down this provides gas-producing microorganisms in the digestive tract with more of what they like – hence more gas is produced. So the first step to solving this problem is to chew well, not eat when you're stressed, reduce your intake of wheat and other foods that you know make the problem worse, and consider supplementing digestive enzymes (see Resources, page 483) with each meal – you may not be making enough enzymes to digest your food properly. Also supplement a high strength multivitamin and mineral containing at least 10mg of zinc because zinc is needed to make stomach acid. If you improve your eating habits you may well find that, within a month, you can stop taking the digestive enzymes and stay well.

There may be other reasons. An overgrowth of candida in the gut, for example, or an excess of 'bad' gut bacteria, can all contribute to excessive wind. People taking antibiotics, which disturb the healthy balance of gut bacteria, often find they pass more wind. Correcting bacterial imbalance with probiotics or beneficial bacteria such as *Lactobacillus acidophilus* and *Bifidobacterium bifidus* often reduces this problem, although it can make matters worse in the first week as the beneficial bacteria re-establish themselves. If these steps don't work, you should see a nutrition practitioner who can assess other potential problems in your digestive system, such as parasites.

Testing

Q *How do I test myself for food intolerances?*

A Food allergies or intolerances are a common cause of fatigue, water retention, digestive problems and more. Wheat and dairy are the most common, though other foods can also be involved – check out foods you eat a lot of. You can check if these foods are a problem by either having a proper blood test or doing an exclusion diet for at least 10 days (that means absolutely no wheat, dairy or whatever you're testing, while being sure to replace them with similar foods, such as soya or rice milk for cow's), followed by a pulse test.

Here's how to do it. Take your resting pulse. Then eat more than normal of the suspect food. Retake your pulse after 10 minutes, then 30, and then 60. If it rises by more than 10 points your body is reacting to the food. Pay particular attention to symptoms over the next 72 hours. Reintroduce foods one at a time, with at least a few days apart. Do not make any other major changes at the same time.

If you do get symptoms or 10-point pulse changes, it would be best to find alternatives for at least three months. Then you can try reintroducing the food, again using the pulse test. This is because the body can 'unlearn' an allergy. Rotating a food, which means eating it every fourth or fifth day, is another way to reduce the likelihood of an allergic response.

My favourite blood test for food intolerances is called an IgG ELISA food intolerance test. This can be done from a 'home test kit' and involves a pinprick test which you then send to the laboratory, which can test it for food intolerance to a wide range of foods (see Resources, page 483, for details on these tests).

Q **I am taking Prednisolone and Methotrexate for rheumatoid arthritis, and Thyroxine for thyroid problems. Would these drugs alter the results of an allergy test?**

A When you take steroids (such as Prednisolone) or immunosuppressants (such as Methotrexate), your immune system will not register a response to allergenic foods. Thyroxine doesn't interfere, but as long as you are taking the others, there's no point in taking a test. However, as almost everyone who suffers from rheumatoid arthritis has food and chemical sensitivities that might make their symptoms flare up, I can understand your desire to do a test.

What I'd suggest therefore is eliminating suspect foods – the most common being wheat, gluten (the protein found in wheat and also barley, rye and to a lesser extent oats), dairy foods, eggs, citrus fruits, tea, coffee, chocolate and soya. Start with one food group at a time, eliminate completely for 10 days, then reintroduce and monitor the results. If all seems to be well, repeat the process with the next food group. You might also have a sensitivity to gas and exhaust fumes, so you could try avoiding these for 10 days to a month to see whether they're exacerbating your condition.

DIG DEEPER: My book *Boost Your Immune System* (Piatkus, 1998), coauthored with immunologist Jennifer Meek, explains allergies in detail and how to reduce your risk by boosting your immunity.

ANTI-AGEING

Ageing is inevitable, but the speed at which you age is not. So it's fortunate that there is a host of ways to put the brakes on wrinkles, degenerative diseases, impaired thinking and many other negative aspects of getting older. Eating the right food, for instance, powerfully affects not only on how you look and the condition of your skin, but also reduces your chances of developing age-related diseases such as diabetes and cancer. For many of us, optimum nutrition can add 10 healthy years to our lives.

Q *I'm 42 years old, and I wouldn't mind ageing a little more gracefully. Any suggestions?*

A There is much you can do to slow the ageing process. And it's quite an issue these days, with a number of gerontologists and other scientists predicting that many of us will soon be living to over 100.

One key to, as you say, growing old gracefully, is large amounts of antioxidants. Professor Denham

Harman of the University of Nebraska Medical School says that there is a 99 per cent chance that oxidants or free radicals, produced during the combustion process (anything from running a car to smoking a cigarette and barbequeing a piece of meat), cause ageing. But antioxidants – vitamin A and beta-carotene, vitamins C and E, bioflavonoids, anthocyanidins and over 100 other protectors – can mop these nasties up. I recommend taking 2g of vitamin C a day combined with two antioxidant complexes, and would increase to 3g of C and three complexes a day if you're older than 50.

Antioxidants, however, are only half the story. B vitamins control a vital process in the body called 'methylation'. This process is vital for keeping your cells young, by protecting DNA and allowing you to build healthy new cells. A high-strength multivitamin should provide optimal amounts of B vitamins.

Another key ingredient in the graceful ageing formula is exercise. Aerobic activity is essential, reducing cholesterol levels in your blood, pulse rate and blood pressure and keeping your mind sharp. So try cycling, swimming and running.

Q *Why are antioxidants so important for anti-ageing?*

A Antioxidants are especially important for ageing because they quench oxidants, often called free radicals, that damage cells and DNA. Oxidants can cause errors in structure and function in cells and DNA that we generally call symptoms of ageing, such as declining vision, wrinkling skin, poor digestion, lack of energy, a decrease in cognitive function, worsening cardiovascular health and so on. You can slow down (perhaps even reverse!) this process from both inside and out using antioxidants. Oxidation occurs from converting food into fuel in the body, and even from breathing, but you speed this process up rapidly by smoking, eating fried and burnt foods or getting too much sun.

You can slow it down by taking in large amounts of antioxidant nutrients – vitamin A from carrots and tomatoes, vitamin C from fruits and vegetables (especially broccoli and peppers), vitamin E from seeds, nuts and fish and anthocyanidins from berries and red grapes. As well as eating these foods it's well worth supplementing an antioxidant complex, the best of which contain all of these key nutrients. You can also take additional powerful antioxidants such as CoQ10 (30–60mg/day), alphalipoic acid (50–60mg/day) and pycnogenol from grape seed or pine bark extracts (50–100mg/day away from food). One of the most powerful antioxidants is the amino acid glutathione. The best antioxidant formulas also contain this.

Q **Do those antioxidant creams really stop you ageing?**

A Yes and no. Depending on the amounts of forms of the antioxidant nutrients in them, they will slow down the ageing process of your skin. But do compare the actual amounts of, say, vitamin E. For a cream to have any real benefit it should provide at least 20mg per gram. One of my favourites is Dermalogica's Multivitamin Power, (see www.dermalogica.com). This is a capsule of highly absorbent antioxidants. After piercing it, you rub the contents into the skin.

The actual ageing process of the body is to do with how perfectly your cells are replaced, since we are permanently renewing ourselves. The skin, for example, is completely new every 20 days. Antioxidants protect your DNA, the blueprint for new cells. That's why it's also important to eat foods rich in antioxidants. I also supplement an antioxidant complex every day that contains vitamin A and E, plus glutathione, which is the body's most powerful antioxidant.

B vitamins, especially B6, B12 and folic acid, also stop DNA from becoming damaged. A good wholefood diet plus a high-strength multivitamin is the best way to keep your Bs up. Strict vegetarians, watch out. There's no B12 in vegetables. You need meat, fish, eggs, dairy produce or supplements to get enough B12. Your supplement should provide at least 10mcg.

Q **Have you got any nutritional suggestions to stop greying hair?**

A The straight, honest answer to that is no (otherwise I myself may not have such distinguished tints at my temples). The colour of your hair is determined by the concentration of the pigment melanin in it. But when the melanocytes die, the pigment is broken down and the hair eventually turns white.

There is some evidence that in prematurely greying hair, a deficiency in B vitamins, especially vitamin B12, may be speeding up the natural process of greying. So it's certainly worth supplementing an all-round multivitamin or B complex supplement. But there could be other factors involved. High levels of stress or a big shock have been known to rapidly speed up greying. What is actually happening in these unusual cases is that people lose more of the non-grey hairs, so they appear to have suddenly gone grey. In truth, it takes many months for a hair to go grey. Both stress hormones and melanin, the stuff that colours hair, are derived from the amino acid tyrosine. Theoretically, reducing stress and supplementing tyrosine (1g a day) might help, but there's no hard evidence. So I would recommend you enjoy your natural, greying hair colour; quite a few women regard it as chic. Or use natural vegetable dyes to hide it, available from healthfood shops.

Q **Why is homocysteine considered an excellent predictor of all causes of death?**

A At least three out of four people die from diseases that are largely preventable. In the main, this means the big five – heart attacks, strokes, cancer, the complications of diabetes and Alzheimer's disease. If you can prevent all of these diseases you are likely to add between 10 and 20 years to your lifespan. If you live in the UK, the average lifespan is 73 if you're a man, and 79 if you're a woman. If you're American, the figures are 76 for a man and 83 for a woman. So an extra decade or two of healthy living would be quite a boon. And probably the best single measure that you are on the right track is your homocysteine level.

But first a word on homocysteine. This amino acid occurs naturally in the blood, but high levels indicate a higher risk for degenerative diseases such as heart disease. Homocysteine is kept in check by a natural process in the body called methylation, which converts it to the essential amino acid methionine. Certain nutrients and natural chemicals boost methylation, notably the B vitamins.

A comprehensive research study at the University of Bergen in Norway measured the homocysteine levels of 4,766 men and women, aged 65 to 67 in 1992, and then recorded any deaths over the next five years. What they found was that the chances of a person of 65 to 67 years dying from any cause increased by almost 50 per cent for every 5-unit increase in homocysteine! This strongly reflects how central homocysteine and methylation (and as a consequence, your nutritional status) are to the underlying causes of the common diseases that kill most of us prematurely in the 21st century. Turn this amazing finding the other way round and we can say that, for every 5-unit drop in your H score, you halve your risk of dying prematurely from all common causes. If, for example, your H score was 15, and you drop it to 6 units or less and maintain it there, you can probably add around 10 years to your life! And it would be a lively decade because, as you will see, if you lower your homocysteine level below 6 units with the proper balance of diet and supplementation, and alleviate your methylation problems, your cells will age slower, you'll have increased vitality and you'll feel younger than your years. There are tests available to check your homocysteine levels.

Q *Human growth hormone supplements are being sold on the Internet to combat ageing. Do they work?*

A Human growth hormone (HGH) is one of the many important 'neurochemicals of communication', along with the likes of DHEA, acetylcholine and serotonin. Also known as somatotrophin, HGH is produced in the pituitary gland and influences the growth of bones, cells, organs and muscles. We produce less of it as we age, hence the interest in it as an anti-ageing treatment.

Taking an optimal amount of the nutrients from which the body builds HGH is unquestionably an effective anti-ageing strategy. They include the amino acids ornithine, arginine, glutamine, glycine and tryptophan, all of which are present in protein foods. Whether or not these specific nutrients actually do create HGH (even when HGH is one of them, as the digestion process often breaks down these structures prior to absorption) is another matter. But there are more pressing concerns to do with taking HGH.

I agree with Dr Michael Colgan, who says in his book *Hormonal Health* that HGH is not candy and is usually irresponsibly recommended. It's very expensive. Some studies have shown no benefits, and side effects can include carpal tunnel syndrome, fluid retention, joint pain, pancreatitis, hyperglycaemia, insulin resistance and full-blown Type II diabetes. There are better ways to increase your growth hormone and insulin growth factor (IGF-1), which is what HGH is really used to increase, than taking HGH. One is exercise, which would also help the conditions HGH is claimed to improve, such as low energy. HGH should only be used by those with a precisely defined deficiency, tested and verified by a good endocrinologist, and only after following a nutrition and exercise programme for six months. I still believe that antioxidants plus B vitamins are the best anti-ageing strategy.

Q *How can I prevent wrinkles?*

A The major cause of skin ageing and the loss of flexibility is oxidation. This happens just from being exposed to air, but the process is really speeded up if you smoke, spend a lot of time in smoky atmospheres or do a lot of sunbathing.

You can slow oxidation down by taking in large amounts of antioxidant nutrients – vitamin A from carrots and tomatoes, vitamin C from fruits and vegetables, vitamin E from seeds and nuts and anthocyanidins from berries and red grapes. As well as eating these foods it's well worth supplementing antioxidants. Another key element is to put on a sunscreen every time you go outdoors on a hot, sunny day. This does mean sacrificing the desire to look 'tanned and healthy', but it will keep you looking younger, longer. Moisturising the skin, and drinking plenty of water, keep the skin supple by preventing dehydration, but they don't really stop the deeper oxidant damage that leads to wrinkles. Most antioxidant-rich skin creams don't penetrate deep enough into the skin to nourish the collagen, which is what stops wrinkles. (See also 'Do those antioxidant creams really stop you ageing?', p 16.)

CHILDREN'S HEALTH

Childhood is the most crucial time for good nutrition, so ensuring your child is optimally nourished is probably the most important thing a parent can do. It also helps the child establish healthy eating patterns that they too can pass on to their children.

As children's metabolism is faster than adults', they tend to respond quicker to changes in diet and nutrient levels. The teenage years are a particularly challenging time, both because of the demands of increased growth rate and sexual development on the body, and because teenagers often end up consuming a lot of junk food, fizzy drinks and alcohol. For them, optimum nutrition offers a way to vanquish acne or overweight – those bugbears of adolescence – and take charge of how they feel, look and think.

Common complaints and illnesses

Q *My teenage son has acne. Is there anything he can take, in addition to eating a healthy diet?*

A Acne is a condition which affects mainly the face, back and chest – those parts of the skin where there are hair follicles and active sebaceous glands, which produce oils or sebum. It shows up as blackheads, whiteheads and redness due to inflammation. The most common type is acne vulgaris, characterised by inflamed, pus-filled spots.

The facts that more teenage boys than girls suffer from acne and that people with no male hormones (eunuchs) do not suffer at all give some insight to the mechanisms behind it. The amount of the male hormone testosterone in the body increases at puberty (in girls too, although not as much as in boys) and triggers the production of sebum and keratin. Keratin is the main constituent of the outer layer of skin, and an excess can block pores, as can too much sebum. It has now been found that it is not just the increase in testosterone – which happens to all teenagers – but excess conversion to an even more powerful version of the hormone called DHT (dihydrotestosterone), which may bring on acne.

With the increase in keratin, a blockage forms which in turn creates a build-up of sebum behind it and shows up as a blackhead. As the pore becomes blocked, it provides an ideal breeding ground for the bacterium *Proprionibacterium acnes*, which normally lives harmlessly on the surface of our skin. *P. acnes*'s ideal party environment is one with no air and plenty of sebum to feed off – so it is easy to see how it has a field day and creates an infection in the skin, causing the inflammation and soreness of a spot. If this inflammation gets out of hand, it can spread through to deeper tissues and, if it does not break through to the surface, it causes a cyst under the skin.

The main consideration diet-wise is to ensure an all-round healthy diet which focuses on plenty of fresh vegetables and fruit, and wholegrains with some protein in the form of fish, lean meat, soya products and beans or lentils. Sugary, processed and fatty foods should be avoided. He should drink six to eight glasses of pure water daily and keep alcohol to a minimum and use a pH balanced skin cleanser. As far as supplements are concerned, make sure he is supplementing at least 3,000mcg (10,000ius) of vitamin A (retinol), 25mg of zinc and 200mcg of chromium daily. Probiotic supplements can also help, especially if your son has been treated with antibiotics.

Q *What's the best way to stop a child from developing allergies?*

A To keep your child allergy-free, you need to start when they are still a baby. Ideally, breastfeed exclusively for at least the first four months (cow's milk formula is more allergenic because its protein molecules are much larger than those in human milk, and so are seen as invaders by the immune system). Don't begin to wean until at least four, and preferably six, months, as your baby's digestive tract is not mature enough to handle solid food and any food can trigger an allergic reaction. At the start of weaning, give your baby food that is very easily digested – cooked, puréed vegetables and fruits are a good start. Also introduce foods one at time to check for any possible reaction. This could be anything from a skin rash or eczema, excessive sleepiness, a runny nose, an ear infection, dark circles under the eyes, excessive thirst, overactivity or asthmatic breathing. If you notice anything amiss, stop giving that food and then introduce another once the reaction has died down. You can doublecheck your observations a few months later when the reaction may have disappeared as the digestive system matures. To help you, here's a list starting with the least allergenic foods to feed your baby. Omit too, for as long as possible, any others that you suspect may not suit your baby – for example, because there is a family history of allergy or because you developed an intolerance while you were pregnant.

From 4 to 6 months
- Vegetables, except tomatoes, potatoes, peppers and aubergines (from the same family as the deadly nightshade)
- Fruits (except citrus)
- Pulses and beans
- Rice, quinoa, millet and buckwheat
- Fish (preferably organic or wild)

From 9 months
- Meat and poultry (preferably organic)
- Oats, corn, barley and rye

- Live yoghurt
- Nightshade family vegetables (tomatoes, potatoes, peppers and aubergines)
- Eggs
- Soya (such as tofu or soya milk)

From 12 months
- Citrus fruits
- Wheat
- Dairy products
- Nuts and seeds (but not peanuts – wait as long as you can before introducing these, and then, only organic varieties)

Once you've established a varied mix of foods that cause no reaction, it's then important to vary the diet as much as possible, especially with commonly allergenic foods such as wheat, dairy, soya and citrus fruits. Eating the same thing over and over again long term can overtax the system and induce an allergy. But also, a varied diet will expand your child's desire for a wider range of foods – and this will ensure they're getting a broader range of nutrients.

Q *My child's asthma is worse in the city. What can I do about this?*

A Apart from moving to the country, there are measures you can take. But first, a look at urban pollution . . .

Pollution in cities is known to exacerbate

asthma and now 1 in 5 children display asthmatic symptoms. Because it is harder to avoid than other contributors such as food intolerances, the first step is to make sure you're easing the burden where you can to reduce your child's respiratory sensitivity. Essential fats are also essential for asthmatic sufferers, so these are your starting points – avoid food intolerances and increase essential fats. Either give him a ground dessertspoon of flax seed on his morning cereal, or three servings a week of oily fish such as mackerel, sardines, organically farmed or wild salmon or trout. (See below for supplementation advice.)

Avoid going out on particularly smoggy days, such as when temperature inversions trap smog-laden air close to the ground. Extremes in temperature can make breathing more difficult, so again, avoid going out in extremely hot or cold weather, when going in and out of vehicles and/or buildings can result in huge temperature fluctuations. Help your child improve their breathing capacity though exercise, especially swimming.

You can also train your child in the Buteyko method of breathing (see www.nwbuteyko.com). Another brilliant way to improve breathing was invented by a life-long asthma sufferer called Frank Goddard. Frank invented a highly effective lung exercise tube that trains you to breathe in a way that helps bring oxygen to the brain and reduce the symptoms of asthma. These tubes cost very little and are available to order from www.diyhealth.co.uk. Follow the asthma supplementation recommendations listed on page 139, especially vitamin C (2g a day), magnesium (300mg a day), and omega-3 fish oils (1,000mg a day). Give a quarter of these amounts to a child under 6, and half these amounts to a child aged 6 to 12.

Q   *Is there anything I can give my child to speed up recovery from an asthma attack?*

A   The mineral magnesium, which is a natural relaxant, has been shown to help some asthma sufferers. It's thought that it helps to relax the restricted airways in the bronchioles leading to the lungs. One study showed that people given magnesium through a drip recovered three times faster from an asthma attack. You can give your child 300mg of magnesium a day to help prevent attacks and pop 300mg if they start to feel wheezy.

It's ideal, of course, to avoid having an attack in the first place. All sorts of foods can trigger attacks, most commonly dairy products, wheat and yeast, so avoiding these could help. Many people with asthma find that taking the omega-6 oil GLA, found in evening primrose or starflower oil, helps because of its anti-inflammatory effects. Give the child 150mg twice a day. Although there is little research on asthma and omega 3 fats, these are very powerful anti-inflammatories and I'd recommend also supplementing 1 gram of fish oil providing 300mg of EPA and DHA. Some supplements combine GLA, EPA and DHA so you can kill two birds with one stone.

Q *My son is four and still has trouble controlling his bladder. Are there any nutritional or alternative therapies that may help?*

A If your son is still wetting his bed, this could be due to a food allergy, a weak bladder or a persistent bladder infection. Diabetes is another possible cause, usually accompanied by excessive thirst. It is worth seeing your GP to discover whether he has an infection. If not, you should see a urologist to rule out the possibility of his having a weak or very small bladder. Try and discover whether he is allergic to a certain food or foods. Bear in mind that wheat, dairy, eggs, citrus, chocolate and soya are among the most common allergens. You could try excluding one group from his diet at a time. Start with one food, eliminate completely for 10 days, then reintroduce it and monitor the results. If all seems to be well, repeat the process with the next food group. You can also test for allergies.

Q *My daughter keeps getting colds or infections. What should I do?*

A Make sure her diet is rich in immune-boosting nutrients. These include foods with abundant antioxidants,

such as sweet potatoes, apricots and carrots for vitamin A; berries, kiwis and green leafy vegetables for
vitamin C; avocados, nuts and seeds for vitamin E; fish
and pumpkin seeds for zinc; and broccoli and Brazil
nuts for selenium. Helping your child eat a varied diet
will also ensure she is getting a wide range of nutrients – not just vitamins and minerals, but also powerful immune-boosting phytochemicals such as
flavonoids, found in berries, and lycopene, found in
tomatoes. If she's fussy (and even if she's not), I'd recommend giving her a children's multivitamin and
mineral formula to ensure she's getting optimum levels of all the nutrients she needs.

As well as putting good stuff in her diet, take any
bad stuff out. This includes refined or processed foods
and anything loaded with sugar or additives, which
all suppress immunity. Instead of fizzy drinks, give
your child plenty of water to drink to help flush out
toxins and stop her from becoming dehydrated,
which can prevent her body functioning effectively.
Also, check her diet for any possible allergens, which
can weaken the immune system. Is she eating or craving lots of wheat, eggs or dairy, for example? If you
suspect she's having a reaction, remove the suspect
foods from her diet (substitute alternatives such as
corn or rye bread instead of wheat, and soya or rice
milk instead of cow's) and see if there's any improvement after 10 days. If not, reintroduce one food at a
time and watch for any negative reaction.

If your child has been taking lots of antibiotics,
her delicate gut flora may be disturbed, and this can

undermine her immune system. So give a daily 'probiotic' supplement for a month or so to replenish levels of healthy bacteria. (See Resources, page 483, for suppliers.)

Finally, when your child succumbs to an infection, help them fight it off quicker with extra vitamin C. Stir 100 to 200mg of vitamin C powder into a glass of water or diluted juice and give it four to six times a day until they are well (and then, gradually reduce the dose over the next few days). If your child develops loose bowel movements (a possible side effect), decrease the dose slightly.

Q *My daughter suffers from chronic constipation, even though she eats plenty of fruit and vegetables and drinks lots of fluid. Any suggestions?*

A If her diet is good – that is, she's eating plenty of naturally high-fibre foods such as fresh fruit and vegetables, beans, lentils and wholegrains such as oats and brown rice, and drinking 1.5 litres of water a day – then perhaps something she's eating is aggravating her digestive tract. The most common suspect is wheat, so try eliminating all wheat from her diet (bread, cereals, crackers, biscuits, cakes and so on), and substitute rye bread, oat cereals, oatcakes, etc., instead. If there's no improvement after 10 days, you could extend this to all gluten grains (that's wheat plus rye, barley and oats) for a further 10 days. Healthfood shops sell gluten-free products to use as substitutes.

Alongside this, you could try soaking a tablespoon of golden linseeds (from healthfood shops) in a glass of water overnight and giving it to her to drink in the morning. A good multivitamin and mineral with magnesium (needed for muscle contractions, so helps with peristalsis) and vitamin C will also help provide the nutrients she needs for a healthy gut. A daily probiotic containing 'friendly' bacteria that aid digestive health would be a good idea too. If there's still no improvement, I'd take her to visit a nutritional therapist, who can do a test to check on the balance of bacteria in her gut and check for parasites.

Q *What supplements would you recommend for a toddler with intestinal colic and loose stools?*

A Since these are both digestive problems I'd start with a probiotic supplement which provides the beneficial bacteria needed for good gut health. These are known to prevent over-loose bowels. Children's needs are slightly different from adults' because they have slightly different strains of bacteria in their digestive tracts, so special probiotics have been made for them. (See Resources, page 483, for suppliers.) The label will tell you how much to give depending on the age of your child. If that doesn't work, try a level teaspoon of glutamine powder dissolved in any liquid, last thing at night, which can help soothe and heal the gastrointestinal lining. You may benefit from seeing a nutritional therapist who could assess the underlying causes of the colic in your child, which could be food intolerance, poor digestion or insufficient fibre.

Q *My son keeps getting ear infections. What can I do about it?*

A It's ironic that ear infections tend to recur after a course of antibiotics – which most doctors will recommend for them. In fact, a child is five times more likely to get another similar infection after taking antibiotics. So instead, I recommend seeking out and dealing with the root cause.

A common trigger for ear infections is an allergy to dairy products. This causes excess mucus to form in the ear, and block the Eustachian tube between the sinuses and the ears. Eventually this will lead to infection. Try cutting milk, yoghurt, cheese, ice cream and anything else made with milk from your son's diet. There are several alternatives to milk, including soya and rice milk. And there are also natural ways of warding off ear infections in their early stages. One is to ensure your son's immune system is doing its job by giving him a good multivitamin that contains zinc; check the label. Dishes that contain onions and garlic, such as pasta sauces, are another excellent immune strengthener. You can also get ear drops that are made from organic aloe or grapefruit seed extract. These can help when he has an infection.

Q *My five-year-old daughter and I both suffer from eczema. Are there any natural remedies that can help?*

A Since you and your daughter both have the condition, suggesting an inherited tendency, an inability to process certain fats properly may be an underlying cause. One way to get round this could be to take supplements of essential fatty acids (EFAs) – either GLA at 250mg daily (in evening primrose and starflower oils) or EPA and DHA, which are fish oils. My favourite essential fat supplements contain all three – GLA, EPA and DHA. Also eat plenty of EFA-rich foods such as fish and seeds (pumpkin, sunflower, sesame and so on). Another important consideration is the possibility of reactions to foods – cow's milk and eggs are two of the most common allergens; others are peanuts and wheat.

Certain drug-free creams can help relieve the soreness and itching. Try an MSM cream or an aloe vera gel, although use this with care, as some people are sensitive to it, especially if the skin is broken.

Q *My one-year-old baby has gastrointestinal reflux and has vomited and had constipation since birth. What can I do?*

A Reflux due to slow formation of the oesophageal sphincter (which separates the stomach from the oesophagus) is common in young infants, but most have grown out of this condition by the age of one. Milk intolerance could be the cause, so I'd suggest eliminating dairy products from his diet. If he's had antibiotics, it would be wise to supplement a probiotic to replenish the good bacteria in the gut that's often knocked out by antibiotics – an imbalance can often cause both nausea and constipation. Children's probiotics differ from adults', and good ones are available – see Resources, page 483.

Q *My son has growing pains and often wakes at night. What can we do to help him?*

A This is not uncommon. From a nutritional perspective, ensure an optimal intake of all the nutrients that help the bones to develop. These are calcium, magnesium, zinc and vitamin D. Eggs and fish are rich in vitamin D, but it is also made in the skin when you're out in the sun. All the others are plentiful in seeds. I therefore recommend you give your son a daily heaped dessertspoon of ground seeds, half flax (rich in omega-3 fats), and half any combination of sunflower, sesame or pumpkin seeds. You can add this to his breakfast. I'd also recommend a children's chewable supplement.

A lack of these essential nutrients could explain why he wakes up at 3 a.m. with pains. Another possibility is that he isn't getting enough food for dinner and is waking up hungry; or is anxious, in which case the magnesium in the seeds will help to calm him.

Q *My child has difficulty getting to sleep. Any suggestions?*

A There are a number of things you can do. First, boost levels of the mineral magnesium, which aids relaxation and peaceful sleep. Dark green leafy vegetables are one of the best sources of magnesium – and that includes chard, kale, broccoli, wheatgrass, watercress, parsley and Chinese greens, but not spinach, as the oxalic acid it contains blocks absorption. Also excellent are organic pumpkin seeds, almonds, molasses, brown rice and other wholegrains, especially buckwheat. In truth, magnesium is found in most vegetables, though the levels have declined by around 24 per cent in the last 60 years according to official UK food composition tables. So buy organic where possible and be sure to include lots of magnesium-rich foods in your child's diet.

Next, limit foods that can interfere with sleep and cause hyperactive behaviour. These include foods or drinks containing excess sugar, artificial colourings or additives. If your child craves sweetness, give them fresh fruit or desserts sweetened with honey or magnesium-rich molasses.

You can also try altering the environment in your child's bedroom with light and smell. We now know that the most powerful sedative drugs, such as Valium, affect smell receptors in the brain. These receptors can be naturally stimulated using essential oils, instead of drugs, with almost instant results and no down side. Most effective are lavender, bergamot, marjoram, sandalwood, rosewood and chamomile, which soothe the senses and help aid peaceful sleep. You can burn any of these in an essential oil burner, mixed with a little water. Ideally do this an hour or so before your child goes to bed so their bedroom is full of the aroma. Blue light is also very relaxing and has been shown to aid sleep, so you may also want to try putting a bulb in a lamp you can use once your child's in bed.

Diet and nutrition

Q *My child refuses food and has a poor appetite. Why is this?*

 First, rule out any possible infection or illness, as children will often refuse food when they are unwell. So visit your doctor or a nutritional therapist who can assess their current state of health. Also check their zinc status. As well as poor appetite, do they also have white marks on more than two fingernails, any stretch marks, a poor immune system (in other words, do they often succumb to infections), or appear listless or depressed? If so, supplement their diet with a multivitamin and mineral formula containing zinc. Biocare produce a good range of liquid supplements formulated for children and will advise on the correct dose for your child's age. (See Resources, page 483.)

If all appears well, next assess whether the food you are giving your child is attractive and appetising. If they refuse whole food groups, for example vegetables, check that you are serving an appealing selection of colours, tastes and textures. A rainbow of stir-fried veg is more likely to whet their appetite than overcooked carrots or limp-looking beans.

Finally, take the emotion out of mealtimes. The majority of food fads are emotionally driven – they are often vehicles for your child to get attention or assert their independence. So the fewer emotions you display at the table, the better. For example, try not to give out lashings of praise for an empty bowl, and don't appear too hurt when your lovingly prepared vegetable casserole goes uneaten. This way your child will learn that eating is something they do for themselves, independently, to satisfy their own appetite.

Q *My son is overweight – what can I do?*

A If you feed your son a wholesome diet that's rich in nutrients and devoid of any refined or sugary foods, as well as encouraging him to be active, then his weight should stabilise. Start his day with a filling breakfast, for example porridge, millet or quinoa flakes (available from healthfood shops) with fruit and yoghurt, or a boiled egg with wholemeal toast. For lunch and supper, give lean meat or vegetable protein (tofu and other soya products, cheese or other dairy), with wholegrains and plenty of vegetables, and mimimise any fried foods. If he craves something sweet, offer fresh fruit. If he feels hungry between meals (and children often need frequent food injections to keep their energy levels up), give snacks that balance carbohydrate with protein, which will slow down their absorption and provide a more sustained level of energy. Try giving an oatcake with some peanut butter or hummus; an apple with 10 almonds; a mini-sandwich of free-range, organic chicken on rye. Instead of sugar and caffeine-loaded fizzy drinks, dilute fruit juice with sparkling mineral water.

But don't deprive your child of all treats – you don't want them to feel as though they are being punished. Just be specific about when and how much they can have. Finally, ensure your child's diet is supplemented with a good multivitamin and mineral providing all the B vitamins and chromium, which work together to manage how much food is burned for energy and how much is stored as fat. If there's any deficiency, this process can become sluggish.

If, after following this advice and doing regular exercise, your child's weight has not stabilised, consult a nutritional therapist who can work with you to rule out other issues such as food allergy or poor digestion.

 How can I get my sons to eat vegetables?

Initially by means of subterfuge. Add grated or mashed vegetables to mince, casseroles, burgers, pasta sauces and soups. As you're doing this, mount a PR campaign to get your children more involved in shopping and cooking so they take a greater interest in the wonderful world of fresh produce. Research by the British Food Council shows that children are more willing to eat the food they themselves have chosen. So try asking your sons to pick out some fruit and vegetables in the supermarket. Children also love colour, so appeal to this sense by introducing them to multicoloured vegetable varieties (but perhaps don't catagorise them as such, just call them by their individual names) – red beetroot, orange sweet potatoes and squash, yellow peppers and courgettes, pink and green chard, white and lime-green chicory. Show them that vegetables mean more than boiled peas.

Q **What should my daughter drink and how much water should I give her a day?**

A Our bodies are made largely of water, so ensuring a regular supply is essential for cells, organs and tissues to function. The brain too is also dependent on water – even mild dehydration can interfere with concentration and cause headaches. Up until the age of two, pure water is the best thing you can give your child – aim to give between 1 to 2 pints of boiled or filtered water each day. But don't wait for your child to ask – by the time she registers she is thirsty, she is already dehydrated.

A diet rich in fruit and vegetables will also provide water in a very available form, so make sure your child eats five or more servings each day. But don't be tempted to give juice – fruit juice is rich in natural sugars but low in fibre (as the flesh and skin have been removed), so can cause a sudden energy surge as well as harming developing teeth. Your child only needs to drink water or milk for the first few years, then can also have juice diluted with 50 per cent water. By this stage, she will also be used to drinking water and so should continue the habit through life.

Drugs and vaccinations

Q *What do you think about giving children antibiotics – and would you recommend any herbal alternatives?*

A From time to time, antibiotics are essential to save life. The problem is that with overuse, bacteria are developing resistance, and there are now superbugs that are resistant to even the strongest antibiotics. Antibiotics also kill off healthy bacteria, so causing an imbalance in the delicate gut flora. Over the long term this can lead to digestive problems and food allergies, and has even been linked with attention deficit hyperactivity disorder (ADHD).

So I recommend that you only give your child a course of antibiotics if they are really necessary (that is, not for a cold). Better still would be to boost their immune system by giving them a nutrient-rich diet. So feed your child antioxidant-rich foods such as sweet potatoes and carrots (vitamin A), berries, kiwi fruits and green leafy vegetables (vitamin C), avocados (vitamin E), fish (zinc) and broccoli (selenium). Ensuring your child eats a varied diet will also ensure he or she is getting a wide range of nutrients – not just vitamins and minerals, but also powerful immune-boosting phytochemicals such as flavonoids found in berries and lycopene in tomatoes. Giving your child plenty of water will help to flush out any toxins and prevent them becoming dehydrated, which can prevent their body functioning effectively. Limit refined carbohydrates and sugar – research shows that sugar suppresses our immune systems. One study published in the *American Journal of Clinical Nutrition* found that participants experienced a 50 per cent reduction in the activity of white blood cells (vital soldiers in the immune army) for two hours after ingesting a sugar solution.

Giving beneficial bacteria such as *Lactobacillus acidophilus* and *Bifidobacteria bifidum* helps the body fight off bugs, especially stomach bugs. There are plenty of probiotic supplements in powder form, which you can mix with water or juice and which are specifically designed for children. (See Resources, page 483.)

 What's your view on the MMR vaccination?

The party line is that there's no good evidence of any risk that the MMR vaccine causes autism in children. And there's some truth to this. The research by Dr Andrew Wakefield at the Royal Free Hospital in

London – which suggests that the vaccine damages the gut and causes toxins to enter the brain, triggering autism – is the first hint of a problem, and it's too early to jump to conclusions. But that doesn't mean it's not important. No one really knows the full consequences of giving a child three immune attacks – mumps, measles and rubella – all at the same time. This simply doesn't occur in nature. Some children with autism do show evidence of chronic measles infection months after the MMR vaccine is given.

I suspect that, in some children whose immune systems are already weakened, perhaps those susceptible to food allergies and infections, these triple vaccines could be the last straw. For most, I doubt it's a problem.

Of course, the last thing the medical profession wants is a whole lot of children not being vaccinated, since that increases the risk of epidemics, yet there's a logical argument for single vaccines from a reputable clinic, if a parent so chooses, especially for children with weakened immune systems. Either way, Dr Wakefield's research should be followed up, not just whitewashed.

Q *Is it safe for my four-year-old grandson, diagnosed with asthma, to have his second MMR vaccination?*

A Personally, I wouldn't recommend it. There is already evidence that some sensitive children become more prone to asthma as a consequence of vaccinations. It is certainly logical that a child whose immune system is already hypersensitive may struggle to deal with three simultaneous infections. If he were my child I would a) insist on separate vaccinations and b) for four days following the vaccination have him avoid both gluten and dairy. This is because introducing an immune reaction, which is what a vaccination does, may theoretically increase the chances of the immune system 'cross-reacting' to other proteins. Gluten and dairy proteins are the most common food proteins to which children become sensitive.

Mental health

Q *My 10-year-old son has been diagnosed with attention deficit hyperactive disorder (ADHD) and prescribed the drug Ritalin. Is there an alternative?*

A One in 10 boys are now diagnosed with ADHD, so this is a widespread condition. You are very wise to seek an alternative to drugs; one study showed that treating ADHD nutritionally was 18 times more effective than using Ritalin.

There are four key considerations. Firstly, ensure he has the right vitamin and mineral intake by giving him a multivitamin supplement. Secondly, keep his blood sugar levels balanced by eliminating sweet foods and drinks (it's surprising how many foods have added sugar), making sure he has three good meals a day providing enough good protein (such as yoghurt, fish or chicken) at each meal. Thirdly, as allergies to certain foods (most commonly wheat, dairy products or eggs) can trigger ADHD, cut these out of his diet for one week and see whether it makes a difference, and cut out food additives (especially E102, tartrazine and E165, monosodium glutamate) altogether.

Last, but certainly not least, give him a daily fish oil supplement. A supplement that contains 1,000mg of the omega-3 fat EPA – which with most brands means he will need to take three capsules a day – has been shown to help children with ADHD, based on research by Dr Alex Richardson at Oxford University. Since fish oils can be contaminated with PCBs, I only recommend those that have been tested and come out PCB-free. (See Resources, page 483.)

Q *My child has been diagnosed with autism. Can nutrition help?*

A Autism is a complex condition sharing many similarities with other conditions such as dyslexia, dyspraxia and ADHD. For a diagnosis of autism to be made, there must be some other symptoms such as difficulties with speech, abnormalities of posture or gesture, impaired understanding of the feelings of others, sensory or visual disperceptions, fears and anxieties, and behavioural abnormalities such as obsessive/compulsive behaviour and ritualistic movements.

Autism appears to be occurring more often, and while it used to occur primarily from birth, over the past 10 years there has been a dramatic increase in late-onset autism, most frequently diagnosed in the second year of life.

Here's what I recommend. Firstly, ensure that any nutrient deficiencies are addressed. Research has shown that taking care of any nutrient deficiencies can dramatically improve symptoms in autistic children. Nutrients of particular importance are vitamins B6, C and A, and zinc and magnesium. A condition called pyroluria should be suspected in children with facial swelling and with a history of frequent colds and middle ear infections and can be tested with a simple urine test. You'll need to see a nutritional therapist to have this urine test done.

Secondly, ensure adequate intake of essential fats. Research has shown that some autistic children have an enzymatic defect that removes essential fatty acids from brain cell membranes more quickly than it should. Consequently, supplementing the omega-3 fatty acid EPA, which not only compensates for the extra need but also appears to slow the activity of this enzyme, may show beneficial effects.

Thirdly, remove allergens. In addition to nutrient deficiencies, the most significant contributing factor in autism appears to be undesirable foods and chemicals that often reach the brain via the bloodstream because of faulty digestion and absorption. The foods which seem to adversely influence a large number of children include wheat and other gluten-containing grains, milk and other dairy products including casein, citrus fruits, chocolate, artificial food colourings, paracetamol, salicylates (prunes, raisins, raspberries, almonds, apricots, canned cherries, blackcurrants, oranges, strawberries, grapes, tomato sauce, plums, cucumbers and Granny Smith apples) and nightshade family foods (potatoes, tomatoes, peppers, chillies and aubergines). The strongest direct evidence of foods linked to autism involves wheat and dairy and the specific proteins they contain – namely gluten and casein. These are difficult to digest and can result in allergy, especially if introduced too early in life.

Finally, supplement probiotics for a healthy gut. A large proportion of parents of autistic children report that their child received repeated or prolonged courses of antibiotic drugs for ear or other respiratory infections during the first year of life. Such broad-spectrum antibiotics kill the good as well as the bad bacteria in the gut, weakening the intestinal membranes. Restoring a healthy gut by supplementing digestive enzymes and probiotics is known to produce positive results in autistic children. The amino acid glutamine is especially important in restoring the integrity of the digestive tract. Drinking 5g dissolved in water just before bedtime can help heal the gut.

Q *What causes autism? Is it the MMR vaccine?*

A As with many conditions, there is a debate as to whether autism is inherited or caused by something like diet or environment. Autism is four times as common in boys as it is in girls. Parents and siblings of autistic children are far more likely to suffer from milk or gluten allergy, have digestive disorders such as irritable bowel syndrome, high cholesterol, night blindness, light sensitivity, thyroid problems and cancer. Being breastfed also increases the risk. At first glance, one might suspect that autistic children may inherit certain imbalances. However, an alternative explanation might be that other family members eat the same food and may be lacking the same nutrients, and there is growing evidence that some of the nutritional approaches used to help correct dyslexia, dyspraxia and ADHD can make a significant difference to the autistic child.

Recently there has been a raging debate over the danger of the MMR vaccine causing autism in children. The official line is that there's no good evidence of such a danger, and it's too early to jump to conclusions about Dr Andrew Wakefield's research at the Royal Free Hospital, which suggests that the vaccine damages the gut and releases toxins to the brain. And for most children, the MMR vaccine is unlikely to be a problem; however, no one really knows the full consequences or giving a child three immune attacks all at the same time. This simply doesn't occur in nature, so there's a logical argument for single vaccines if a parent so chooses, especially for children with weakened immune systems. Perhaps for children with nutrient deficiencies, lacking essential fatty acids, susceptible to food allergies and/or gut problems, these triple vaccines are the last straw. My opinion is that MMR is a small part of the overall picture for most children with autism.

Q *Do autistic children ever get better?*

A Yes, without a doubt. But it takes a lot of work to identify all the contributing factors and then make the necessary changes. Most autistic children have food sensitivities, especially to gluten grains and to dairy produce. They often have gut infections and need more vitamins, minerals and essential fats.

One four-year-old diagnosed with autism was a case in point. He had serious speech and language problems, was severely behind in social and emotional development and attended special education classes for children with developmental delay. He had shown some improvement with the use of special multivitamins, minerals and DMG (dimethyl glycine) prior to visiting the clinic. He was then given comprehensive biochemical testing for deficiencies and imbalances, and was found to have low levels of five vitamins (A, beta-carotene, B3, B5 and biotin) and three minerals (magnesium, zinc and selenium). He also had low levels of omega-3 fats and GLA, an omega-6 fat, and the amino acids taurine and carnitine. His digestion was poor, he had abnormal gut flora and indications of a yeast infection. Food allergy testing showed clear sensitivity to milk products and some other foods.

He was given a special diet free from milk and

casein, a personalised supplement programme, and later some nystatin, which is an anti-fungal drug. He also started a programme of applied behaviour analysis, working with a therapist. He improved steadily and was able to attend his local primary school from the age of six. According to the Autism Research Institute's evaluation list, his improvements were: speech/language from 36 to 89 per cent; sociability from 13 to 68 per cent; sensory/cognitive awareness from 22 to 97 per cent; health/physical behaviour from 64 to 96 per cent, where 100 per cent means non-autistic behaviour.

When he was five, this child had had absolutely no interest in presents or visitors. One year after the evaluation, just before his eighth birthday, he made a list of eight presents he would like to have, including a computer. His parents told him the evening before to wake them at 7.30 a.m. on his birthday, and that's exactly what he did. During the day he couldn't wait for his friends to arrive and celebrate the special day.

I hear of many similar stories about children diagnosed with autism making incredible recoveries. But it isn't easy. It takes a lot of perseverance and good detective work to reverse this condition. A child psychologist can advise on applied behaviour analysis.

Q *Why do autistic children not look you in the eye?*

A Paediatrician Mary Megson from Richmond, Virginia, believes that many autistic children lack vitamin A. Otherwise known as retinol, vitamin A is essential for vision. It is also vital for building healthy cells in the gut and in the brain. There is no real doubt that something funny is going on in the digestive tracts of autistic children. Could this be related to vitamin A deficiency, she wondered?

The best sources of vitamin A are breast milk, organ meats, milk fat, fish and cod liver oil, none of which are prevalent in our diets. Instead, we have formula milk, fortified food and multivitamins, many of which contain altered forms of retinol such as retinyl palmitate, which doesn't work as well as the fish or animal derived retinol. Dr Megson wondered what would happen if these children weren't getting enough natural vitamin A. Not only would this affect the integrity of the digestive tract, potentially leading to allergies, but it would also affect the development of their brains, and disturb their vision. Both brain differences and visual defects have been detected in autistic children. The visual defects, she deduced, were an important clue because lack of vitamin A would mean poor black and white vision, a symptom often seen in the relatives of autistic kids.

If you can't see black and white, what you lose is shadow. Without shadow you'd lose the ability to perceive three-dimensionality and, as a consequence, you can't make sense of people's expressions so well. This might explain why autistic children tend not to look straight at you. They look to the side. Long thought to be a sign of poor socialisation, it may in fact be the best way they can see people's expressions because there are more black and white light receptors at the edge of the visual field than in the middle! They are trying to compensate for the fact that their whole visual world is fragmented snapshots.

Of course, the proof is in the pudding. Dr Megson has reported rapid and dramatic improvements in autism simply by giving cod liver oil containing natural, unadulterated vitamin A. Often she has seen results within a week. Here are some of the comments her patients have made after cod liver supplementation. 'Now I know where my fingers are.' 'Now I can see my arms at the same time I see my fingers!' 'My box is getting bigger every day. Now I can see emotion on the faces on TV.'

Q *What would you recommend for my 14-year-old grandson, who has poor concentration and short-term memory skills?*

A Impaired concentration can blight the teenage years. The problem is often down to an imbalance in blood sugar, and a diet poor in omega-3 fats. So first off, ask your grandson to take an honest look at how many sugary and starchy snacks he's eating. Like many teenagers he could be overdosing on refined carbohydrates such as potato-based snacks, or munching regularly on sweets. Stimulants are another bugbear, so he'll need to look at his tea, coffee and cola intake. All these can send blood sugar into orbit, then as suddenly cause it to crash, jeopardising his ability to concentrate as he teeters between a sugar high and total exhaustion. Try to wean him off these baddies and on to a diet higher in fresh vegetables and fruits, slow-release carbohydrates such as whole-wheat or rye bread and pasta, and high-quality proteins such as fish and free-range organic chicken. Snacking on a combination of seeds and nuts with fruit can help by balancing his protein and carbohydrate.

As for omega-3s, upping his intake of oily fish such as mackerel, herrings and salmon (organically farmed or wild) is ideal. Three times a week is a good rule. Or he can have a dessertspoon of ground flax seeds on his cereal in the morning. In addition to a good multivitamin, I would recommend a 'brain food' supplement and additional essential fats, either as a supplement or by using a blend of essential oils in/on food. (See Resources, page 483.)

DIG DEEPER: My book *Optimum Nutrition for the Mind* has several chapters on children's mental health issues, including dyslexia, dyspraxia, ADHD and autism. Also see the website www.mentalhealthproject.com

---

Supplements

Q *Should I be giving my kids supplements, and which are the best?*

A In a word, yes. As long as you remember that they are *supplementing* a good diet and not replacing one, vitamin and mineral tablets are ensuring that your child has a good supply of the full spectrum of nutrients to optimise good health and growth and minimise illness. Studies have shown that children given a good supply of nutrients perform better at school.

It's important to start out with a good-quality chewable multivitamin that contains a broad range of nutrients at adequate doses. Most brands are too low in zinc (it has a nasty taste), calcium (it makes the tablet chalky) and vitamin C (it takes up a lot of space) for my liking. But all are vital: the mineral zinc, for instance, is essential for growth and a strong immune system. So choose a multi that contains at least 6mg of zinc, the recommended amount for three- to four-year-olds, and then increase the dosage by giving more multis as your children get older. See Resources, page 483, for my favourite multis.

To take up the slack for vitamin C, I recommend giving children fresh fruit; strawberries, kiwi fruits and oranges are rich sources, as are tomatoes. Peppers and broccoli contain more vitamin C than oranges so keep feeding them their greens. An easy way of topping up their calcium is to add ground almonds or seeds to their morning bowl of cereal.

Q *I want to supplement my young children's diet with flax oil but someone told me recently that children cannot convert it to DHA and EPA. Is this true?*

A There is a difference in the way the body can use fish oils, compared to flax seed oil. The body converts the original type of omega-3 fat, known as (alpha)linolenic acid, which is the principal fat in flax seeds, into EPA and DHA, which are both found in fish oils, but not in flax. So by eating fish or taking fish oils, you are saving the body from having to do the conversion. What's more, the efficacy of the conversion is dubious in many people. The enzymes that convert linolenic acid into EPA and DHA are very underdeveloped in babies which is why breast feeding is so important and why supplying children with a direct source of EPA and DHA is essential.

Another problem with relying on taking flax seed oil is that, for an unknown reason, the linolenic acid appears to convert more readily to EPA than DHA. On average, 15 per cent of linolenic acid coverts to EPA, while only 5 per cent converts to DHA. Indeed, vegetarians have been shown to have lower levels of DHA, even if their EPA levels are adequate. Since DHA is literally a building component of the brain it is most vital in pregnancy, infancy and early childhood. It is also important to ensure a good supply of the nutrients on which the conversion enzymes depend, i.e. vitamins B3, B6 and C, biotin, zinc and magnesium, which is easily achieved by giving your child a good multivitamin and mineral supplement.

DIG DEEPER: To find out more about optimum nutrition for infants and children, I recommend my book *Optimum Nutrition Before, During and After Pregnancy* (Piatkus, 2004), coauthored by Susannah Lawson, and Lucy Burney's *Optimum Nutrition for Babies and Young Children* (Piatkus, 1999).

DETOX PROGRAMMES

The body, and most of all the liver, is permanently detoxifying. It makes safe all the breakdown products that result from 'burning' carbohydrate for energy and from utilising proteins, as well as all the potentially harmful substances that we both make and consume every day. The body spends a vast amount of time and energy keeping you safe, not only from the 'exhaust' from your normal body processes, but also from toxins in food, water and air. Much of this is done by the body's intelligent chemistry by rendering a harmful substance harmless by effectively handcuffing it to other molecules through a process called conjugation, which can then be escorted out of the body. But when you have too many toxins and an overworked liver, you start to suffer all sorts of minor, then major health problems. A detox programme that supports your liver can get you back on track.

Q **What symptoms can one expect to experience during a detoxification programme?**

A During a detox your body is 'throwing off' a lot of toxins and you can feel worse before you feel better. Some people mistakenly think they're doing the wrong thing when their symptoms worsen, though this is a short-term stage in the process and may actually be a good sign.

Common symptoms include headaches, acne, general malaise, fatigue and joint pain, though I should say that it will manifest differently in different people. If you have blood sugar problems, leaving out sugar, alcohol and other stimulants will result in blood sugar imbalance symptoms such as tiredness, poor concentration and memory, cravings, dizziness and a need for frequent meals. Detox diets aren't recommended for people with diabetes unless they include carefully measured amounts of carbohydrates. Be aware that detox symptoms should not persist for more than three to five days and often don't happen at all if you take in enough nutrients, especially antioxidants, which help the liver detoxify.

Q **What do you think about liver detox regimes?**

A At least half the body's energy is spent in detoxifying the toxic substances it makes, plus those we consume from food, water and air. So you do need to give your body a rest from its burdens and support the liver with certain detoxifying nutrients. Some regimes on the market are gimmicky, but alongside cutting out 'toxic' foods and drinks such as coffee, alcohol, sugar and white bread, many foods are a blessing for your poor liver.

A good detox regime should emphasise glucosinolate-rich foods such as broccoli, Brussels sprouts, kale, cauliflower and cabbage, and sulphur-rich foods such as onions and garlic, with a big emphasis on fruits and vegetables and away from animal products, to help restore the body's acid/alkaline balance and provide antioxidant nutrients such as vitamins A, C and E. You also need to supplement the amino acid glutathione and/or the herb milk thistle – major players in the liver's detox systems. Also excellent for assisting liver detoxification is a form of sulphur called MSM; you'll need to take 1 to 3g a day. Remember to drink 1.5 to 2 litres of water a day, too.

Q *Could my liver be affected by my long-term regular intake of medicinal drugs, and need a detox?*

A Yes, medicinal drugs can be a burden on your liver and you may need to assess your liver function and perhaps undergo a detox. Here's a typical diet for a one week detox:

DOs
- Begin your detox at the weekend or during a time when you don't have too much going on.

- Walk for at least 15 minutes every day.
- Drink at least 2 litres of purified, distilled, filtered or bottled water a day. You can also drink dandelion coffee or herbal teas.
- Every day have half a pint of fruit or vegetable juice – either carrot and apple juice (you can buy these two separately and combine with one-third water) with grated ginger, or fresh watermelon juice. The flesh of the watermelon is high in beta-carotene and vitamin C. The seeds are high in vitamin E, and antioxidant minerals zinc and selenium. You can make a great antioxidant cocktail by blending watermelon flesh and seeds in a blender.
- Eat in abundance:
  Fruit – the most beneficial fruits with the highest detox potential include fresh apricots, all types of berries, cantaloupe, citrus fruits, kiwi fruits, papaya, peaches, mango, melons and red grapes.
  Vegetables – especially good for detoxification are artichokes, peppers, beetroot, Brussels sprouts, broccoli, red cabbage, carrots, cauliflower, cucumber, kale, pumpkin, spinach, sweet potato, tomato, watercress and bean and seed sprouts.
- Eat in moderation :
  Grains – brown rice, corn, millet or quinoa, not more than twice a day.
  Fish – mackerel, sardines, or organically farmed or wild salmon, not more than once a day.

Oils – use extra-virgin olive oil for cooking
and in place of butter, and cold-pressed seed
oils for dressing.

Nuts and seeds – one handful a day of raw,
unsalted nuts and seeds should be included.
Choose from almonds, Brazil nuts, hazelnuts,
pecan nuts, pumpkin seeds, sunflower seeds,
sesame seeds and flax seeds.

DON'Ts

- Avoid all wheat products, all meat and all milk
  and dairy products, eggs, salt and any foods
  containing it, hydrogenated fats, artificial
  sweeteners, food additives and preservatives, fried
  foods, spices and dried fruit.
- Limit potatoes to one portion every other day and
  bananas to one every other day.

Don't be surprised if you feel worse for a couple of
days before you feel better. This is especially likely if
you are eliminating foods to which you are allergic/
dependent.

Commonly used non-steroidal anti-inflammatories
(NSAIDs) may also have been damaging your gut
lining, so you may need to detoxify your bowel. You can
help restore the health of your gut lining by supplementing 5g of glutamine powder before bed. I would
also recommend you work under the guidance of a nutritional therapist, who could assess why you have needed
to continue taking medications long-term, and explore
ways of improving your overall health.

Q *What's the best way to detoxify after Christmas?*

A The festive season can be a marathon for your liver, and giving your body an early spring-clean can be a great start to the new year. First off, drink at least 1.5 litres of water a day: water is the best detoxifier of all, so stay with this. Come right off all alcohol as well as other things that put a burden on your body's cleansing processes, such as coffee, tea, sugary foods, sweet drinks, fried foods, cheese and fatty meat. Eat plenty of fresh fruit and vegetables, organic if possible (especially broccoli, cabbage, onions, garlic and kale). Fresh vegetable juices are very cleansing – carrot juice is widely available these days, or invest in a juicer. And eat fibre-rich foods such as beans and wholegrains like brown rice.

To support your system while you're doing this, I'd recommend having a shot of aloe vera juice every day, upping your vitamin C intake and also adding in the herb milk thistle. Take three 1g vitamin C tablets a day for one week, then cut back to one a day. Milk thistle capsules are readily available from healthfood shops. Your liver's other best friend is sulphur. A highly bio-available form of sulphur called MSM can certainly help you detoxify, while also improving your skin, hair and nails. Take three 1g MSM tablets daily for a week, then cut back to one a day. Combining MSM with vitamin C and water is great for hangovers, but the best thing of all is to stir a heaped teaspoon, about 5g, of glutamine powder into a glass of water and drink this before going to bed.

Glutamine not only helps the liver to detoxify; it also heals the digestive tract, which is seriously damaged by alcohol.

Q *How long should a detox last?*

A There are many ways to detoxify and many programmes you can follow. Your needs will differ depending on your toxic load, and some people, such as women who are pregnant or breastfeeding, or those using medical or recreational drugs, should be very careful and only go for mild forms of cleansing such as two to three-day detoxes and skin brushing. This is because drugs and other toxins are stored in the body, usually in fat tissues, until they can be safely released; and that may be years down the line, and in some cases, only released when you detoxify. This is why some people feel worse for a few days when on a detox diet, or on a weight-loss diet, as toxins are released from fat cells as they break down.

For most people a standard detoxification program lasts one week, and can be done perhaps twice a year such as at the beginning of spring and autumn. Start on the weekend, or do it at a time when you don't have too much going on. However, provided the detox diet you are following is well balanced, there's no reason why you can't follow it in principle full-time. It has to be said that the best way to keep your detoxification potential at its best is to not consume foods and drinks containing toxins.

DIET AND NUTRITION

We live in an age of discovery, nutritionally speaking. The science of nutrition is constantly refining and defining what an optimal diet actually means. Gone are the days when the goal was simply to achieve enough protein, fat and carbohydrate, plus fibre. Not only have we discovered new nutrients, from omega-3 and 6 fats to antioxidants, but we now realise that most natural foods contain hundreds of active ingredients. On top of this, some staple foods, most notably dairy produce and gluten grains, don't suit many people – and of course, our differing body chemistry means there is no one 'ideal' diet. Finding your own optimum nutrition is both a science and an art, involving plenty of educated trial and error along the way. Here you'll find answers to a vast range of questions on this consuming passion.

Eating habits

Q *What are your basic guidelines for an optimally healthy diet?*

A To achieve optimal nourishment and wellbeing, here's the essence of what you need to eat.

Every day, have 1 tablespoon cold-pressed seed oil (you can buy top-quality essential oil blends) or 1 heaped tablespoon ground seeds (ideally, half flax seeds and half sesame, sunflower and pumpkin seeds). Eat two servings of protein (beans, lentils, quinoa, tofu, peas, broad beans, organic meat or chicken, fish, cheese or free-range eggs); one serving of mineral-rich foods such as kale, cabbage, root vegetables, yoghurt, seeds or nuts, as well as fresh fruit and wholefoods such as wholegrains; three servings of dark green, leafy and root vegetables (watercress, carrots and broccoli, to name just three); three servings of fruit (citrus, apples, pears, berries, melon or bananas); four servings of whole carbohydrates such as wholegrains (rice, millet or rye, for example); fibre from wholefoods; 1 to 1.5 litres of water; and a good-quality, high-strength multivitamin and mineral.

Q *Can you get all the nutrients you need from a well-balanced diet?*

A This is the greatest lie in nutrition today. Even if you consider the recommended daily allowances (RDAs) enough, over 90 per cent of people who think they eat a balanced diet fail to achieve these levels. For example, the RDA for zinc is 15mg and the average intake is 7.6mg. This is, in part, a consequence of today's farming, food processing and storage, which leave much of our food depleted of nutrients.

If, however, you're after optimum health – that is, feeling great rather than OK and rarely getting sick, as opposed to merely avoiding deficiency diseases such as scurvy (which is what the RDAs are based on) – then think again. Modern life places extra demands on our bodies. Stress, pollution, medications, food additives, food processing – all increase our need for nutrients. So if you're up for boundless energy, sharp brain function and minimal illness, including reducing your risk of cancer, heart disease and other killers, supplementing a good diet with nutrients is essential. That's why I recommend everybody take at least a high-strength multivitamin every day and an additional 1g of vitamin C. See Resources, page 483, for a list of good multivitamins.

Q *How do I know if I'm getting enough protein?*

A Apart from growth and development, protein is used in the body for energy and is needed in the manufacture of hormones, antibodies and enzymes, as well as helping to maintain the proper acid-alkali balance in the body. If someone is deficient, they will have generally poor health. That means poor wound healing, depression, apathy, frequent infections, hormonal imbalance, imbalances in blood sugar, fatigue, an under-functioning liver and more, depending on which amino acids are lowest, as they each have different functions in the body.

Obtaining enough protein is not difficult. Ideally it should make up at least 15 per cent of the calorific intake, and that's easily achieved by having at least two daily servings of beans, lentils, quinoa, tofu, eggs, fish, cheese, seeds or nuts. If your energy is poor, eating protein whenever you eat carbohydrates can really help to stabilise blood sugar. Snack on pumpkin or sunflower seeds when you eat a piece of fruit, and balance out baked potatoes with grilled free-range chicken, mackerel or a bean stew.

Q **What is the truth to the saying 'Breakfast like a king, dine like a pauper'?**

A There's a lot of truth to this old saying, with a little modification. First, you need food for energy during the day, so it doesn't make sense to eat half your day's food in the evening. Also, it is definitely not a good idea to go to bed still digesting your dinner. As a general rule, eat dinner early and leave at least two hours before going to sleep. Similarly, we are not designed to eat as soon as we wake up. It is better not to eat until you are totally awake, perhaps an hour after waking. Breakfast is the most important meal of the day and, as such, should be substantial (say, a boiled free-range egg with wholemeal toast, or seed-rich muesli with yoghurt, milk or soya milk). Having said that, if you are eating three meals a day, plus two pieces of fruit as snacks in between, no meal need be vast. It is better to leave a meal feeling satisfied, not stuffed.

Q *What's a good diet for me? I'm a teenage schoolgirl.*

A That depends a lot on your current health and lifestyle. Aside from following my recommendations for an optimal diet (see 'What are your basic guidelines for an optimally healthy diet?', page 65), there are a few other points you might consider.

Ensuring your hormones are healthy involves eating enough fat – but the right kind. Less meat, dairy, fried food, damaged fats (in many processed foods), and more seeds, nuts, avocados and oily fish – sardines, mackerel, and organically farmed or wild salmon. Avoiding acne involves many things, but the vital elements are reducing sugar and junk food in your diet, drinking plenty of water and eating plenty of fresh fruit and vegetables to cleanse your system (see also 'My teenage son has acne . . .', page 24).

Controlling your weight is *not* about skipping meals, but instead eating small amounts of healthy food regularly throughout the day – breakfast, lunch and dinner, with a fruit snack mid-morning and mid-afternoon. And exercising. This keeps your metabolic rate up, so you burn energy faster, whereas skipping meals or dieting slows it down and makes it much harder to lose weight.

These tips – eating good fats, eating small meals frequently, plenty of fruit and vegetables, less sugar and junk food, and so on – will also help your brain function well to get you through the stresses of school work.

Q *What's the healthiest working snack lunch?*

A You are halfway through the day. Your brain and your energy need a boost. Here's how to do it.

Number 1 – don't overeat. You'll get better energy by snacking on a piece of fruit mid-morning and mid-afternoon, preferably an apple or pear, and keeping lunch relatively light. Number 2 – you want to eat some protein, some 'slow-releasing' carbohydrate and some fresh veg. Imagine your plate divided in half. Half should be salad or fresh vegetables. The remaining half should be half protein, such as fish, chicken, eggs, beans or tofu, and the other half slow-releasing carbohydrate such as wholewheat bread, pasta or brown rice.

A chicken sandwich with wholemeal bread and loads of salad would hit the mark. Alternatively, egg and cress, but ideally you want double the cress contained in a standard sandwich. A bean and rice salad with some vegetables would be great for a vegetarian. Or, if you're on the road, try a small tub of hummus (chickpea spread), a raw carrot and half a dozen oatcakes.

Don't drink a fizzy drink. Either have water (still or naturally carbonated), apple juice or best of all an Optio, which is a blend of fruit juices with optimal amounts of nutrients. These are available in supermarkets.

Q *I entertain a lot as part of my job. Can you translate the ideas of optimum nutrition into haute cuisine?*

A Absolutely. Healthy, whole, fresh organic foods, which are the ingredients of optimum nutrition, are inherently great-tasting ingredients. The trouble is that many people don't know what to do with beans, lentils, seeds, herbs and other cornerstones of optimum nutrition. Also, most celebrity chefs pay lip service to healthy eating, using high-sugar and high-fat sauces to add flavour, and frying far too much. For cream and the like, I often substitute coconut milk or coconut cream, tahini (sesame seed spread), tamari with crushed ginger and lemon juice or cashew cream, and I tend to steam rather than fry food.

I asked several hundred nutritionists trained at the Institute for Optimum Nutrition to give me their best-tasting, most interesting recipes and then got the great cookery writer and gastronomic expert Judy Ridgway to try them out and pick the best recipes for taste, look and health. The result was the *Optimum Nutrition Cookbook* (Piatkus, 2000). I strongly recommend you use this for your healthy haute cuisine.

Q *What's the difference between nutritional therapists and dieticians?*

A Both nutritional therapists and dieticians are experts trained to give you a dietary programme to keep you healthy. A dietician is probably trained more conservatively, basing nutrient requirements on the recommended daily allowances and often working with people who have serious health problems and are on medication. GP practices and hospitals often refer people to dieticians to help manage their diet.

A nutritional therapist looks at your *optimum* levels, that is, what you need to maximise your potential. Nutritional therapists also take into account your lifestyle and environment as well as what you eat and drink. Nutritional therapists are generally well up on the subject of supplementation and dieticians are not. When you visit a nutritional therapist, make sure they have had three years of training.

The organisation representing dieticians is called the British Dietetic Association (BDA). Meanwhile, the British Association of Nutritional Therapists (BANT) acts on behalf of nutritional therapists. I think there is a need for regulation of the profession, and it is, in fact, moving towards standardisation and self-regulation to ensure that good standards are set and maintained in nutritional therapy. Nutritional therapists from recognised colleges, such as the Institute for Optimum Nutrition that I founded, are trained to a very high standard. But these fields of nutrition, nutritional therapy and dietetics should really all be one.

Q *I drown my food in pepper – is it bad for me?*

A Happily, no. Unlike salt, pepper is positively good for you. This is because it contains piperine, which increases the absorption of nutrients in your food. So effective is piperine at improving the uptake of nutrients that you might literally double the nutrients you take in from food simply by going heavy on the pepper. Piperine is particularly high in black pepper, not white, and it's not present in the other so-called peppers, such as chilli, paprika and cayenne; these are all fruits from the capsicum family with their own interesting properties. Chillies, for example, are one of the richest known sources of vitamin C. Some people are allergic to these 'capsicum' peppers, but allergy to black pepper is rare. It can, however, make you sneeze.

Q *Isn't chargrilled or barbequed food better for you than fried?*

A It isn't. Frying has long been suspect, but so has meat charred or burnt by barbequeing. For some time it was thought that the main danger of frying and barbequeing was that fats, cooked at high temperatures, produce oxidants – powerful cancer-promoting chemicals. And of course frying can also mean more fat and more calories.

To add fuel to the fire, however, alarming research has found another cancer-promoting substance, acrylamide, in foods cooked at high temperatures, with or without fat. While the safe limit set for acrylamide in food is 10 parts per billion (ppb), chips and crisps have been found to contain more than 10 times this amount. The worst foods are chips sold in fast-food outlets, crisps and crispbreads. Ryvita contains between 1,340 to 4,000ppb. According to UK research, Walker's crisps average 1,250 and Pringles 1,480. In the US,

McDonald's French fries, followed by Burger King, come out worst. However, even home-cooked chips have been found to be high. Acrylamide is produced by frying, barbecuing, baking and even microwaving.

So, the honest answer is that anything browned or burnt, or cooked or processed using high heat, is likely to be bad for you. The bottom line is to eat more raw food and if you cook it, steam-fry or boil it rather than stir-fry. To steam-fry foods add a very small amount of olive oil to a pan and sauté the ingredients for literally a minute, just enough to generate enough heat so that you can then add a water-based sauce, such as equal amounts of soya sauce, lemon juice and water. When you put on a lid, this liquid then steams the food. The result is hot food that's full of flavour, but not full of oxidants or acrylamide because nothing is burnt.

Food charts and indices

Q *I am confused about the different glycaemic indices.*

A The glycaemic index ranks foods by how much your blood sugar increases after eating them. But there is more than one such index, and the confusion over them arises for two reasons.

Firstly, the index to what? Originally, one gave glucose a score of 100 as the fastest-releasing of all sugars. Another used white bread, meaning glucose would score over 100 in that index. But now, everyone has agreed to use glucose as the index.

Secondly, the effect measured is the effect produced by feeding people the amount of any given food required to give 50g of carbohydrate. Here lies a more significant problem. That's a lot of carrots (which are largely water) or a very tiny amount of, say, chocolate. This tends to create the impression that fruits and vegetables have a high GI score and hence should be avoided when, in truth, the amount we eat would not have a pronounced effect on blood sugar.

There would be some merit in giving the GI for a serving of a food, rather than the amount required to achieve 50g. This is becoming more popular and is sometimes called the 'glycaemic load' of a food. I have done this in some instances in the charts in my books to give a more publicly realistic view. It is also worth pointing out that not all researchers (hence individuals) respond in the same way, so a GI for a food is an average response, usually of a relatively small number of people.

Q *Where can I find the most up-to-date and comprehensive list of acid- and alkali-forming foods?*

A What effectively makes a food alkaline forming is the presence of the minerals calcium, magnesium, potassium and sodium. Fruits and vegetables are very rich in potassium and magnesium and are therefore alkaline (except asparagus, cranberries, plums and olives). What makes a food acid forming is the presence of amino acids. So proteins such as meat, fish, eggs, cheese and nuts (except almonds) are acidic, and grains such as rye, oats, wheat and rice slightly less so. Butter or margarine, sugar, tea and coffee are considered neutral. In terms of lists, I compiled the one below, reproduced from the *Optimum Nutrition Bible*, on the basis of all the research to date.

Which foods are acid, alkaline and neutral

ACID		NEUTRAL	ALKALINE	
High	*Medium*	Butter	*Medium*	*High*
Edam	Brazil nuts	Margarine	Almonds	Avocados
Eggs	Walnuts	Coffee	Coconuts	Beetroot
Mayonnaise	Cheddar	Tea	Milk	Carrots
Fish	cheese	Sugar	Beans	Potatoes
Shellfish	Stilton cheese	Syrup	Cabbage	Spinach
Bacon	Herrings		Celery	Dried fruit
Beef	Mackerel		Lentils	Rhubarb
Chicken	Rye		Lettuce	Berries
Liver	Oats		Mushrooms	Cherries
Lamb	Wheat		Onions	Figs
Veal	Rice		Root	Grapefruit
	Plums		vegetables	Grapes
	Cranberries		Tomatoes	Lemons
	Olives		Apricots	Melons
			Apples	Oranges
			Bananas	Peaches
				Pears
				Raspberries
				Tangerines
				Prunes

Food families

Eggs and dairy products

Q *Should we avoid eggs because they are high in cholesterol?*

A It's a complete myth that eggs raise your blood cholesterol. True, eggs do contain cholesterol but they are also an excellent source of protein, vitamins, minerals and, more interestingly, unsaturated fats, especially if you feed the chicken seeds. Of the 5g of fat in an egg, half is monounsaturated (as in olive oil), which actually helps lower the risk of heart disease. The egg yolk also contains the richest known source of choline, which helps the body make good use of fats – including cholesterol.

The trouble is, if you fry them you destroy these beneficial nutrients and damage these good fats. Also, an egg is only as healthy as the chicken that laid it, so if possible buy nothing but organic, free-range eggs, laid by chickens that have been fed grains and seeds, rather than battery chickens fed who knows what. Nowadays you can even buy eggs high in omega-3 fats. These eggs may be positively good for people with raised cholesterol. My advice, if you have raised cholesterol, is to have no more than seven healthy eggs a week, and don't fry them.

Q *Is drinking milk good for the bones?*

A It's true that milk is a great source of calcium, the mineral needed for healthy bones. But bone health demands other minerals that are not abundant in milk, particularly magnesium and boron. Vegans (who avoid milk) can get adequate calcium *and* magnesium from seeds, nuts, beans and vegetables. So drinking milk is not strictly essential for bone health if you eat these wholefoods – after all, our ancestors weren't milking wild buffaloes. You may lack vitamin D if you avoid milk but you can get that from fish and eggs, or exposure to sufficient amounts of sunlight. Again, this was not a problem for our ancestors, but it may be difficult for northern Europeans and people who spend too much time indoors.

And drinking too much milk can actually be bad for your bones. One 10-year study in the US involving thousands of women surprisingly found that women who drank two or more glasses of milk had a 45 per cent *increased* risk of hip fracture. This may have been because eating too much protein, found in meat and milk, actually decreases the health of the bones. The underlying reason is that protein is made from amino acids and when the bloodstream is too acidic the body releases calcium from bone to neutralise it. So you need to strike a balance between your protein intake and calcium intake.

Q *I eat soya products and try to avoid dairy. Is there any nutritional value in soya yoghurt, or would I be better off eating live dairy yoghurt?*

A Soya has been shown to benefit our health in many ways. Researchers have found that it can protect us from heart disease by raising 'good' cholesterol and lowering 'bad' cholesterol. No less than six anti-cancer compounds have been found in soya beans, and high soya consumption is thought to be one of the factors helping Japanese men and women enjoy much lower rates of cancer than people living in Western countries (see 'Why are soya products good for cancer?', page 143). Soya is one of the few plant sources of 'complete' protein, containing well-absorbed iron and calcium, B vitamins and lecithin. For women, soya can be very helpful in balancing hormonal levels naturally (see 'I read that soya is dangerous because it interferes with hormones', page 100)

Fruit yoghurts, whether diary or soya, are often laden with sugar, so go for plain live soya yoghurt and add your own fresh fruit. It's important, though, not to rely too heavily on soya – people can become sensitive or allergic to it, and it's also known to slow thyroid function if you eat too much of it.

Fats and oils

Q **Which is better – butter or margarine?**

A I'd go for butter any day – both on the taste front and because it's generally better for you. Butter has been much maligned for its high saturated fat content but it is also a good source of the important fat-soluble vit-amins A and D. Compared with most commercial margarines, its fats are not actually that bad for you.

Most margarines are made from highly processed

vegetable fats called hydrogenated fats, in which the chemistry of the oil has been altered so that it becomes solid. These hydrogenated fats can actually be harmful because they still have the hallmark of the original vegetable fat as far as the body and brain are concerned, for example linoleic acid in sunflower oil, but have been altered so that the body can't use it. This 'bad fit' can alter the way fatty membranes work in the body for the worse. So although the essential fatty acid content of cold-pressed sunflower oil, for example, is good for you, highly processed versions of it are not. New brands of margarine, free from hydrogenated fats, are emerging, some with specified amounts of the essential, highly beneficial omega-3 and 6 fats. So I would recommend these, or butter – as long as it's organic.

Q *Is cholesterol bad for you?*

A This is one of the biggest, most lingering myths about diet, and it made eggs a four-letter word. What is often forgotten is that cholesterol is essential for good health – your brain contains it and it is used to make the sex hormones oestrogen, progesterone and testosterone. What's more, staying away from cholesterol-rich foods such as eggs does very little to reduce body cholesterol levels, as most of it is produced in the liver anyway. The problem is not cholesterol as such, but damaged or oxidised cholesterol, because this can accumulate in the arteries.

So two things are important here. Firstly, avoid eating oxidised cholesterol such as that found in fried food. A boiled egg is fine, but fried eggs and bacon are off the agenda – bad news for the classic British fry-up. Secondly, a good intake of antioxidant nutrients such as vitamins A, C and E is important because they protect cholesterol in the body from being damaged.

Q **Is olive oil good for you?**

A Any fat or oil should be eaten in moderation and while olive oil is no exception to this, it certainly is one of the 'healthiest', especially if it's the extra-virgin, cold-pressed kind. Firstly, it contains 7 per cent omega-6 fats which, in a cold-pressed olive oil, will still have all their healthy properties such as keeping blood thin, improving hormone and immune function and reducing inflammation. Studies have also shown that people in Mediterranean countries who consume a lot of olive oil have less risk of heart disease (although this may be due also to other dietary factors, such as eating more vegetables). Olive oil is a mono-unsaturated fat, which means that when used for cooking, it is less susceptible to being damaged by heat and turning into a harmful 'trans fat', which is what happens to some other oils such as sunflower oil. Trans, or altered, fats can't be used properly by the body and are more likely to accumulate.

Q *I don't eat fish. Is there any advantage in taking fish oils?*

A Definitely. Fish oil is proven to have amazing health benefits, not least in the brain. It's also good for your heart, your immune system and your skin. That's because omega-3 fats, a kind of essential fatty acid, are a vital nutrient that is often missing in the modern diet. Fish oils are also natural painkillers and anti-inflammatories. So vital are omega-3 fats that the amount in an infant's blood correlates with their IQ at age five. If you don't eat fish, take a fish oil supplement rich in omega-3 fats. You need about 400mg a day of the omega-3s, of which cod liver oil is a very rich source.

There are two highly important kinds of omega-3 fats – DHA and EPA. DHA is more structural and is used to build the brain. Hence, it is proving important in pregnancy and infancy, although there is now research showing that it may also help reduce dementia. EPA is more functional and is coming up trumps in research on ADHD, dyslexia, depression and schizophrenia.

I'd recommend getting equal amounts of both, ideally 400mg of each a day. Flax seed oil is the best alternative for strict vegetarians. It is rich in a type of omega-3 fat called alpha-linolenic acid, which the body can convert into EPA and DHA. However, supplementing directly with EPA and DHA does tend to work better in terms of health benefits, as it's 'ready for action' straight from the jar.

Q **Do we need more omega-3 essential fats in winter?**

A Yes, upping your intake of omega-3 fatty acids in the winter can be important, especially if you live in northern Europe or other less sunny parts of the world. Omega-3 fats are highly concentrated in our brain and nervous system, and essential in all the cell membranes that send and receive messages, where they help to improve learning, memory and mood. So we need omega-3 fats all year round, but in winter, we produce less serotonin – the 'happy' brain chemical – because of the relatively short days and decreased exposure to sunlight, which can lower our mood and motivation (see 'I suffer from seasonal affective disorder', page 193). Omega-3 fats help produce more serotonin in the brain, as well as increasing the efficiency of the serotonin you have, so can really help maintain mood and motivation throughout winter. I'd recommend supplementing an omega-3 rich fish oil giving 400mg of both EPA and DHA. With most brands, this means two capsules.

Fruits and vegetables

Q **Why are certain vegetables so hard to digest?**

A The plant fibres in vegetables are a great source of roughage, but they are also hard for our digestive systems to break down. Leeks, onions and garlic contain a type of fibre called inulin, and cruciferous vegetables such as broccoli, cauliflower and cabbage contain glucosides that are also hard to digest.

There are two main ways to make them easier for

your gut to process. One is to lightly cook them. If you either briefly steam them, or quickly stir-fry or steam-fry them to keep their nutrient content, you'll help break down the fibres and make them more digestible. (In steam-frying, use a very small amount of oil, stir-fry the vegetables for a minute, then add a bit of water, or a mix of water, soy sauce and lemon juice, cover and steam for three minutes or so.) The other way is to supplement with enzymes. Our bodies produce digestive enzymes to break down the food we eat, but sometimes stress or poor diet slows or disrupts the process. So try taking a digestive enzyme supplement that contains amyloglucosidase (sometimes called glucoamylase) with your meals, to break down the glucosides. (See Resources, page 481.)

Q *How are blueberries good for you?*

A Not only do blueberries taste great, they are one of nature's superfoods. All fruits with a purple-blue colour are especially rich in a flavonoid called anthocyanidins. These natural plant chemicals are very powerful antioxidants that help combat the effects of pollution and toxins in general. They are also anti-inflammatory, help reduce allergic reactions and have been shown to keep blood capillaries healthy, which is useful in conditions such as varicose veins or if you find you bruise easily. Flavonoids also help potentiate the qualities of vitamin C, which is another nutrient in blueberries, and because of this they are helpful for boosting your immunity. Blueberries are a good source of fibre too. And they're very versatile, equally good in smoothies, with yoghurt, in fruit salads, on cereal or as a snack.

Q **Why are carrots good for your eyes?**

A In the retina – the special tissue at the back of your eyeball – are light-sensitive chemicals that convey what you see to the brain. These chemicals are made from retinol, or vitamin A. While you can get retinol from meat, much of the vitamin A we receive comes from fruits and vegetables in the form of beta-carotene. This is especially abundant in carrots and other orange foods such as sweet potatoes, apricots, melons and tomatoes. Deficiencies in vitamin A make you more prone to long and short-sightedness, glaucoma, eye infections, night blindness and watery or itchy eyes.

The RDA of vitamin A is 600mcg, but this is not enough to keep your eyes optimally healthy. Our hunter-gatherer ancestors obtained something like 10,000mcg. A good diet, including a carrot a day, can give you the equivalent of 7,000mcg, in the form of beta-carotene. I'd recommend supplementing a further 2,000 to 3,000mcg (6,600 to 10,000ius). B vitamins and eating enough protein are also important in eye health. The herb eyebright helps too, and is effective at combating eye infections and cataracts. Lutein, found in spinach, kale and other dark green vegetables, is another eye-friendly substance – and yet another reason to eat your greens.

Q *What are cruciferous vegetables and why are they good for you?*

A The cruciferous family of vegetables includes any whose leaves grow in a cross shape – broccoli, cabbage, cauliflower, Brussels sprouts, cress, horseradish, kale, kohlrabi, mustard, radish and turnip. They are all laden with vitamins (broccoli, for example, is a richer source of vitamin C than oranges), minerals and other health-promoting nutrients, including fibre. Cruciferous vegetables also contain a range of powerful antioxidant substances that help counteract pollution and support the body's own detoxification process. They're particularly rich in natural chemicals called glucosinolates that appear to detoxify all sorts of toxins, including carcinogens, substances that can trigger cancer. One piece of research showed that eating cruciferous vegetables three times a week might cut your risk of getting colon cancer by 60 per cent. So to increase your resistance to illnesses and to boost your body's detox capacity, include a range of the above vegetables in your meals at least three or four times a week.

Q *Is it true that fruit juice rots your teeth?*

A Yes. Both fruit and fruit juice contains acids which are the major cause of tooth erosion, thinning the enamel on teeth, both at the front and back. Worst of all are sweetened fizzy fruit juices, as the carbonation makes even more acids. Tooth-rotting acids are also made by bacteria that turn sugars into acids.

Fruits that aren't properly ripened and taste sour are bad news – that sour taste is acid. Blackcurrants, grapes and citrus fruits are the worst. Grapes are particularly bad because their sweetness masks the sour taste of the high tartaric acid level in them. That's why wine drinkers tend to have more tooth erosion. Pears and bananas are the least harmful to teeth.

But of course, both fruit and fruit juice have other health benefits, so here's what you can do to get the best of both worlds. If you're going to drink fruit juice, dilute it at least half and half with still water. Accompany your apple or pear with a few almonds; they're high in calcium and so good at neutralising acids. And have yoghurt with your fruit. If the fruit is hard, like a Conference pear, but not sour, the fibres will actually benefit your teeth by giving them a good wash.

Q *Is garlic good for your heart?*

A For thousands of years people have been aware of the beneficial properties of garlic. Garlic contains around 200 biologically active compounds, many of which play a role in preventing heart disease as well as another major killer, cancer. Garlic lowers cholesterol in the blood and prevents the formation of atherosclerosis – deposits on artery walls. It also thins the blood – a safer way to prevent blood clots than an aspirin a day, which can cause stomach bleeding. One study has also shown that garlic can lower your homocysteine level, another known risk factor for heart disease. So all in all, it's not surprising it's been shown to reduce the risk of a heart attack.

If you choose a supplement go for either garlic pearls (garlic oil) or brands that use 'Pure-Gar', a concentrated form of garlic particularly rich in allicin, the phytochemical that is responsible for so much of garlic's dramatic healing properties.

Q *Are oranges the best food for vitamin C?*

A Although they've practically become synonymous with vitamin C, oranges aren't actually the richest source. That honour goes to the Australian billy goat plum, which has been eaten by the Aboriginals for over 1,000 years. With over 100 times more vitamin C than an orange, the billy goat plum even exceeds another big contender, the acerola cherry. A glass of acerola cherry juice provides a whopping 3,872mg of vitamin C, while a glass of orange juice contains 121mg and the juice of a lemon provides 83mg.

On a more practical note, when you're out at the supermarket opt for kiwi fruits, strawberries, grapes, grapefruit, melons, pineapples and mangoes, all front runners in the vitamin C stakes. And don't pass the vegetable bins by. Top of the class are broccoli, peppers, Brussels sprouts, cauliflower, peas and asparagus. Broccoli and peppers contain more vitamin C than oranges and kiwi fruit: a serving of broccoli provides 110mg, the equivalent of two oranges. But the hottest source of vitamin C is raw, hot chilli peppers – a cup of these provides 364mg!

Q **How are prunes good for you?**

A Your granny was certainly on to something with her morning serving of soaked prunes, but not just for the reason you're thinking of. Yes, prunes are a very rich source of fibre and fibre is good for keeping your bowel movements regular. But prunes are also the richest source of antioxidants, essential for countless processes in the body, from keeping your skin healthy to boosting your ability to detoxify, and generally protecting you from disease and ageing. And there's more. Prunes are fat-free and high in the important minerals potassium and iron.

Luckily, they're also delicious. Have them on cereal or yoghurt or in a smoothie for breakfast, as a snack, in a loaf instead of raisins, or make a prune fool by blending them with fromage frais and drizzling lightly with maple syrup.

Q **Is spinach good for you?**

A Popeye knew his stuff. Spinach is very rich in all sorts of nutrients, including iron, sulphur, beta-carotene, magnesium and calcium. There are, however, a couple of drawbacks on that front. First, the iron in spinach is not that easily absorbed, certainly compared to iron in meat. One way of helping to improve that is to eat it with a squeeze of lemon juice – vitamin C helps make the iron more available for absorption. Secondly, spinach is high in oxalic acid, which binds itself to minerals such as calcium, leaving them less available for absorption in the body.

Leaving all that aside, Popeye's favourite vegetable has qualities that can compensate for these problems. The rich green colour in spinach is from chlorophyll – a highly cleansing substance that helps bring life-giving oxygen into cells. It contains high amounts of antioxidants such as beta-carotene, and it is also high in fibre. So, all round, yes, spinach is good for you – as long as you don't count on it for your iron and calcium.

Q *How are watermelons good for you?*

A Apart from the refreshing juiciness, the crunch and the taste, watermelon has a lot to offer. The flesh is very rich in powerful antioxidant nutrients such as vitamin C, lycopene and beta-carotene – all important for helping your body detoxify, fight infections, slow down ageing and counter inflammation. The seeds are loaded with more antioxidants – zinc, selenium, and vitamin E, as well as essential fats. All in all, it's an extraordinary food. The best way to have it, so that you not only get the goodness from the flesh, but also the seeds, is to make a delicious, simple smoothie by whizzing up large chunks in a blender. This cracks the seed husks, which sink to the bottom, leaving all the goodness in the drink and giving you a powerful nutrient boost. There's yet another plus: it's also great for hangovers.

Q *Are frozen vegetables really better than fresh, vitamin-wise?*

A Arguably so. That's because there is a marginal loss of vitamins from freezing a food, and slight loss on storing and then defrosting a food – say 10 to 20 per cent of nutrients depending on storage time. There's then an additional loss of perhaps 20 per cent from boiling the vegetable. So, the total loss might be as much as 40 per cent from pea, to frozen pack, to plate.

So, fresh peas eaten raw would be best, but how long is it between you eating a food and the farmer picking it? Unless you eat very fresh vegetables and eat them raw or lightly cooked, the chances are your frozen vegetables are as fresh if not fresher than the so-called 'fresh' food you buy in a supermarket. This is partly because vegetables are frozen very soon after picking. I certainly think that buying frozen is an excellent alternative when a vegetable is out of season.

Q *Can you name your top 10 healthy fruit and vegetables?*

A I decided to run the equivalent of the 'best vegetable of the year' from a nutritional point of view, and obtained analyses of vegetables using five main criteria: glucosinolates; antioxidant power using the overall oxygen radical absorption capacity (ORAC) rating; vitamin C; zinc; and folic acid. Glucosinates are the main anti-cancer nutrient in vegetables and help the liver detoxify. The ORAC rating is the best measure of a food's antioxidant potential. Vitamin C helps support the immune system, as does zinc, which is important for the skin. Folic acid is associated with maintaining a healthy cardio-vascular system and brain.

Here's what I found:

Vegetable	Glucosino-lates	ORAC rating	Vitamin C	Zinc	Folic acid	Total score
Tenderstem	5	4	4	5	3	21
Curly kale	3	5	5	3	4	20
Spinach	3	4	2	5	5	19
Asparagus	2	3	1	4	5	15
Broccoli	3	2	3	3	3	14

Tenderstem is a cross between broccoli and Chinese kale that has very tender and tasty stems, a bit like asparagus, and heads like broccoli. This hybrid vegetable has double the glucosinolates found in broccoli, making it the best vegetable for cancer protection, as well as for detoxification, since glucosinolates substantially enhance liver function. It is also a good all-rounder for anti-ageing antioxidant nutrients and homocysteine-lowering folic acid. (High levels of the amino acid homocysteine are associated with increased risk for a number of degenerative diseases, including diabetes and coronary disease.) All this makes it my first choice of vegetable, followed by kale. My recommendation is to eat at least three servings of vegetables a day, including any two of the above.

As far as fruit is concerned my all-time favourites are berries – strawberries, raspberries and blueberries. These are very high in antioxidants and slow-releasing sugars, so by eating them you keep your blood sugar stable while giving your energy a boost. I recommend two servings of fruit a day, with one preferably berries.

Meat and fish

Q **Is it true that fish makes you brainy?**

A Fish is the best brain food on the market. The dry weight of your brain is 60 per cent fat, but only special types of fat make it work well. Most vital of these is DHA, a member of the omega-3 fat family, of which fish is a particularly rich source. DHA not only improves learning and age-related memory, but is also a prime mood enhancer. So important are these omega-3 fats that the amount in an infant's blood correlates with their IQ at age five. Fish – and especially sardines – are also good sources of two other important brain nutrients, choline and pyroglutamate.

You're best off eating fish three times a week, but if you don't like it, at least take a fish oil supplement rich in omega-3 fats DHA and EPA. You need at least 400mg a day of the omega-3s (that's EPA plus DHA). Cod liver oil is a very rich source; pick the high-strength kind that contains these amounts of EPA and DHA.

Q *Why is oily fish so good for you?*

A Not all fats are created equal. There are fats that kill, sure, but there are also fats that heal, and omega-3 fats are essential nutrients. They are vital throughout your body – your brain contains large amounts and needs them to function properly, they reduce inflammation, thin your blood, lubricate skin and joints, help in the making of hormones, and are in fact a part of every cell in your body. While seeds and oils like flax and hemp are good sources, the best are cold-water fish like mackerel, herring and sardines, as well as salmon (either organically farmed or wild – not ordinary farmed salmon, as this can have high levels of contaminants). Fresh tuna needs to be sourced carefully and eaten rarely, as it can have a high mercury content.

The problem is that many people don't get nearly enough omega-3 fats. The average person today gets a sixth of the amount found in the diet of those in 1850, partly due to food choices, but mainly due to food processing that tends to remove or damage it. Boosting your level of omega-3s by eating a minimum of three portions of oily fish every week can improve skin conditions, boost mental clarity, reduce your risk of heart disease and aid inflammatory conditions such as arthritis, asthma, eczema, allergies and hay fever, and can actually help you burn stored fat more efficiently. If you're on a no fat/low fat diet and suffer from allergies, hay fever, dry skin or hair, cracked lips, poor memory or concentration, excessive thirst, or joint problems, chances are you need more omega-3s. Try supplementing fish oil; you'll need 400mg a day of both DHA and EPA, the omega-3s so many of us are deficient in.

Q *Didn't our ancestors eat a lot of meat, and far fewer carbohydrates?*

A My understanding is that the composition of our ancestors' diet depends entirely on which ancestors in which period of evolution you're looking at. More broadly, we have evolved the digestive system of an omnivore, not a carnivore. And our body chemistry suggests a very long period of substantial fruit intake, not unlike the eating habits of our cousins, the jungle-dwelling primates.

At the moment, some nutritionists are suggesting that a high animal protein/fat diet is healthier. Yet all the meta-analyses indicate that larger intakes of fruit, vegetables and fibre mean substantially less risk for both digestive cancers and cardiovascular disease, while increased meat consumption is clearly linked with an increased risk of developing both conditions. This is hardly surprising since all meat putrefies and, unlike carnivores, we have a digestive system more geared to larger amounts of fibre. Any unbalanced diet leads to micronutrient deficiencies. However, both meat-oriented and vegetarian-oriented diets can be adapted to provide enough.

However, it is true that grains, our current major source of carbohydrates, were introduced into our diets relatively recently. This is probably why so many people are allergic to them. Yet the number of people sensitive to grains is much lower in cultures such as Egypt, where grains have been grown the longest. In northern countries where grains are not grown but imported, the incidence of gluten sensitivity is very high. It is likely that, in ancient days, those less adapted to eating grains were weaker and hence died off younger, leaving a genetic pool of people who were better adapted.

So, I favour a diet containing fresh fruit, vegetables, seeds, nuts, fish in preference to meat and less grains. This is most consistent with large periods of our ancient history.

Q **Is meat the best food for protein and iron?**

A The best foods to eat for protein are not simply those that are highest in protein. Although meat has a high percentage of calories as protein, its actual usability in the body – which depends on the balance of amino acids it contains – is not as good as that of soya or quinoa. Quinoa (pronounced 'keen-wa') is a grain-like food from South America, available in healthfood shops.

A food's other nutritional constituents also have to be taken into account. Most meat is actually as much as 50 per cent fat, mainly saturated, whereas a vegetarian source of protein like tofu provides, percentage-wise, a lot less fat, mainly polyunsaturated, and more than enough protein. As for iron, other foods such as spinach, beans, lentils and pumpkin seeds are richer in this important mineral than meat, but the iron in meat is more absorbable. So overall, for iron at least, meat probably is best.

Q **What do you think of meat replacement products such as Quorn?**

A Quorn is a microprotein produced from mushrooms that some people are allergic to or that can aggravate yeast intolerance. But if you have no reaction to it, then there should be no problem eating it. However, I'd advise that you don't eat it every day, but mix in other sources of vegetable protein – for example, soya products such as tofu and tempura, pulses (such as lentils and beans) mixed with rice, quinoa (the protein-rich South American grain), seeds or fish.

Nuts, seeds and pulses

Q *I am always reading that beans are good for you. Does this mean all types of bean including runner, French (dwarf) and broad beans?*

A Beans means not just green beans, but beans in the pulse family such as kidney beans, mung beans, black beans, lima beans, pinto beans ... Other pulses include lentils and chickpeas. The reason they are so good is that they contain protein, nutrients and lots of natural fibre. They are delicious mixed with rice or added to soups or casseroles.

***

DIG DEEPER: For a range of recipe ideas, see my book *The Optimum Nutrition Cookbook*, coauthored by Judy Ridgway (Piatkus, 2000).

***

Q *I would prefer not to eat meat all, but I don't really like beans and pulses. Would I get enough protein from fish, eggs, nuts and dairy products?*

A Yes, as long as you make sure you eat protein regularly and try to vary the sources. For instance, don't forget the protein-rich vegetables such as broccoli, peas, spinach and potatoes, plus grains such as quinoa, which has as much protein as meat (you can buy this from your healthfood shop). Tofu is wonderfully versatile, and you can obviously ring the changes as much as you like if you include fish (sardines are an excellent source, as is cod), eggs, nuts (cashew nuts, peanuts and almonds are good) and dairy products such as yoghurt and cottage and hard cheeses.

Q *How are flax seeds good for you?*

A Native Americans have used flax seeds, also known as linseeds, for years for a wide variety of health problems. They are the richest plant source of the essential omega-3 fat that balances hormones and helps with PMS, menopausal problems, male infertility, and the working of the brain, immune system, heart and arteries. The most common sign of deficiency is dry skin. In most cases, a daily tablespoon of flax seed oil, either in orange juice or added to salad dressings, soups or cereals, improves dry skin within a week. Alternatively, take capsules – three 1,000mg capsules a day.

Best of all is to eat the seeds. As well as all the beneficial omega-3 fats, the seeds are an excellent source of minerals, vitamin E and protein. You get more out of them by grinding them, since they are so small that they can pass through the digestive system undigested. Whole flax seeds are also excellent for digestive health – soak a dessertspoonful overnight in a glass of water and drink the mixture in the morning. This can not only alleviate constipation but help cleanse the gut of toxins.

Q *Weight-Watchers say nuts are fattening.*
Do you agree?

A While it's true that nuts contain a high percentage of fat, that's not the whole story. Eliminating all fat from the diet is unwise: the essential fats omega-3 and 6 actually help you burn fat more efficiently. Raw nuts contain useful levels of these good fats, as well as providing a source of protein to slow down the release of sugar from carbohydrates. This is important because controlling weight requires controlling blood sugar, and balancing carbs to protein 2:1 is an important part of this. For most people this means eating more protein, for example having a small handful of nuts or seeds with a fresh fruit snack. See how useful nuts can be?

Roasted nuts contain damaged fats, and therefore fall into the category of those you want to avoid when trying to lose weight; others are saturated (animal), hydrogenated and fried fats. But raw nuts, for both their essential fatty acid and protein content, eaten in moderation, are a useful part of a calorie-restricted, exercise-including, supplement-supported weight loss programme. And their rich taste makes them a satisfying as well as healthy alternative to biscuits or chocolate.

Q *Are peanuts good for you?*

A Peanuts do, indeed, have a lot going for them. They are a rich source of protein and a healthier snack than a sugary chocolate bar. Some people steer clear of peanuts because of their high fat content (almost 50 per cent) but half of it is oleic acid, an omega fat that also boosts the healthy qualities of olive oil, and 30 per cent is omega-6 fats. Many people are low in such essential fats, which help keep the brain, nerves, hormones and skin healthy.

Another reason why some people avoid peanuts is that they can trigger allergic reactions – from poor digestion or eczema to full anaphylactic shock. This may be a reaction to the protein in peanuts or a poison that is commonly found on the surface of the nuts, aflatoxin. If you do eat peanuts, choose the fresh, unsalted ones in their shells, rather than the dry-roasted or flavoured ones.

Q *I read that soya is dangerous because it interferes with your hormones. Is this true?*

A Soya does indeed contain substances called phyto-oestrogens which research has shown to affect hormonal function – but positively. These natural chemicals – mainly two called genistein and daidzein – act as weak oestrogens in the body but in a very special, balancing way. So if your natural oestrogen levels are low, they will lock onto oestrogen receptor sites on cells and act as weak oestrogens, thereby raising levels, which could be particularly useful during the menopause. Conversely, if your oestrogen levels are high (which can cause premenstrual symptoms), they lock onto the receptors and actually block them from receiving excess oestrogen or toxic chemicals from the environment such as pesticides or plastics which have oestrogen-like effects. Only one study I know of has shown soya extracts to be harmful. In this experiment, rats were fed extremely high amounts. Eating soya products regularly has been shown to reduce menopausal symptoms, PMS and hormone-related cancers such as prostate cancer.

I would not, however, recommend giving infants large amounts of soya, for example by feeding them soya milk formula exclusively. This is simply because we don't know the effects of a large amount of phytoestrogens during such a vital growing phase. Note also that adults eating excessive amounts of soya can develop an allergy to it, especially if their digestion isn't good. There is also some evidence that allergy to soya can run in families, so be careful if other members of your family are allergic to soya.

Q *I've heard soya contains high levels of aluminium. Is this true?*

A Processed soya products *can* contain aluminium as they are often stored or processed in aluminium tanks. But this will not always result in high aluminium levels, any more than in any other processed food. So I don't recommend avoiding soya, and missing out on all the other benefits, such as balancing hormones, staving off cancer and lowering cholesterol, unless you know you have a problem with high aluminium levels.

To save yourself unnecessary worry, you could have a hair mineral analysis done which will show you whether or not you have a high aluminium level (see Resources, page 483). I've seen over 5,000 such tests and haven't noticed a link between aluminium and soya consumption.

Q *Why are pumpkin seeds so good for you?*

A Pumpkin seeds are an absolute superfood. Rich in so many nutrients, they make an excellent snack, or can be sprinkled generously on cereals, soups or salads. As with all seeds, they contain abundant calcium for bones and teeth, but additionally carry a large amount of other minerals, such as iron, zinc and magnesium. Their reputation as a male sexual tonic lies in their high zinc content, protecting the prostate gland and enhancing sperm health. Organic pumpkin seeds have a darker green colour, revealing a higher content of magnesium, a key mineral component of the green plant pigment chlorophyll. Magnesium aids the absorption of calcium and is an excellent muscle relaxant.

But it doesn't stop there. Pumpkin seeds are a good source of protein and omega-3 essential fats, great for lubricating skin and joints and soothing inflammatory conditions like asthma, eczema, hay fever and arthritis – and keeping your brain on an even keel. Eat them every day. Raw is best, though a delicious, moreish alternative is to dry-roast them in a pan till they start to brown, then add a dash of soy sauce that sizzles off and coats the seeds.

Salt

Q *How much salt does a person need?*

A Sodium is eaten mainly in the form of sodium chloride (salt). Of the 92g of sodium in the body, more than half is in the fluids surrounding cells, where it plays a vital role in both nerve transmission and the maintenance of the body's normal water balance. Too much sodium means you retain too much water, which can be a reason for weight gain. Most of this excess will come from eating salted foods or adding salt to foods as a flavour enhancer. You only need about 2g of salt a day. The following table shows how much salt 100g of common foods contains.

Salt content of common foods

Food (100g serving)	Salt content (in mg)
Prawns	2,300
Olives	2,020
Ham	1,500
Celery	875
Cabbage	643
Cottage cheese	405
Kidney beans	327

Deficiency is exceedingly rare both because excess amounts are added to foods and also because the body tends to keep hold of it. Sodium is present in most natural foods in small amounts and we get most of our intake from processed foods. So there is no need to add it to food and good reasons not to since too much is associated with high blood pressure, oedema and kidney problems.

Q **Why is salt bad for you, and is potassium salt a better alternative?**

A Minerals are like electricity couriers for the body and brain. As they move in and out of cells they control whether or not the cell 'fires'. But they need to be in balance. Too much sodium, and not enough magnesium or potassium, makes you hyperactive in more ways than one. Muscles contract, resulting in physical tension and cramps or spasms. Nerve cells become overstimulated and you get more anxious and can't get to sleep. Since arteries are surrounded by a layer of muscle, too much sodium and a lack of magnesium and potassium makes them contract, raising your blood pressure. So, in general, if you want to be healthy, you need less sodium and more potassium and magnesium.

Not all salt, however, is bad for you. Traditional salt is simple sodium chloride. Sea salt contains other minerals, but is still predominantly sodium. An alternative is potassium salt, which is much better for you but doesn't taste so good. Another alternative is low sodium Icelandic salt, known as Solo Salt.

This is quite different from regular sea salt. Its sodium content is 60 per cent lower, plus it has significantly more potassium and magnesium. In fact, there's more potassium (21 per cent) than sodium (16 per cent) in it, and considerably more magnesium. Some 17 per cent of the salts in Solo Salt are magnesium salts. A double-blind controlled study carried out on 100 men who had high blood pressure averaging 157.5/90.8 mm Hg gave them either regular salt or Solo Salt over 24 weeks. The result was a significant reduction in blood pressure in those using Solo Salt, with the systolic blood pressure falling by 7.6 mm Hg and the diastolic blood pressure falling by 3.3. Solo Salt is therefore a healthy alternative to regular salt and should be positively recommended for those with hypertension.

Sugars, sweets and sugar substitutes

Q *What effect does brown rice syrup have on blood sugar?*

A Brown rice syrup is roughly 50 per cent soluble complex carbohydrates, 45 per cent maltose and 3 per cent glucose. The glucose is absorbed into the bloodstream immediately, the maltose takes up to one and a half hours to be digested, and the complex carbohydrates take from two to three hours, providing a steady supply of energy. This means it has a much less marked effect on your blood sugar than eating other sweeteners, including sugar and honey.

Q *I'm weaning myself off sugar. Any ideas?*

A You're on the right track: cutting out sugar is important, as it plays havoc with your blood sugar and can lead to degenerative diseases such as Type II diabetes. Begin by cutting sugar out completely, and start substituting fresh fruit as a sweetener for other foods, such as your breakfast cereal, and as a snack (best with a small handful of nuts). In due course you will find yourself gradually losing your sweet tooth. One day you'll discover that you simply don't need any sweetness beyond the natural flavour of fruit, wholegrains and the like.

To help the process along, it is a good idea to

gradually dilute fruit juice and go easy on the dried fruit. If you absolutely have to sweeten something, I'd use fructose, as this is a natural fruit sugar that does not have a disturbing effect on your blood sugar. You can buy this in any healthfood store. In time, you'll be astonished at your former need for supersweetened food, and you'll have the energy and sense of well-being that balanced blood sugar gives.

Q *What's your view on artificial sweeteners such as Nutrasweet?*

A One of the major problems with artificial sweeteners is that they constantly stoke your cravings for sweetened foods and drinks. But there are more serious drawbacks to Nutrasweet, or aspartame.

Aspartame has been linked to a variety of health problems including birth defects, diabetes, emotional disorders, epilepsy or seizures and migraines. Recent research from Japan has indicated that very low doses reduce sperm count quite considerably in mice. Mice given very low amounts of aspartame had almost a 10 per cent decrease in healthy sperm.

While this, and other reports of negative effects, can be criticised, I don't see the point of encouraging any artificial sweeteners. Sugar itself contributes to diabetes, obesity, heart disease and probably cancer, and artificial sweeteners aren't much better. If you are addicted to adding or eating something sweet my advice is to wean yourself off both sugar and artificial sweeteners, and sweeten cereal and desserts with fruit instead. Fructose is OK if you're desperate to add something to drinks, but you'll find a sweet tooth will disappear with time.

Q ***What will happen if I eat too many sweets?***

A Compared to some habits, a daily encounter with a bag of sweets might seem innocent enough. But consider this. Concentrated, refined sugar of the type you find in sweets is literally a 'sweet nothing', practically devoid of vitamins and minerals and classified as empty calories. Sugar even uses up valuable nutrients while the body digests it. More: eating too much of it boosts glucose levels in the blood so much that the excess glucose is stored, eventually emerging as fat. So sugar can pile on the weight.

The sudden surges in blood sugar that bingeing on sweets causes also send you on an energy rollercoaster – from sugar highs to exhausted slumps. You end up with an energy imbalance, which triggers a host of symptoms. When your blood sugar is low, for instance, you may experience anything from fatigue to irritability, poor concentration, nervousness, headaches and sweating. If your consumption of sweets is really out of control you can even be at risk of Type II diabetes, which is after all just an extreme form of blood sugar imbalance. Sugar can also upset the balance of beneficial bacteria in your gut. So think twice before reaching for that bag or bar: the bitter truth is that you'd be doing your body no favours.

Q *Why do I crave chocolate?*

A It's not just psychological and it's not just because it tastes so good – chocolate can really be addictive. It contains a mood-enhancing substance called phenethylamine. Even experimental, alcoholic rats will forego some alcohol for chocolate, given the choice. Chocolate also contains the stimulants caffeine and theobromine, so along with phenethylamine, it boosts levels of one of the body's mood-enhancing chemicals, dopamine. Researchers have found that dopamine triggers a chain reaction producing hormones that make women interested in sex. Another major ingredient in chocolate is sugar, which lifts mood, energy and concentration temporarily, before it sends you crashing down again. So, if you're tired or stressed out, it's not surprising that you would crave chocolate.

If your chocolate cravings have spiralled out of control, you should consider weaning yourself off it. Try replacing it with healthy snacks such as fruit, nuts, a yoghurt or a muesli bar. And to help stabilise your energy levels, supplement 200mcg of the mineral chromium a day.

Q *I keep reading that chocolate is good for you. Is this true?*

A Chocaholics will rejoice to know that their passion does indeed contain substances that not only make you feel good, but that are also good for you. But this isn't a signal for ripping into a big bar of the stuff.

It's well known that chocolate contains caffeine and theobromine, addictive stimulants that raise your energy and give you a mental lift, and sugar, which boosts the mood-altering hormone serotonin as well as dopamine. Along with the flavour, this accounts for chocolate's popularity. But there is more. Chocolate contains magnesium, and there is a theory that women get premenstrual chocolate cravings to correct deficiencies in this mineral. Scientists have also found that chocolate, especially the dark variety, contains antioxidants vital for protecting against pollution and heart disease. All this said, I still wouldn't start calling chocolate a health food. Fruits and vegetables give you better value for antioxidants, and the energy boost chocolate provides is short-lived and leaves you craving more. It's good for the soul to have the odd indulgence, so keep it as just that.

Wheat and other cereals

Q *How is quinoa good for you?*

A Quinoa (pronounced 'keen-wa') is a staple food in the high Andes and is reputed to have been the source of the Incas' strength as they worked at high altitudes to build an empire. Known as the 'mother grain' for its unique sustaining properties, it contains significantly more protein than any other grain, with a quality of protein better than that in meat. It's also rich in vitamins and minerals, providing almost four times as much calcium as wheat, plus iron, B vitamins and vitamin E. Not technically a grain, but a seed, as such quinoa is rich in polyunsaturated oils, providing essential fatty acids. So it's about as close to a perfect food as you can get.

You can buy quinoa in most healthfood shops and even some big supermarkets. To cook it, first rinse it well. Then boil it for 15 minutes in twice as much water and serve it as you would rice. It is exceptionally versatile, excellent in tabbouleh-like salads with beans and chopped vegetables, or served hot, as its nutty taste goes very well with tomato-based sauces and stews.

Q *I keep hearing mixed reports – should we eat wheat?*

A Wheat in itself is no bad thing; it has, after all, proved a staple food for thousands of years. The main reason people need to cut down on wheat is that many people are sensitive to it and overconsumption is making matters worse. Consider a typical day's meals of toast, a sandwich and pasta. That's a lot of wheat.

Why is it problematic? Gluten, the protein in wheat, is sticky and hard to digest. It can clog the gut and trigger reactions – from constipation and bloating to grogginess and depression. What's more, much wheat is now hybridised to contain more gluten because high-gluten flour produces a larger loaf with less flour. About 1 in 100 people are sensitive to gluten, a condition called coeliac disease, although this frequently goes undiagnosed. Gluten is also in rye, barley and oats. However, there is a sub-fraction of gluten, called gliadin, which seems to be the major allergic culprit for many people, and which is not in oats.

Another down side is wheat fibre, which contains phytates that attach themselves to minerals such as calcium and prevent them from being absorbed. So I recommend you don't have wheat every day – instead, eat rye bread, oat or rice cakes, corn or oat-based cereals, less pasta and more rice.

Q *Why does wheat cause bloating?*

A Wheat is the number one culprit if you suffer from bloating and flatulence. This is because modern wheat has been hybridised over the last 2,000 years to contain more gluten, a sticky protein in wheat that produces a larger, fluffier loaf with less flour. The very high gluten content in modern wheat makes it hard to digest and can reduce the absorption of other nutrients in your intestines by turning into a sticky, gluey substance not unlike papier-maché which is, after all, just flour and water. But not all wheat is bad. Spelt, the grain sometimes called 'Roman wheat', is how wheat was before selective breeding. Spelt has a much lower gluten content, and is now widely available in healthfood shops as flour, bread, pasta and more. And *kamut* is an ancient Egyptian form of wheat, going back 3,000 years.

Studies in the *Journal of Gastroenterology* have shown that up to 20 per cent of dietary starch (such as wheat) escapes absorption in the small intestines. This is then completely digested by the bacteria living in your intestines, which produce various gases, causing bloating and flatulence. If you're plagued by these problems, try cutting wheat out completely for 10 days, replacing it with other grains like rye, oats or rice. Then reintroduce it (and have a lot), and see what happens. If this shows you that wheat is causing bloating and flatulence for you, reduce it as much as possible, and in time (a few months, say) if you have it occasionally it shouldn't cause you too much of a problem.

DIG DEEPER: The book *Dangerous Grains* (Avery Press, 2002) by Dr James Braly is the most comprehensive book on the subject of gluten sensitivity, for those who want to find out more.

Q *Is wholewheat bread good for the bowels?*

A Sure, brown bread is likely to contain more fibre than white bread, but this does not necessarily mean it's better for the bowels. Insoluble fibre, which is the kind brown bread contains, is generally important for keeping the digestive tract clean and preventing constipation. It does this by absorbing water and bulking out the stools, which stimulates the movement of the guts. However, wheat bran can be very irritating to the gut wall, causing inflammation and pain.

Then there is wheat intolerance, which is all too common: consuming too much wheat from bread (or pasta, cereals, pastry and biscuits) is associated with constipation, bloating, flatulence, irritable bowel syndrome and diarrhoea. If you experience any of these, avoid wheat for 10 days – have rye, oats, rice, corn and potatoes instead – and see if you notice any difference. If you do, avoid wheat strictly for three months, which is the time it takes for the immune system to forget it's sensitivity (that's if you have an IgG sensitivity – if you have an IgE sensitivity you'll need to avoid wheat for life). After that, reintroduce it and, if you get no return of symptoms, only consume wheat periodically, ideally no more than every four days, spacing it out with other grains.

Q *Why are we told that white or refined products are bad? What does this mean in essence?*

A We're talking here about refined carbohydrates – sugar and grains mostly, including white sugar, bread, rice and pasta. A grain is made up of three key parts – the germ, which contains the plant embryo; the starch, which feeds it; and the bran, which surrounds it all, inside the husk (which we don't eat). The bran and germ have been removed in white rice, bread or pasta, leaving just the white-coloured starch. The problem with this is that the bran and germ contain almost all of the nutrients – fibre, B vitamins, minerals, vitamin E – while the starch part provides little more than simple sugars and a small amount of protein. White rice, bread and sugar contain 80 to 90 per cent fewer minerals, vitamins and fibre than brown rice, wholemeal bread/pasta or raw sugar. Nutritionists generally consider refined carbohydrates to be 'bad' foods because they provide a lot of calories but very few nutrients, whereas the path to optimum health and longevity is generally fewer calories and more nutrients.

Wholegrains are known to reduce the risk of heart disease, improve digestive function, help balance blood sugar levels and lower homocysteine (indicating a reduced risk of developing degenerative diseases). If you consider the standard food pyramid, think of wholegrains in the large bottom section, and refined ones in the very top section with sugars and fats, labelled 'eat sparingly'.

Q *Is white basmati rice refined? I thought it was better for you than normal white rice.*

A Basmati rice is a long-grained rice named after the tropical basmati blossom in Southeast Asia. It's aged for a year after harvest to fully develop its nutty flavour, and its grains elongate when cooked rather than fatten like most other rices.

Basmati rice comes in both brown and white versions just like normal rice, and yes, white basmati is refined. However, basmati is lower in overall starch and higher in a particular kind of starch called amylose than other rices, and consequently has a lower glycaemic index of around 58. Brown rice has a similar GI, while white rice is much higher, meaning it causes a greater spike in your blood sugar after you eat it. That can disrupt your blood sugar balance, erode energy levels and often contribute to weight gain (as unused glucose in the blood is stored as fat). For a tasty white rice, basmati is a good choice, though it's still had much of its minerals and fibre removed (see 'Why are we told that white or refined products are bad?', page 113). So ideally, brown basmati is the one to go for.

Food processing and modification

Q *What's your view on genetically modified food?*

A It's natural for plants, animals and microorganisms to change. The trouble with genetic modification is that, by inserting a gene into a plant or animal, it creates a significant and rapid shift, the long-term consequences of which are unknown. Of course we'll find out, but at what cost?

And in fact, I foresee some major problems with genetically modified foods. The pro lobby argues that GM crops increase food production. Whether this is done for social or commercial interests is a matter of opinion. In any case, it has often been bad agricultural practice in the first place that has caused poor plant yields by stripping soil of nutrients and forcing food growth with chemicals. Organic farming practices aim to restore healthy soil and plant growth. I think the government should be promoting organic farming more than GM technology.

But my real objection to GM food is twofold. First off, GM crops affect the environment: they can contaminate other plants. This is a major concern because, in the broader sense, what we would be doing is interfering with the fundamental ecological balance that has evolved over millions of years. The real question for me is, whom do I trust more here? Nature or the food industry?

Recently, scientists in Britain have reported the results of trials in which the fields with GM crops had fewer weeds and insects; this was seen as a threat to the country's already depleted wildlife. And in Canada, one of the first countries trying out GM strains of seeds, the consequences have been diabolical. The seeds were genetically modified to be resistant to herbicides so that the fields could be sprayed with them and only the crop would grow. The promise was greater yields, but the reality has been the opposite. The genetic modifications have spread, creating 'superweeds'. The GM strains have travelled much further than expected, contaminating organic farms and, in essence, threatening to put them out of business.

Secondly, there's very little research on the effects on humans who eat the crops, in either the short or long term. The first human blunder happened in 1989, when a GM organism was used to produce cheap tryptophan, a constituent of protein. Thousands of people who consumed it got sick, and 17 died. This alone is good reason to proceed with extreme caution.

If genetic alterations can easily jump from plant to plant, as we've seen in Canada, they can also theoretically jump to the humans who eat them, or at least, alter biochemical reactions to what are, in essence, new foods.

Q **What's your view on irradiated food?**

A Irradiated food is not sold in the UK. The controversy surrounding irradiation laid to rest plans to make it legal about 10 years ago and until three years ago, only a few irradiated herbs and spices were sold. Irradiating food would be a quick answer to any food hygiene and preservation problems – it zaps nasty bugs like salmonella and listeria, takes away the need for excess pesticides or additives and gives food a longer shelf life. A supermarket's dream perhaps, but a consumer's nightmare. Although there appears to be no residual radiation on irradiated foods, the process itself creates highly reactive oxygen molecules – oxidants – that are known to be at the root of heart disease and cancer. What's more, irradiating food has also been shown to reduce its vitamin content by as much as 96 per cent, and make the essential fats in foods such as vegetable oils and nuts go rancid.

Q **What's your view on foods fortified with vitamins?**

A I am always wary of foods with 'added vitamins', since most fortified foods, such as breakfast cereals, are full of refined foods and sugar. Some refined foods, such as white flour, have to have certain nutrients (B1, B2, B3, iron, calcium) added back in by law. In the US there are moves to extend this list to include B12, folic acid and B6.

Why not just stop refining flour, which is the cause of the deficiency in the first place? Many refined foods have lost other key nutrients such as zinc, selenium or chromium. The foods often state that they contain 100 per cent of the RDA of every vitamin, but what about these minerals? It is far better to choose wholefoods, unrefined and without sugar, and then supplement meaningful amounts of a wide range of vitamins and minerals in a high-strength multi.

Organic and wholefoods

Q *How important is it to eat organic?*

 There are more reasons to eat organic that most people realise. First, organic food is free from herbicides and pesticides. On average, a gallon of these is sprayed on the fruit and vegetables eaten by one person in a year. No one really knows what the effect of this is, but it certainly isn't good for you.

Organic food has 26 per cent more 'dry matter' and less water in it than non-organic foods grown with fertilisers. The effect of these chemicals is to get more water into the plant. In other words, two organic carrots fill you up the same as three non-organic carrots. So, if the organic carrots are 20 per cent more expensive they are still better value for money. On top of this, organic produce tends to have 50 to 100 per cent higher mineral levels.

The most important organic foods to eat are grains and cereals. This is because each non-organic grain is sprayed with herbicides and pesticides and the net residue in things like breakfast cereal is considerable. On the other hand, if you buy something you can peel, like a banana, most of the chemicals are in the skin, not the flesh.

Q *Are all so-called organic foods grown to the same standards? Can I trust the organic food in the supermarket?*

A The term 'organic' is actually a legal definition, so anyone breaching the standard set by the government, say, by using chemicals or GM ingredients, can be prosecuted. Organic products grown or made in the UK must carry a certifying body's mark (such as the Soil Association or the Organic Farmers and Growers) and licence number. Produce from within the EU is covered by the same stringent regulations and anyone wanting to import products from elsewhere has to get a UK licence, so local standards are always checked first. True, a small percentage of the feed of animals raised to produce organic meat can be non-organic, but even this is being phased out. What's more, organic animal production takes into consideration the animals' welfare and doesn't routinely use veterinary products. So no wonder organic sales are up by 40 per cent for the second year running.

DIG DEEPER: For further information see
www.soilassociation.org.

Q *Is organic food worth the money?*

A Yes, it is. The most comprehensive review of the scientific evidence published last year showed that compared to non-organic produce, organic produce contains fewer pesticide residues, fewer food additives, less water (so more carrot in your organic carrot!), more minerals and vitamin C, and more protective phytonutrients. If you want to be healthy you need to both avoid the bad guys and eat the good guys. That's why organic food is an important part of a healthy diet. Organic food is not a luxury; it is how food is supposed to be.

Buying things on the cheap often proves more costly in the long run, and food is no exception. So while you can save money now by buying cheap food, it may cost you your health later. Even organic crisps, cola, ice cream, cakes, biscuits and so on, while not healthfoods themselves, should contain fewer additives and cannot contain harmful ingredients like hydrogenated fats. So they're usually better choices than their non-organic equivalents, as long as they are enjoyed in moderation.

Q **What is a wholefood?**

A A wholefood is a food that hasn't been refined. Foods such as wheat and rice were traditionally refined into white flour and white rice so that they would be less prone to infestation by weevils: refining removes the nutrients the insects need to survive, allowing these staples to be stored longer. This was necessary during the Industrial Revolution to feed workers in cities before improved transport systems and refrigeration made it possible for everyone to eat fresh food.

So, if you eat a lot of refined food you're eating food that wouldn't support the life of a weevil! Instead, eat wholefoods – beans, lentils, seeds, nuts, and wholegrains such as oat flakes, wholewheat or whole rye bread or pasta. Basically, if a food you buy is recognisably near its original condition, when it was plucked from a tree or pulled out of the ground, it's a wholefood. If not, the chances are it's been refined or processed in some way that has reduced its nutritional value.

Vegetarian, vegan and other specialised diets

Q **Do different blood types really need different kinds of food?**

A The 'blood type' diet, advocated by Dr Peter D'Adamo in his book *Eat Right for Your Blood Type*, is valid and backed up by serious scientific research. And yes, many people find they feel better and maintain their ideal weight when they eat the foods recommended for their specific blood type. However, there's a snag. The blood type diet is based on giving foods that were available when each blood type was most prevalent. For example, type O is associated with hunter-gatherer eating, and people with this blood type tend to do better on more meat protein, while As are essentially peasant farmers, doing better on grains. The trouble is that in the 21st century we have other factors to take into account, such as consuming antioxidants to protect us from the effects of pollution, or eating beans such as soya to stave off cancer. In the nutritional principles I lay out in *The Optimum Nutrition Bible*, I take account of these factors. So most people would be better off starting with these as the basics, and then using the blood type guidelines to 'fine-tune' their diet.

Q *Is combining proteins and carbohydrates really bad for your health?*

A So-called 'food combining', or the Hay Diet, is actually food separating. In this diet you avoid having protein-rich and carbohydrate-rich foods at the same time. Some people find that when they eat like this they digest their meals better, lose weight and have more energy; and in fact, anyone with digestive problems would be wise to try it.

A great many more people, however, would

benefit from having some protein at every meal, no matter what they combine it with. The reason for this is that protein helps balance blood sugar levels, which affect energy, mood and weight. Meals low in or devoid of protein and high in carbohydrates are more likely to leave your energy and mood in tatters, and over time are also likely to encourage weight gain. But ultimately, we are all very different, so it's a matter of working out which diet is best for you.

Q **Does a high-protein diet raise or lower testosterone?**

A Testosterone is a powerful sex hormone found in both men and women. Deficiency leads to a lower sex drive and motivation in both men and women. Excess in women can lead to facial hair and less feminine features. In men it can lead to too high a sex drive and increased aggression.

The balance of evidence is that meat increases testosterone, although the mechanism is not fully understood. It may have little to do with the protein, and more to do with the cholesterol content. Perhaps this is why there are conflicting views on the effects of protein on testosterone. Hormones, including testosterone, are made from cholesterol; so increasing one's intake of cholesterol may increase one's production of testosterone. A low cholesterol, vegetarian diet is known to lower testosterone.

> **DIG DEEPER:** The most authoritative voice on this subject is Dr Malcolm Carruthers, and for more information you may wish to read his excellent book *The Testosterone Revolution* (Thorsons, 2001).

Q *What's your view on macrobiotic diets?*

A Macrobiotics is based on the principle that all life can be viewed as a balance of two energies: yin and yang. For example, men and daytime are yang, while women and nighttime are yin. Foods are also classified as yin and yang. Meat, for example, is yang. In practice, macrobiotics recommends eating unrefined wholefoods with an emphasis towards vegetarian foods. As such it is consistent with current views of optimum nutrition. It also recommends avoiding sugar, alcohol and stimulants. There are, however, some differences. Macrobiotics recommends little fruit, especially in the winter, on the basis that these fruits are out of season. In this respect a macrobiotic diet is unlikely to provide optimal intakes of vitamin C and other antioxidants.

Q *Are raw food diets better for you?*

A There are many advantages to eating plenty of raw food daily. Fresh fruit and vegetables, seeds and nuts are full of nutrients, undamaged by heating or processing. On a more ethereal level, raw foods are still laden with the energy from the earth and sun. In fact, many people say they have more energy when they eat some raw food regularly.

There are, however, a few drawbacks to eating nothing but uncooked foods. Some people find them difficult to digest because heating has not softened the fibres. Cooking also makes some of the nutrients more available. And it is certainly good for the body to keep it well warmed in the winter with hot, cooked foods. So keep cooked and uncooked food in healthy balance. Avoid frying in fats or cooking for long periods of time, and steam away: steaming foods is a great cooking method that leaves the nutrients intact. Green beans, cauliflower and broccoli, for instance, all take kindly to a quick steaming.

Q *Is a vegan diet healthy?*

A There's no reason why vegans should get any fewer nutrients than carnivores, although there are some that they need to take care to include. The most obvious is protein – make sure you eat enough soya produce, beans, lentils, nuts, seeds and sprouted seeds. You'll need two servings of protein a day. You also need to ensure you get a good supply of essential fatty acids – for healthy brain, skin and hormones. Nuts and seeds are good sources of these, particularly flax seeds, because they are the only vegetarian food that has high amounts of omega-3 fats. I recommend a dessert-spoon of flax seed oil a day. Nuts, seeds and beans are also good sources of calcium, a mineral that new vegans are often afraid to miss out on because they'll be giving up milk. One nutrient that vegan diets can fall short on is vitamin B12, which as far as food goes is only really available in animal products; so I'd suggest taking a good multivitamin containing B12.

Q **How do I stop losing weight on a vegan diet?**

A A vegan diet can be very helpful for those wishing to lose weight. But if you are already underweight, it's important to have an adequate dietary intake of all the macronutrients – protein, carbohydrates and fat. While you *can* get all the protein you need on a vegan diet, many vegans don't. Ensure a healthy intake (two daily servings) of nuts, seeds, tofu, beans, lentils, wholegrains and pulses – mixing them up over each day or two to ensure an adequate amino acid intake. Fat sources are important, and your vegan choices are seeds (sunflower, flax, hemp and pumpkin) and their cold-pressed oils, both of which should be regular features of your diet. Finally, be sure you're eating enough carbohydrates – the complex, not refined type – to satisfy your energy needs. Balance them with half as much protein at each meal/snack to avoid glucose intolerance from excess carbohydrate intake.

DIG DEEPER: See the Vegan Society's website (www.vegansociety.com) for more tips.

Q *To what extent do I need to combine grains, pulses and nuts/seeds to optimise protein intake on a vegetarian diet?*

A Combining these foods certainly makes a difference in terms of protein utilisation, but you don't need to do it at every meal. The body has a pool of amino acids that don't become depleted with each meal, but over a day where you eat no essential amino acids, levels might get low. So try to have a mix each day and throughout the week.

For example, eat seeds and grains for breakfast, and then some beans, nuts, lentils or tofu for lunch and/or dinner. Don't just eat grains at each meal. This should be sufficient. Soya/tofu and quinoa are really complete in their own right, so you should make a point of having them regularly.

Q *I'm a strict vegetarian. Are there any nutrients I'm missing out on?*

A The most obvious nutrient to watch out for is protein – many veggies either eat too little or rely heavily on cheese. So make sure you get two servings of soya produce, beans, lentils or eggs a day. Eggs are also a great source of iron and other important nutrients. You need a good supply of essential fatty acids – for healthy brain, skin and hormones. While these are abundant in oily fish, flax seeds are also rich in them so I recommend a tablespoon of flax seeds or a dessertspoon of flax seed oil a day. If you do tend to be more vegan, also make sure you are having a good multivitamin that contains vitamin B12, as this is only really available in animal products.

Q *I am a vegetarian suffering from anaemia. How do I improve my iron intake?*

A The optimum intake of iron is 15mg a day, which can increase up to 25mg if your deficiency is very serious. Pumpkin seeds, parsley, almonds, prunes, cashew nuts, raisins, Brazil nuts and dates are all, in descending order, good sources of iron. Organic eggs are also rich in iron. Eating iron-rich foods with vitamin C-rich foods increases absorption, so pair your seeds and nuts with an orange, a handful of strawberries or a few chunks of kiwi fruit.

In terms of supplements, some are absorbed better than others. I recommend either iron bisglycinate or a 'truefood' iron, which is iron within a food matrix. (See Resources, page 483.) But you shouldn't focus on iron alone. Other nutrients are needed to make blood cells – Vitamin B12 or folic acid, and zinc, for example – so you should take a good-quality multivitamin and mineral supplement. And if you have low stomach acid or a lack of other digestive enzymes, you may not be able to absorb iron or other minerals from your food. In this case taking a digestive enxyme that contains betaine hydrchloride can help.

Q *Many of your articles recommend omega-3 fish oils. As a strict vegetarian can I assume that omega-3 oils from seeds are just as effective?*

A Omega-3 oils are also found in flax, hemp and pumpkin seeds. You can take the first two as seed oils – which you can mix into salad dressings or drizzle over vegetables – or as whole seeds, ground in a coffee grinder, then sprinkled on cereals, soups or salads. Pumpkin seeds can also be ground, or eaten whole, again on cereals or as a delicious snack; it's best to eat them raw, not toasted. Ideal quantities are 1 tablespoon of seed oils or 2 tablespoons of flax seeds, or 4 tablespoons of pumpkin seeds.

All these vegetarian sources of omega-3 oils contain alpha-linolenic acid. This has to be converted by the body into EPA and DHA, the most powerful and biologically active omega-3 fats. However, the conversion is not that great, usually less than 10 per cent. This is why omega-3 fish oils, which are a direct source of EPA and DHA, work better, especially for those who need much larger amounts, for example for people with arthritis, cardiovascular disease or mental health problems. If you have a particular need for EPA and DHA, it's up to you whether you're willing to compromise by taking fish oil.

Water

Q *To minimise the intake of harmful oestrogens, is it better to drink filtered tap water or mineral water from a plastic bottle?*

A If there are oestrogens in your tap water I doubt that a simple jug-type filter, say, could remove them. Bottled water is usually a good choice. There is no evidence that oestrogen-like or other chemicals in the plastic leach into the water.

If you want to be absolutely sure of getting no oestrogens in your water supply, you should consider having an under-sink water filter installed. Your options are the Fresh Water Filter Company's ceramic filter, which can remove around 90 per cent of the synthetic oestrogens, though not natural ones, or the Pure H20 Company who sell reverse osmosis filters. (See Resources, page 483.) This system produces medically pure water that would have absolutely no oestrogens in it. I recommend you call any water filter company and ask them about their filters' abilities to remove oestrogens before choosing your preferred option. Also, don't forget that pesticides can also be xeno-oestrogenic and therefore buying organic produce where possible is important.

Q *I've heard fizzy water is bad for you. Is this true?*

A Yes and no. Fizzy water is carbonated, and carbon grabs hold of minerals. Naturally carbonated mineral water, such as Badoit, contains carbonated minerals that are absorbed into the body. The carbon in artificially carbonated water, however, could theoretically grab hold of minerals in the body and take them out. Being potentially concerned about this, I've investigated the evidence and don't think there's any real problem with carbonated mineral water.

The problem really lies with fizzy drinks that contain caffeine and phosphoric acid – many of which are sparkling. Too much phosphorus can hinder the absorption of calcium, which is essential to bone health. It is therefore these other ingredients that are present in some sparkling soft drinks and not the carbon dioxide that may be the cause of problems in those cases where absorption difficulties have been identified.

People who drink loads of artificially fizzy drinks tend to have less bone density as a result. So the best mineral water to drink is naturally carbonated, followed by still or artificially carbonated. Most important of all is to drink enough water: you need 1 to 1.5 litres of water a day. Drinking this much water keeps the skin hydrated, detoxifies the liver and protects the kidneys by diluting toxins in the blood.

Q *I have been told to drink 2 litres of water per day. Is it really necessary for me to try and force down more water than I feel my system can cope with?*

A Drinking water can be difficult when you are not used to it, so build up slowly. Try having a large mug of hot water with lemon juice in the morning, then take a 1-litre bottle with you, either at home or on your desk at work, and sip it gradually during the day. As soon as you feel able, switch to a 1.5-litre bottle. Obviously don't force more down than you can manage. Also make sure you are supporting your liver and kidneys with other measures – that is, a stimulant and alcohol-free diet with plenty of nutrient-rich vegetables and fruit.

Rather than forcing yourself to drink a specific amount, I'd be guided by your own body. Any combination of the symptoms below could be a cry for water, and recognising them can help you become more in tune with that.

- Are you prone to constipation?
- Are you often thirsty?
- Do you have joint problems?
- Do you feel tired?
- Are you having difficulty concentrating?
- Are you overheating?
- Do you have dry skin, mouth or lips?
- Do you get frequent infections?
- Do you have dry, brittle hair?

The other way to judge is by the colour of your urine. If your urine is a very strong, dark yellow, you're not drinking enough. This simple gauge is, however, complicated by the fact that riboflavin (vitamin B2) makes the urine a fluorescent kind of yellow. Ideally, your urine should be a light straw colour. If, however, it is often clear, like water, you may be drinking too much water and not taking in enough nutrients.

Q *I drink up to 6 litres of water a day because I thought it was a healthy thing to do. I have to go to the loo four times per hour, yet my urine is still pretty dark in the mornings.*

A It sounds like you are drinking too much water – so it's not surprising you are going to the loo so often! While most people don't drink enough, it is also possible to overload your kidneys. Drinking 1.5 to 2 litres of water a day should be enough, and of course more if you exercise, but only an extra litre or so. Your urine could be stronger in the morning because your body slows down water release overnight, so urine is usually much more concentrated. Taking supplements, particularly B vitamins, can also colour your urine and give it a distinctive smell, and this may be more pronounced in the morning, especially if you're taking supplements before bed. However, if you have any pain or discomfort, or your urine has an unpleasant smell, you should go to your doctor to test for any infections.

DISEASES, AILMENTS AND INJURIES A–Z

One of the most remarkable and heartening aspects of optimum nutrition is that it can be tailored to treat conditions ranging from the common cold to thyroid problems, heart conditions to cancer. Over the years, many of the questions I've received have focused on specific health problems. If you're on medication, the right foods can complement the treatment. In some cases, diet alone is enough. Whatever your needs, this section offers useful advice on a broad range of conditions.

Anaemia

Q *I'm always tired and look pale. Is this anaemia?*

A Yes, you may be deficient in iron. Iron is needed in the body to make haemoglobin – a key part of blood responsible for the delivery of oxygen and other nutrients to your tissues, brain, muscles and organs. If you're low in iron you can't make enough red blood cells, hence the pale appearance; and with fewer red blood cells, your brain and body don't get the levels of oxygen and other nutrients they need. The result? You feel perpetually tired.

Red meat is a well-known source of iron, and a good source too. The problem is that it's also rich in saturated fat, so go for an alternative: eggs, spinach and other greens, beans, lentils, prunes, dried apricots, molasses and pumpkin seeds. Two simple tests of your iron status involve your eyelids and fingernails. The area under your lower eyelids should be a rich pink/red colour; and if you press on the end of your fingernail, turning the bed white, and then release it, it should turn red again quickly, not stay pale.

Anaemia can also be caused by B12 or folic acid deficiency. A blood test can determine if you have either of these. Just in case, I'd recommend that you supplement a B complex or a multivitamin containing B vitamins. (See Resources, page 483.)

Q *I've been given iron supplements for anaemia but they are making me constipated. Any suggestions?*

A The minerals contained in food supplements are bound with various other substances, and some forms are better absorbed than others. Ferrous sulphate, inorganic iron, appears in many multi-mineral or straight iron supplements because it's inexpensive, but it is not well tolerated by many and can cause constipation. One of the most assimilable forms of iron is the amino acid chelate form. It's well absorbed, without any gastrointestinal irritation or constipating effects. Look out for iron supplements with titles such as 'gentle' or 'organic' iron, and the label will usually tell you it's also 'non-constipating'. Also good are those called 'true food' iron.

Arthritis

Q *Can diet affect arthritis – and alleviate joint pain?*

A Yes, it most certainly can. A diet high in meat tends to encourage pain and inflammation, while a diet high in fish and seeds calms it down. Many people with arthritis also have food allergies. Of course, different people have different allergies, but two of the most common foods associated with arthritis are gluten grains such as wheat, and milk. These are certainly worth avoiding for 10 days to see if it helps you, but it's best to have a food intolerance test so you know what your specific intolerances are (see Resources, page 483, and 'How do I test myself for food intolerances?' on page 11).

Foods such as fish and flax seeds are good because they provide essential fats, especially omega-3s, which are natural anti-inflammatories. Try adding a ground dessertspoon of flax seeds to your cereal or in soups. Seeds are doubly good because they are very high in bone-building minerals such as calcium, magnesium and zinc.

Ginger is a natural anti-inflammatory, as is turmeric, the yellow spice in curry powders. Black pepper also has some benefits. So too do fruits and vegetables high in antioxidants – especially anything orange, red or blue, so raspberries, blueberries and carrots are great. These kinds of foods can make a tremendous difference to arthritis pain.

Q *What supplements can I take to help repair cartilage damage and prevent arthritis in my knee?*

A There is evidence that glucosamine and omega-3 fatty acids can aid joint health and help repair damaged cartilage. Glucosamine is a building block of cartilage that both stimulates rebuilding and inhibits deterioration, while omega-3 fats help to reduce any inflammation. You can buy glucosamine in supplement form – look for a formula combined with just sulfate rather than chondroitin sulfate, which can be harder to absorb. Omega-3 fatty acids are the healthy fats found in oily fish such as sardines, wild salmon and mackerel. Unfortunately, you'd need to eat around 10 portions a week to get sufficient quantities, so I'd advise taking a good-quality, high-dose omega-3 fish oil supplement as well. You need the daily equivalent of at least 1,000mg of combined EPA and DHA, if not double this amount, for maximum effectiveness. (See Resources, page 483.)

Q *I suffer from rheumatoid arthritis. What do you recommend?*

A Rheumatoid arthritis is an autoimmune disorder in which antibodies are formed against your own tissues – in this case, your joints. There are many possible reasons for this, including genetic susceptibility, lifestyle, nutritional deficiencies, food sensitivities and bacterial infections. Rheumatoid arthritis does not exist in isolated communities eating primitive diets, with lots of fruits and vegetables and very little salt, wheat, refined sugars and alcohol; so eating in this simple way is a good place to start. You should have yourself checked for food intolerances (see Resources, page 483) and eliminate or rotate any foods that cause an immune response.

If you have a wheat intolerance but still want to eat wholewheat pasta or wholewheat bread from time to time, you can try supplementing NAG (N-acetyl-glucosamine), as it blocks the inflammatory reaction to wheat fragments in the blood. You'd do well to avoid other foods that cause inflammation, such as citrus fruits, nightshade vegetables (tomatoes, potatoes, peppers, aubergines and chillies), meat and diary products. Drink plenty of bottled or filtered water daily, and eat oily fish (mackerel, sardines, wild salmon and trout) for their anti-inflammatory omega-3 content at least three times per week. Other excellent natural anti-inflammatory foods include ginger, turmeric, pineapple and papaya, which should all be regular features of your diet.

Asthma

Q *What's the nutritional solution for asthma?*

A Asthma is caused by inflammation, and this means that your body is in a state of 'alarm' because of an overload of harmful factors. These usually include pollution, food allergies, inhalant allergies and stress. The most common food allergies are to dairy products and wheat, and it's worth avoiding these for 10 days to see if that makes a difference. Any additional burden on the body's immune system could tip the scales over into asthma, which is probably why triple vaccines, which are like having three infections at once, can increase the risk of developing the condition.

In addition to decreasing your total load of such factors, certain nutrients and herbs help to calm down the inflammation that constricts the air passages in the lungs. These include vitamin C (2g a day), magnesium (300mg a day), omega-3 fish oils (1,000mg a day) and the herbs curcumin, boswellia and ginger. (See

Resources, page 483.) (For treating asthma in children, see page 27 in the Children's Health section.)

Athlete's foot

Q *How can I get rid of athlete's foot?*

A Athlete's foot is caused by a fungal infection, and can be treated with grapefruit seed extract, a very powerful natural anti-fungal available in liquid or capsule form. Put 10 to 15 drops of the extract in a basin of water and soak your feet for a few minutes. Alternatively, squeeze a few drops onto a damp piece of cotton wool and rub it over your feet.

This is the ideal solution for the occasional bout, but if you are getting athlete's foot repeatedly and also suffer from bloating or lethargy, it is worth checking whether you have a more extensive fungal infection in your body. A nutritionist would be able to help you work out whether this is your problem. In the meantime, avoid sugary foods, as they tend to feed fungal infections.

Cancer

Anti-cancer nutrition

Q *Which are the best traditional anti-cancer diets in the world? I've heard amazing claims for the Mediterranean and Japanese diets.*

A The Japanese have, traditionally, had very low risk for breast and prostate cancer. This is also true for parts of China and may be ascribed to a high intake of beans, especially fermented soya produce.

The Mediterranean diet, high in high-fibre wholefoods and fresh fruits and vegetables, is likely to be protective against cancers of the digestive system, notably of the colon. They also use olive oil, which some studies have shown contains fatty acids that have anti-cancer properties.

I think we can take the best factors from diets all over the world to make the best anti-cancer diet. The most important rules are to eat at least five servings of fruits and vegetables a day, organic if possible; cut back on meat and choose fish or soya products instead; reduce alcohol intake; and avoid frying. You can 'steam-fry' by briefly stir-frying a panful of, say, vegetables and tofu in a small amount of oil, then adding a smallish amount of water, or a water/soy sauce/lemon juice mix, to the pan. Put the lid on tight and steam briefly to heat through and cook lightly.

I recommend you:

- Avoid or at least limit your intake of red meat to a maximum of 80g (3oz) a day.
- Avoid or rarely eat burnt meat – be it grilled, fried or barbecued.
- Minimise your intake of fried food. Boil, steam, steam-fry, poach or bake food instead.
- Limit your intake of dairy food, choosing organic whenever possible.
- Don't drink alcohol and, if you do, certainly limit your intake to two drinks a day and ideally limit

your intake to three or four drinks a week, preferably choosing red wine.

- When you eat meat, opt for organic low-fat, game or free-range chicken.
- Eat fish (herring, mackerel, wild salmon or trout) instead of red meat.
- Eat plenty of fruit and vegetables – at least five servings a day, organic whenever possible.
- Have a 'rainbow' of fruits and vegetables, including something orange every day such as carrots, sweet potato, tomatoes, peaches or melons, and something red/purple such as berries, grapes or beetroot.
- Have a serving of cruciferous vegetable every day. This includes broccoli (including the tenderstem variety, which is excellent), Brussels sprouts, cabbage, cauliflower and kale.
- Have a clove or two of garlic every day, use shiitake mushrooms when you next have a stew or steam-fry and spice up dishes with turmeric. These all contain anti-cancer agents.
- Have some soya milk or tofu every other day.
- Add flax seeds to your breakfast cereal and use flax seed oil in salad dressings. Generally avoid refined vegetable oils – use only cold-pressed.
- Eat wholefoods, such as wholegrains, lentils, beans, nuts, seeds and vegetables, all of which contain fibre. Some of the fibre in vegetables is destroyed by cooking, so eat something raw every day.
- Drink green tea and 'red' herb teas rich in antioxidants. If you must have it, drink regular

tea in preference to coffee. However, for general health, don't drink excessive amounts of either.

- Ensure you drink six to eight glasses of water, diluted juices, or fruit teas each day. An excellent choice would be cat's claw tea sweetened with blackcurrant and apple concentrate.

Q *Why are soya products good as an anti-cancer food?*

A Collaborative research between Hong Kong's Chinese University and Manchester University indicates that the soya bean may protect people from developing prostate and breast cancers.

Soya beans contain large amounts of phyto-oestrogens which may have a protective effect. The traditional East Asian diet is particularly high in isoflavonoids, one type of phyto-oestrogen. Levels of isoflavonoids in the blood have been found to be 7 to 110 times higher in Japanese men with a low incidence of prostate cancer, compared to Finnish men. However, just how phyto-oestrogens help is not yet fully understood. Professor Norman Blacklock from Manchester University believes they may exert a 'weak oestrogen effect': there is evidence that phyto-oestrogens may block oestrogen receptor sites, thereby lowering body levels of active oestrogen. If this proves to be so, it is consistent with accumulating evidence that many modern diseases, including breast and prostate cancer, are the result of too much oestrogen.

There is also evidence that a protease inhibitor in soya, Bowman-Birk Inhibitor (BBI), may be another key anti-cancer compound. A study at the University of Pennsylvania School of Medicine added BBI to the diet of rats that had previously been fed a substance known to induce colon cancer. None of the rats developed tumours. In another similar study, BBI suppressed the formation of tumours by 71 per cent.

Whatever the mechanism, phyto-oestrogens have consistently been associated with reduced cancer risk. Women whose diets are abundant in soya beans have a lower risk for breast cancer, while men with a high soya intake have a substantially lower risk of prostate cancer. Research is beginning to focus on two isoflavonoids – genistein and daidzein. Japanese women, who generally have a lower risk of breast cancer than women in other industrialised societies, have been found to have higher levels of these in their bodies. They may protect against the harmful effects of unopposed oestrogen. In fact, a recent study from Singapore, which monitored a group of women for early signs of breast cancer, found that the more soya a woman ate, the less chance there was of having pre-cancer changes in breast cells.

A likely ideal intake for cancer prevention is around 5mg a day of genistein and daidzein, which you can get from a 12oz serving of soya milk or a serving of tofu. Soya milk can be used in drinks and on cereal like cow's milk, while tofu is excellent in stir-fries. Tofu is the richest source of isoflavones, while very processed soya products are the poorest source.

However, I don't advise having more than this. Even plant oestrogens could be oestrogenic in excess, and you can develop allergies to soya if you eat too much of it.

Breast cancer

Q *Two family members have had breast cancer. How can I prevent it?*

A Eighty per cent of breast cancers are termed 'oestrogen positive'. There is a high likelihood that hormone-disrupting chemicals play a major part. Diets high in meat and saturated fat may mean more exposure to such chemicals, which can store in body fat. Other associated risks are oral contraceptive use, hormone replacement therapy containing oestrogens or synthetic progestins, a high percentage of body fat, alcohol consumption above one or two drinks a day, smoking, a low intake of fruit and vegetables, exposure to herbicides and pesticides and low dietary fibre. The chances are that family risk relates not to genes, but to similar diets and lifestyle factors.

That said, a small percentage of women do have genes that increase the likelihood of breast cancer. These include the BRCA1, BRCA2 and CERB genes. The genes themselves don't cause cancer, but encourage growth of breast cells if they are activated. If they are over-activated this can lead to the overgrowth of cells, resulting in cancer cells. This activation can be triggered by hormone replacement therapy, or by dioxins, PCBs or DDT, which are examples of oestrogen-mimicking pollutants that might be found, say, in non-organic meat.

Therefore, it's important to eat loads of fruit and vegetables, organic whenever possible. Beta-carotene-rich vegetables such as carrots, broccoli and sweet potatoes, and fruits such as cantaloupes and apricots, are excellent choices; anything with high levels of vitamin C, such as peppers, watercress, cabbage, tomatoes, oranges and kiwi fruits, is important. It's good to eat garlic, which clears toxins and has antioxidant properties. Choose fish instead of meat, especially mackerel, herring, trout, sardines and wild salmon that are rich in omega-3 fats, which keep your hormones, skin and brain in top condition. (Flax seeds and their oil are the best vegetarian source of omega-3 fats.) Regular consumption of beans and soya in, say, tofu or soya milk, means you'll keep your isoflavones topped up, which will lower risk. Or you can take daily isoflavone supplements. (See Resources, page 483.)

Q *Why is breast cancer on the increase?*

A As you say, breast cancer is very much on the increase, and is now estimated to affect 1 in 10 women during their lives. And this is happening despite improved cancer diagnosis and treatment, which are failing to save many more lives than in the past.

Essentially, there are two main kinds of breast 'cancer': invasive breast cancer, and 'ductal carcinomas in situ' (DCIS for short), which are detected much more frequently these days due to mammogram screening. DCIS is not really cancer as we know it and is considered '99 per cent curable'. However, because more DCISs are picked up these days, due to mammograms, the survival rates look better. Conventional treatments for breast cancer – surgery, radiation and chemotherapy – do nothing to address the major underlying cause, which I believe is 'oestrogen dominance'. New drugs that block oestrogen sites in order to reduce oestrogen dominance are becoming more and more popular. But if a doctor prescribes such a drug, they should also tell you about what you can do to stop oestrogenic dominance in the first place.

Too much oestrogen makes breast cells overgrow, potentially resulting in cancer cells. Oestrogen is normally balanced by the hormone progesterone, but an excess can occur for a number of reasons. You can amass environmental oestrogens from pesticides and plastics; from too much dairy and high-fat meat products; from using the Pill before breasts have fully matured; from undergoing hormone replacement therapy that contains either oestradiol or progestins; from prolonged stress or obesity; or from a lack of beans in the diet – beans are high in phytoestrogens that block oestrogen receptors, thereby countering the effects of strong oestrogens. These are all risk factors that you can easily minimise. (For dietary advice, see 'Two family members have had breast cancer . . .', page 145.)

> **DIG DEEPER:** There's an excellent book on this subject by Dr John Lee called *What Your Doctor May Not Tell You About Breast Cancer* (Thorsons).

Q *Do you think there's a link between antiperspirant and breast cancer?*

A No one has really substantiated the supposed link between antiperspirant and breast cancer, although there is obviously logic to the idea that it's unwise to block your body's sweat glands, especially with those products containing aluminium salts. Many antiperspirants contain undesirable chemical preservatives called parabens. These can be absorbed and have been found in breast tumours, according to research by Dr Phillippa Darbre at the University of Reading.

If you perspire heavily and want to fix this, however, be aware that heavy perspiration is usually due to stress and blood sugar problems, or indicates a need to detoxify your body.

There are three things you need to do to balance your blood sugar and reduce stress: cut right back on sugar and stimulants such as tea and coffee; eat foods that release their sugar content slowly, such as oat-based foods (porridge, oat cakes, etc.), wholegrains, vegetables and fruit; and supplement 1g of vitamin C, a B complex and 200mcg of chromium.

To detoxify your body, exclude meat, dairy products, refined foods, stimulants such as coffee and tea, and alcohol. Eat lots of specific detoxifying fruits and vegetables plus wholefoods, and drink plenty of water (1.5 litres), for about 20 days. The best fruits are fresh apricots, berries, cantaloupe, citrus fruits, kiwi fruits, papaya, peaches, mango, melons and red grapes; among the top vegetables are peppers, beetroot, broccoli, carrots, spinach, tomatoes, watercress and beansprouts. White potatoes and avocado can be eaten in moderation.

As far as antiperspirants are concerned, avoid those with aluminium-based chemicals, which block the sweat glands or parabens. You'll find plenty of choice in your local healthfood shop.

Cervical cancer

Q *What is the best nutrition for fighting cervical cancer?*

A Cervical cancer is not linked to nutrition, but in the majority of cases to the human papilloma virus. The preinvasive form is almost always curable and early diagnosis has led to a 70 per cent reduction in mortality.

Therefore, you should follow an anti-viral diet, paying particular attention to getting a good intake of vitamins D and E and the minerals selenium and calcium. Also eat organic wherever possible and have lots of soya (in tofu and soya milk), beans and lentils – although don't overdo the soya, as this can encourage allergic reactions in some people. Supplement antioxidant nutrients and at least 3g of vitamin C a day. Also, avoid anything that weakens your immune system such as smoking, alcohol and fried foods. I recommend that you see a nutritional therapist who can help you find the perfect diet and supplement programme for you. For where to find them, see Resources, page 483.

Prostate cancer

Q *What are the nutritional recommendations for preventing and combating prostate cancer?*

A Prostate cancer is the most rapidly increasing cancer in men. It's predicted to become the most common within 20 years, possibly affecting as many as one in four men at some point during their life. Its causes are very similar to those of breast cancer, and the nutritional approach to both preventing and treating it is much the same, too. This involves avoiding the known risk factors: a diet high in saturated fat, regular consumption of dairy products and meat, low fibre intake, obesity, smoking, high cadmium levels, exposure to hormone-disrupting chemicals and pesticides, and high levels of testosterone.

The lowest risk diet is a vegan diet (no meat, no dairy). Eat organic wherever possible. If you don't go for the vegan option, fish, especially mackerel, herring, trout and wild or organically farmed salmon that are rich in omega-3 fats, lower your risk. Flax seeds and their oil are the best vegetarian source of omega-3 fats. Regular consumption of beans, lentils and specifically soya such as tofu or soya milk (two servings a day maximum is adequate) and pumpkin seeds also lowers risk. Tomatoes, rich in cancer-combating lycopene, are also recommended. Make sure your supplement programme includes 3,000mcg (10,000iu) of vitamin A, 400mg (600iu) of vitamin E, and 12mg of beta-carotene, plus the minerals selenium and zinc. Consider supplementing genistein and daidzein, the protective factors found in soya, and possibly the herb saw palmetto (300mg a day), which helps enlarged prostates. (See Resources, page 483.)

Risk factors

Q **Can beta-carotene give you cancer?**

A While there are hundreds of studies that show that beta-carotene (the vitamin A in carrots), either in food or supplements, reduces cancer risk, there are two studies that found a slightly increased incidence in lung cancer in heavy smokers supplementing beta-carotene. These studies also found a decrease in risk among non-smokers. A recent study may explain why.

Researchers from the National Cancer Institute in the US gave people who had had colon cancer beta-carotene on its own, vitamin C and E on their own, or all three versus a placebo. Each vitamin, on its own, or in combination, reduced incidence of colo-rectal polyps – except for smokers taking beta-carotene on its own. They had an increase in polyps, which is an indication of increased risk for cancer of the colon.

So, what does this mean? Smoking delivers a massive amount of cancer-causing oxidants. A 'team' of antioxidants, including beta-carotene, C and E, normally disarms these. When an antioxidant, such as beta-carotene, disarms an oxidant it becomes an oxidised, in other words becomes an oxidant in its own right. This is almost certainly what's happening by giving smokers beta-carotene on its own. However, the antioxidants 'oxidised' by smoking are then effectively 'reloaded', or turned back into good guys, by other members of the antioxidant team. Provided beta-carotene is given with other antioxidants such as vitamin C and E the effect is only positive. It's a case of 'united we stand, divided we fall'.

So, beta-carotene, either in foods that contain other vitamin C and E (that is, in fruits and vegetables) or in antioxidant supplements containing vitamin C and E, will reduce your risk of cancer. However, it may be wise not to supplement beta-carotene on its own if you are a smoker.

Q *I read that chromium can increase the risk of cancer. Is this true?*

A We've got the UK Food Standards Agency to blame for this myth. In a recent report they referred to a trial published almost a decade ago that implied that one form of chromium, chromium picolinate, could cause DNA damage.

Many people supplement chromium because it helps to stabilise blood sugar, hence helps to keep both your energy and your weight on an even keel. Chromium supplementation is especially important, and highly recommended, for anyone with diabetes for this very reason. Even the FSA agree that chromium is non-toxic in amounts 10 times higher than supplements, which usually provide 200mcg.

The question on cancer risk only related to chromium picolinate. However, even this has since been proven to be a red herring. A decade of research has failed to find any evidence of potential harm. One animal study gave several thousand times more chromium picolinate than is available in supplements and found no evidence of danger. There are now 35 human trials involving 2,000 people that have shown no safety issues. In the US the National Toxicology Program investigated chromium picolinate and found no evidence of 'genotoxicity' or any other ill effects. The fact is there is no evidence that supplementing chromium picolinate, let alone any other form, has the potential to cause cancer in either animals or humans. So for people with chronic fatigue, weight problems or blood sugar problems such as diabetes, chromium remains a beneficial, and safe, supplement.

Q *Is it true that cancer is largely genetic?*

A Scientific research categorically shows that cancer is largely caused by diet and lifestyle choices rather than inherited risk. A recent study published in the *New England Journal of Medicine* found that identical twins – who have the same genetic make-up – had no more than a 15 per cent chance of developing the same cancer. This shows that most cancers are at least 85 per cent due to environmental factors such as diet, lifestyle and exposure to toxic chemicals. A report by the World Cancer Research Fund found that you could halve your risk by eating lots of fruit and vegetables, and severely limiting alcohol or red meat. Also supplementing antioxidant nutrients and avoiding known carcinogens can probably cut your risk by 85 per cent or more.

So it's up to you, not your genes – increase your fruit and vegetable intake, take antioxidant supplements, avoid toxins by eating organic and not smoking and you'll be optimising your protection from one of the biggest killers.

Treatments

Q *My sister is having chemotherapy for cancer. Is there anything to help reduce the side effects?*

A The good news for anyone having chemo is that nutrition *can* help reduce the unwanted effects and improve their general wellbeing. Dietary changes like reducing animal fat intake, eating plenty of fruit and vegetables, drinking 1.5 litres of water a day and avoiding coffee, tea, alcohol, sugar and processed foods help optimise your nutrient intake and reduce the load on your body.

Antioxidants, which help protect against the toxicity of the drugs, are particularly helpful, so I recommend taking an all-round antioxidant complex. I recommend one that contains Co-enzyme Q, since some types of chemotherapy drug deplete this important antioxidant. (See Resources, page 483.) The digestive enzyme bromelain, found in pineapple, has been shown to improve tumour regression, given alongside chemotherapy. The researchers found that 2g a day was the most effective.

Other nutrients can help reduce any nausea, vomiting and diarrhoea. Try vitamin B6 (50mg). Glutamine is another possibility: not only has it helped on the digestive front, but it also has been shown to speed up recovery from chemo and to reduce the incidence of infection. But as it can also enhance the effectiveness of chemotherapy, note that it should only be used under medical supervision. If you're given the go-ahead, you can find glutamine powder in healthfood stores. Take 5 to 10g in water last thing at night; a well-heaped teaspoon is about 5g.

Q *What are your views on the use of laetrile (B17) for cancer treatment/prevention?*

A Laetrile, an extract from the apricot kernel, has often been used in aggressive anti-cancer strategies. It acts more like chemotherapy, but is claimed to target only the cancer cells. When laetrile is broken down by the body, one of its components is cyanide. Normal, non-cancerous cells contain an enzyme that converts this to thiocyanate, a non-toxic substance used by the body to make vitamin B12 (cyanocobalamin). Cancer cells lack this enzyme and are effectively poisoned. Another breakdown product of laetrile – benzoic acid – is said to act as a natural painkiller.

The California Medical Association were critical of its value as an anti-cancer substance, although their report did state, 'All the physicians whose patients were reviewed spoke of an increase in the sense of wellbeing and appetite, gain in weight and decrease in pain.' It continues to be used, with reported success, as part of various natural anti-cancer regimes. Like shark cartilage, it is not a necessary part of a prevention strategy.

Q *Do you have any recommendations for people who have had lymph glands removed and suffer from swollen limbs?*

A Regular exercise helps to stimulate the flow of lymph, and lymphatic drainage massage can aid lymphatic flow and drain excess fluid from your limbs. A lot of cancer care clinics will be able to refer you to someone who does this kind of massage. You may find that exercises like yoga and Psychocalisthenics (see Resources, page 483) will help.

A diet low in salt and high in potassium (which is abundant in all fruits and vegetables) is a good idea. Watermelon is particularly high in potassium. You can make a delicious and easy-to-drink smoothie by blending slices of watermelon with ice in a blender (including the seeds, which are very nutritious). Also drink lots of pure water, aiming for 8 to 10 glasses a day.

Q *What supplements might help recovery from radiotherapy, surgery and high doses of steroids given as treatment for cancer?*

A Cancer, radiotherapy and surgery are all considerable stresses on the body, and antioxidants can help you deal with them. Although many people are advised not to take vitamin or mineral supplements during radiotherapy, several studies have shown that antioxidants can not only protect against the toxicity of the drugs and radiation but also enhance their cancer-killing effects. Supplementing 50mg of vitamin B6 can also prevent nausea and vomiting caused by radiotherapy.

Especially important is vitamin C. Thin skin, easy bruising, frequent infections and difficulty in shifting infections are all symptoms of vitamin C deficiency. I recommend a minimum of 3 to 4g of vitamin C per day. You may need more, but this should be done under the guidance of a nutritional therapist.

Q *What's your view on Tamoxifen for breast cancer? Is soya an alternative?*

A Most, but not all, breast cancers are oestrogen-positive. Tamoxifen was one of the first drugs used that binds to oestroegen receptors, hence blocking them. While there is some evidence that it reduces the recurrence of breast cancer, the positive effects of the drug wear off after five years. It also increases risk for a number of other problems, including uterine cancer and pulmonary embolism. In one trial where women without breast cancer were divided into a control group and a group given Tamoxifen, fewer of the women on Tamoxifen developed breast cancer, but more of them experienced pulmonary embolism, deep vein thrombosis and strokes. So Tamoxifen can have mild benefits and considerable down sides.

Soya beans contain isoflavones which are weak plant oestrogens. By occupying oestrogen receptors, but not delivering a strong oestrogenic 'message', these too are touted as protecting against oestrogen dominance. And there is evidence to support this (see 'Why are soya products good as an anti-cancer food?', page 143.) But since even plant oestrogens could be oestrogenic in excess, I wouldn't encourage women to eat vast amounts of soya foods.

The relatively low incidence of breast cancer among women in East Asia is likely to be due partly to eating soya, and partly to other positive factors in their diet – more vegetables, garlic and ginger, and less meat and milk, for instance. So my advice is to eat a diet containing soya, but not more than 12oz of, say, soya milk and tofu a day. And eat beans, lentils and chickpeas too, as these are good sources of phytoestrogens. Overall advice on anti-cancer diets can be found in 'Which are the best traditional anti-cancer diets in the world?', on page 140.

Is a total anti-cancer diet, backed up with supplements, a valid alternative to Tamoxifen? I'd say so.

DIG DEEPER: For more information on preventing and fighting cancer naturally, see my book *Say No to Cancer* (Piatkus, 1999).

Colds, flu and related infections

Q *How can you prevent getting colds through the winter?*

A There are plenty of natural substances for your anti-cold arsenal. Thirty-seven out of 38 studies have shown that supplementing 1g of vitamin C a day reduces the incidence, duration and severity of cold symptoms. Other immune-friendly nutrients include zinc and the herbs echinacea and cat's claw, which can be taken as preventives. Drinking a cup of cat's claw tea or 10 drops of echinacea tincture in water every day during the winter months can really help stave off the sniffles. Berries contain anthocyanidins that boost your immune system, and black elderberry extract has been shown to halve the recovery time from flu. These are also worth supplementing to keep your immune system strong. Some vitamin C supplements contain combinations of these. (See Resources, page 483.)

Q *What's the quickest way to kill a cold?*

A Up your vitamin C intake to 3g every four hours. This level of vitamin C supplementation saturates the

bloodstream in it and simply stops viruses from surviving. This is for short-term use only, however; while
it isn't dangerous, you may get loose bowels. Once your
cold has gone, go back to taking 1 to 2g of vitamin C
a day to prevent colds. Another cold killer is black
elderberry extract, available in healthfood stores.
Black elderberry effectively stops viruses from getting
inside your cells and multiplying. I'd also drink two or
three cups of tea made from the Amazonian herb cat's
claw. The bitter taste can be improved by adding in
some blackcurrant and apple concentrate. Also effective is 10 drops of echinacea two or three times a day.

Putting all these together is the quickest way to
kill a cold. Beyond this, eat lots of fruit, avoid dairy
products and take it easy.

Q *I've heard that echinacea is a wondercure for
colds. What's your view?*

A It is. I always keep a bottle of echinacea close at hand,
and take it at the first sign of an infection. Echinacea
(*Echinacea purpurea*) is an old Native American remedy for purifying the blood, and that is quite literally
what it does. Blood contains white blood cells called
macrophages and lymphocytes, which go around cleaning up viruses, bacteria and other unwanted material.
Echinacea has been well proven to strengthen the
immune system by helping these cells do a better job.
It is also an effective anti-viral agent against flu and herpes, and can even destroy cancer cells in the test tube.

However, not all echinacea does the trick. This is because there are many species of echinacea, and many immune-boosting active phytochemicals within the plant, such as echinosides, alkamides, cichoric acid and so on. Some cheaper echinacea products contain none of these, making them virtually useless for fighting off infections. So it's one of those cases where you really do get what you pay for. You need a standardised, full-potency extract of the herb, which will guarantee certain levels of the phytochemicals. It's best taken as capsules of the powdered herb (2,000mg a day) or drops of a concentrated extract – you'll need to use up to 20 drops three times a day. Be guided by the instructions on the label. You can also get echinacea syrup, which is especially good for children.

But echinacea isn't just something to take when you've got an infection. One study of a group of healthy men found that after five days of taking 30 drops of echinacea extract three times a day, their white blood cells had doubled, which indicates more immune power.

Q *Aside from echinacea, are there any other herbs that cure colds?*

A Cat's claw, the bark of the *Uncaria tomentosa* plant from the Peruvian rainforest, is a particular favourite of mine. Cat's claw is so called because the thorn on the plant resembles the claw of a cat. A woody vine, it can wind its way over 100 feet up through the trees in its search for light in the dense forests. The Native Americans have long used it to treat cancer, joint problems and many other diseases.

Although research on the plant is still in its infancy, the studies that have been done has been so convincing that the plant has been overexploited. It is now an endangered species, and in 1989 the Peruvian government banned the harvesting and use of the root of the two main species, which would of course kill the living plant. In any case, the bark contains most or all of the medicinal properties, and harvesting some of this will allow the plant to grow back afterwards. It is still feared that worldwide demand for this bark exceeds production so, as with ginseng, the purchaser needs to be aware of substitutes.

Components of cat's claw have been shown to increase the ability of white blood cells to carry out phagocytosis, that is, to engulf, digest and so destroy an invading bacterium or virus. It has also been shown to contain other chemicals which reduce inflammation. It is potentially a super-plant, with immune-stimulating, antioxidant, anti-inflammatory, anti-tumour and antimicrobial properties.

Austrian researchers have also identified extracts which they have been using to treat cancer and viral infections. One problem they have come across is that different samples contain different amounts of these therapeutic chemicals, which makes dosage difficult to calculate; it is not yet known whether this is due to variations in location, season or species.

Cat's claw comes either as capsules, with 2g a good daily dose for a cold, or as tea (loose or in teabags) – two cups a day should be sufficient. You can get more out of the loose tea by boiling it for five minutes and then adding a little blackcurrant and apple juice concentrate to improve the taste.

Q *I keep getting sinus infections. What can I do?*

A If the sinuses, which are chambers in the cheek and forehead area, get blocked and can't clear, they are prone to infection. This can happen as an aftermath of a cold or because your mucous membranes are irritated (pollen and alcohol do this), or perhaps because you are allergic to something, the classic being milk products. Once the sinuses are infected it's hard to get rid of the infection without anti-biotics. The trick is to stop them from getting blocked up.

If you've got the first signs of an infection, avoid all milk products, including cheese. Eat lots of fresh fruit and supplement 3g of vitamin C a day, which boosts your immune system, until you are back to normal (some people get loose bowels from taking this amount of vitamin C, so adjust as necessary). Saline or seawater sprays, which are used a lot in Europe, can also help clear and clean out the sinuses. Ask for Sterimar, Rhinomar or Prorhinol brands in your local chemist and use three or four times a day.

Q *I have to take a short course of antibiotics for a sinus infection, but I usually get an upset stomach whenever I have them. Is there anything I can do to stop this?*

A Taking a probiotic supplement will help to repopulate your gut with the healthy bacteria that antibiotics can wipe out, which is what may be the cause of your stomach upsets. The two most prevalent strains of beneficial bacteria are *Lactobacillus acidophilus* and *Bifidobacterium bifidus*. Some fermented products such as *kefir* contain these bacteria, but probiotic supplements are a more direct way to boost levels (see Resources, page 483). It's best to take probiotics on an empty stomach – one tablet first thing in the morning and again before you go to bed. Start when you begin the antibiotics and continue for one week after you finish the course.

Q *I've had a minor sore throat and catarrh for weeks now. What can I do?*

A You may well have a low-lying, low-grade infection that your body's defences just can't shift. If you are particularly stressed, overexercising, drinking too much alcohol or eating badly, these will burden your immune system, so you'll need to deal with that. To give your immune system a boost, eat plenty of fruit and vegetables and take a supplement which contains vitamin C, zinc and berry extracts three times a day. Also take the herbal remedies cat's claw and echinacea (see other questions in this section). Some people find that avoiding milk products when they have catarrh helps by reducing mucus, so give that a go too.

Q **I keep getting sore throats. What can I do to stop this?**

A Sore throats can be a sign of streptococcal infection or allergy, both of which weaken your immune power. Antibiotics don't work well for sore throats, according to a study published in the *British Medical Journal*. Over 700 patients with sore throats were given either antibiotics for seven days, or after three days if symptoms persisted, or nothing. Regardless of the group they were in, there was no difference in the number of people feeling better after three days or the overall length of illness. Due to the overuse of antibiotics there are now antibiotic-resistant strains of streptococci bacteria.

A better strategy is to boost your immune system by supplementing cat's claw and echinacea; see other questions in this section for the lowdown on these herbs. In addition, take 1 to 3g of vitamin C a day (the higher amount may make your bowels loose, so adjust as necessary). Zinc lozenges also help, while ginger tea can soothe the throat, as well as being anti-inflammatory.

Colitis

 Q *I suffer from colitis. Are there any nutritional remedies that can help?*

A In colitis, the large intestine is inflamed, so reducing inflammation is key. Fish oils rich in omega-3 fatty acids are natural anti-inflammatories. But that's only part of the jigsaw. Many colitis sufferers also find relief by avoiding foods they are sensitive to – most commonly wheat, milk and yeast, although coffee, tea and spices can add to the problem. Easily digested foods, such as steamed vegetables, rice, fish and fruit, plus digestive enzyme supplements, often help.

You also need to replenish beneficial bacteria in the gut, which will help protect the gut wall, by taking a supplement such as acidophilus. Doctors have found that people with colitis are likely to have what is called a 'leaky gut' – an overly porous intestinal wall. This is a fairly serious condition that demands a dual approach: avoiding foods you are sensitive to, and repairing the gut lining with nutrients such as glutamine. It's best to work with a nutritionist who can design a programme to meet your particular needs. (See Resources, page 483.)

Crohn's disease

Q *Have you got any dietary tips for dealing with Crohn's disease?*

A Crohn's disease is an inflammatory bowel disorder that responds very well to nutritional therapy. First, a few factors should be considered. Sensitivity to certain foods, most commonly gluten (the protein found in wheat, oats, rye and barley) and milk, can aggravate Crohn's, so avoiding them can help. Also avoid coffee, alcohol and sugar, drink 1.5 litres of water daily and eat fresh wholefoods that are naturally high in fibre, such as lentils, beans, ground seeds, fruits and lightly cooked vegetables. Be careful, however, with the introduction of fibre-rich foods, as the digestive tract of Crohn's sufferers is very sensitive. The amount of good bacteria in the gut is likely to be low, so restore the balance with a probiotic supplement such as acidophilus. Taking some omega-3-rich fish or flax oil helps calm the inflammation. The herbs boswellia and curcumin are also good anti-inflammatories, while slippery elm and marshmallow are very soothing to the gut lining. The amino acid glutamine, taken last thing at night (mix 5 to 10g of the powder in a glass of water), also helps to repair the gut.

Q *I was told to avoid fibre in my diet when I was diagnosed with Crohn's. But what will not eating fibre do to my general health?*

A You can't avoid fibre completely and wouldn't want to. Fibre is a natural constituent of a healthy diet high in fruits, vegetables, lentils, beans and wholegrains, and by eating this way you have less risk of bowel cancer, diabetes or diverticular disease, and are unlikely to suffer from constipation.

But there are different kinds of fibre. *Insoluble* fibre, found in bran and wholegrains, is harsh on the bowel and doesn't suit a sensitive or inflamed digestive system. *Soluble* fibres, on the other hand, found in oats, lentils, beans, fruits, vegetables and flax seeds or linseeds, are a whole other story. Soluble fibres are very water-absorbent, and by bulking up foods and slowing the release of sugars, can help to control appetite and play a part in blood sugar control and weight maintenance. They make faecal matter bulkier, less dense and easier to pass along the digestive tract, decreasing the amount of time food waste spends inside the body and reducing the risk of toxins being reabsorbed by the colon.

Soluble fibre-rich foods contain many other nutrients as well, so are an important part of any healthy diet, even in Crohn's sufferers. So don't stop eating soluble fibre, cut out bran and go easy on the wholewheat.

Diabetes and insulin resistance

Q *I'm a diabetic on tablets, not injections. What dietary advice do you recommend?*

A Diabetes is an extreme form of blood sugar imbalance. It arises when your body can no longer produce sufficient insulin, a hormone that helps to carry glucose (the breakdown product of carbohydrate) out of the blood and into cells, where it's made into energy.

From a nutritional point of view, the following factors are most important to help balance blood sugar:

- Eat more fibre in wholefoods, particularly soluble fibre found in oats, beans and vegetables.
- Eat foods which release their sugar content slowly – that means wholegrains, oats, lentils, beans, apples and raw or lightly cooked vegetables.
- Eat protein with every meal or snack – so have brown rice, potatoes, or pasta with chicken, tofu, lean meat or fish; fruit with a few nuts or seeds; oatcakes with hummus, and so on.
- Eat oily fish such as wild or organic salmon, mackerel and herring three times a week, and pumpkin or flax seeds, for their omega-3 essential fatty acids.
- Severely limit refined or processed carbohydrates: don't eat white flour or foods made from white flour, biscuits, sweets or cakes.
- Every day, supplement vitamin C (1g), vitamin E (400mg/600iu), magnesium (400mg), chromium (200mcg) and the essential fats, especially the fish oil EPA. Be aware that supplementing chromium may enhance the effectiveness of the drug you are taking, hence you may temporarily experience a blood sugar low and need to reduce the amount of the drug. Therefore, I advise you to let your doctor know that you want to try this strategy.

Q **I have Type II diabetes. Can you recommend any supplements?**

A In addition to following a diet designed to reduce the damage caused by high blood sugar (which is what Type II diabetes is) – wholefoods rich in fresh vegetables and wholegrains, balanced with good-quality protein and essential fats – an array of supplements can help. The mineral chromium can help to regulate blood sugar, but you will need to consult your doctor to ensure it doesn't affect your medication. If he or she gives you the go-ahead, take 200mcg of chromium a day. An essential fats supplement will help to reduce inflammation to the eye area. Magnesium, manganese and zinc also help to stabilise blood sugar, and you will get these from a good-quality multivitamin and mineral supplement. Lipoic acid and vitamin E help to reduce the effects of the damage caused by the excess blood sugar, and these can be found in a good antioxidant formula. (See Resources, page 483.)

Q *Is there a supplement programme that can prevent further deterioration from diabetic neuropathy?*

A Diabetic neuropathy is a nerve disorder caused by diabetes, which can affect the eyesight (leading to double vision, for instance), legs and feet (causing tingling, numbness, pain or ulceration), and the digestive tract. Following the right diet for balancing your blood sugar is essential (see 'I'm a diabetic', page 168), and taking vitamin B6 plus 200mcg of chromium may help. I would also recommend having your homocysteine level tested and then supplementing therapeutic levels of B vitamins if it's high; in addition to 100mg of B6, that means 100mcg of B12 and 800mcg of folic acid. Also supplement 15mg of zinc and 300mg of magnesium daily. Homocysteine is an amino acid made in the body, and high levels have been linked to more than 100 different diseases, including diabetes. Homocysteine is also the best indicator of your ability to 'methylate' which is an essential way in which the body repairs and maintains the nervous system. So, if your homocysteine level is low you are giving yourself the best possible chance to prevent and hopefully reverse neuropathy. See Resources, page 483, for information on the homocysteine tests available.

Q **My sister has recently been diagnosed with insulin resistance and put on Metformin to try to regulate glucose uptake. Is there a nutritional alternative?**

A Ordinarily, insulin conveys glucose, or blood sugar, to where it can provide energy. But habitual stress and a diet centring on refined carbohydrates flood the blood regularly with glucose, which triggers the production of more insulin. The more insulin you produce, and the more often, the more your body becomes resistant to insulin – hence the condition of insulin resistance. This means that the blood sugar the insulin is carrying is 'turned away', and stays in the bloodstream. Over time this can lead to Type II diabetes and other serious conditions.

The way to deal with insulin resistance is to stabilise both blood sugar and the stress response. The right diet can regulate blood sugar. Your sister should start by eating more fibre in wholefoods, particularly soluble fibre such as that found in oats, beans and vegetables. She should also concentrate on foods that release their sugar content slowly, such as wholegrains (including brown rice, millet, rye, quinoa as cereal, wholewheat in moderation and maize), lentils, beans, apples and raw or lightly cooked vegetables. With every meal or snack she should eat some protein, so with brown rice, potatoes or pasta she needs to eat chicken, meat, fish or tofu; with fruit, she needs to add in a few nuts or seeds; with oatcakes, she should have hummus; and so on. Finally, she should supplement vitamin C (1,000mg), vitamin E (400mg/600iu), magnesium (400mg), chromium (200mcg with breakfast and 200mcg with lunch) and the essential fats, especially the omega-3 fatty acid EPA found in fish oil. You need at least 600mg of EPA to have any significant effect.

However, if your sister continues to take Metformin, it is very important that she lets her doctor know that she is taking chromium, as it may boost the effectiveness of the drug, hence necessitating a lower dose. After two months of following this diet, she might like to be re-tested.

Q *I have just been diagnosed as having insulin resistance. I eat reasonably healthily, but I drink white wine daily. Is this OK?*

A Unfortunately, alcohol can contribute hugely to blood sugar imbalances such as insulin resistance, simply because it converts to glucose very fast in the body. So in addition to following the right diet (see 'My sister has been diagnosed with insulin resistance', page 171), and taking chromium, you really need to cut most alcohol out until you no longer test positive for insulin resistance. Give yourself a couple of months. In the meantime, I would recommend just having a couple of glasses a day at weekends only.

Q *On a packet of ginseng I bought it said not to use it if you are diabetic without first consulting your doctor. Could you explain this please?*

A Ginseng helps stabilise the adrenal hormone cortisol. Cortisol also interacts with the body's blood sugar control. I am not aware of there being any danger for diabetics in taking, say 1g of ginseng a day, but neither would I specifically recommend ginseng for people with that condition. The best way to take ginseng if you are diabetic is by starting with a low amount, say 500mg, and increasing up to no more than 3g. But do let your doctor know you are trying this.

Digestive complaints (see also Colitis, Irritable bowel syndrome)

Constipation, diarrhoea and related problems

Q *I suffer from chronic constipation and nothing seems to help. Any suggestions?*

A It's very important to deal with long-term constipation because the knock-on effects can be legion: hormone imbalance, poor cholesterol processing, skin problems and general fatigue.

First, make sure you are drinking at least 1.5 litres of pure water daily to lubricate the gut and keep the stools from drying out in the large intestine. The next step is to take a look at what you're eating. Foods naturally high in fibre are vital, as they help keep the bowel muscles moving, bulk out and soften the stools and sweep the gut like a broom. So your daily diet has got to include fresh vegetables and fruit (which have a beneficial high water content too), beans, lentils and wholegrains such as brown rice and oats. I don't suggest you take laxatives, even herbal ones, because they do not deal with the underlying problem. Nor do added fibres such as wheat bran, which simply irritate the gut. A good alternative is to soak a tablespoon of organic golden flax seeds, available in healthfood stores, in a glass of water overnight, and drink the mixture in the morning. If you've been constipated for a long time, do a colon cleanse using colon-cleansing herbs and fibres. Aloe vera is also good. (See Resources, page 483.)

Q *What do you recommend for diarrhoea, and what's your view on anti-diarrhoeal medications?*

A Anti-diarrhoeal medications don't address the underlying cause and can stop the body from trying to rapidly clear toxins, if that's why you have diarrhoea. As far as treating the condition naturally goes, it's important to avoid irritants such as spicy foods, and eat more soluble fibre. Insoluble fibre such as wheat bran is harsh on the bowel and does not suit a sensitive and often inflamed digestive system. A much better alternative is soluble fibre, found in fruit and vegetables. It's a good idea to eat more of these. To really knock the problem on the head, though, try psyllium husks *or* flax seeds, both available from your local healthfood shop.

Here's how you use them. For psyllium husks, take 1 teaspoon morning and afternoon (away from food supplements) in a full mug of water, building after one to two weeks to 1 dessertspoon two times day in at least a mug, better a pint of water. This should dramatically increase your stool bulk and formation. If you choose to use flax seeds, soak a dessertspoon overnight in a glass of water and drink the lot in the morning.

If increasing your fibre and water intake doesn't work, consult a nutrition practitioner who can explore other possible reasons such as intestinal parasites, imbalanced gut bacteria or irritable bowel syndrome (IBS).

Diseases, ailments and injuries A–Z

 How can intestinal parasites, probably picked up while travelling abroad, be eliminated?

A Some one in four people in Britain carry parasites in their digestive tracts. These parasites can cause no symptoms at all, or all sorts of problems, from bloating, abdominal pain and digestive upset to constipation, diarrhoea, irritable bowel syndrome and anal irritation. If you suspect you've got a parasitic infection it's a good idea to find out which one it is by having a stool parasitology test, which a nutritional therapist can arrange for you. The most common parasites are *Blastocystis hominis*, *Dientamoeba fragilis*, *Entamoeba species* and Giardia.

Once you know which kind you have, you can target that species with either natural anti-parasitic herbs such as garlic, wormwood, fenugreek and goldenseal, or strong antibiotics. There are different types and dosages depending on the parasite. In my experience, and I don't usually recommend taking them, antibiotics are most effective and get the job done quickly. Afterwards, however, you'll need to replenish the beneficial gut flora felled by the antiobiotics with high-strength probiotics like acidophilus. Whichever approach you take, heal the gut lining with glutamine (2 to 4g a day) and aloe vera juice (as directed). An anti-parasitic programme should be undertaken under the guidance of a qualified health practitioner.

Q *What does pain before I need to empty my bowels mean and what can I do about it?*

A First, see your doctor to eliminate any serious underlying reasons for the pain. If you get the all-clear, start by gently increasing your fibre intake with fruit and vegetables, drinking plenty of water, and avoiding any potential food intolerances (wheat and dairy are common culprits). Try soaking a dessertspoon of flax seeds overnight in a glass of water and drink the lot in the morning. Another possible reason for pain could be some kind of infection in your digestive tract. A stool analysis test can check this out. (See Resources, page 483.) Mucus in the stools can indicate inflammation in the bowel, which may be a response to a food allergy or intolerance.

   I would recommend seeing a nutritional therapist, as well as your doctor, who can investigate these possibilities.

Q *I would like to know what the different stool colours mean in terms of health.*

A The colour of your stools largely depends on your diet. Very light stools may be so coloured because of undigested fat, for instance. Fatty stools are greasy and may sometimes float – and this is not healthy. Stools that float may also be due to excessive gas in the digestive tract. Dark stools may be the result of eating a lot of red meat. But if they are blackish, or look as though the colour may be caused by blood, you must see a doctor.

Flatulence and bloating

Q *What do you recommend for flatulence?*

A Flatulence is a sign that your digestion isn't working as well as it should and the 'bad' bacteria in your gut are feasting on your undigested food, producing gas. There are three key steps to getting rid of the gas. Firstly, chew more thoroughly: this is the number one way to improve your digestion. Secondly, check for food intolerances – wheat is the big culprit if you suffer from bloating and flatulence. Try cutting it out completely for 10 days, and replacing it with other grains like rye, oats and rice. Then reintroduce it (have a lot) and see what happens. If this shows you that wheat is a cause, reduce it as much as possible, and in time (a few months, say), if you have it on occasion, it shouldn't cause you too much of a problem.

Thirdly, consider taking digestive enzymes. If you often feel bloated, get indigestion after meals or suffer from excessive flatulence, you may not be making enough enzymes to digest your food properly. It's a vicious circle, because with fewer enzymes you absorb fewer nutrients and with fewer nutrients you make fewer enzymes. If this is your problem, there's a simple solution. Supplement a digestive enzyme tablet with each meal. The good ones contain lipase (for digesting fat), amylase (for digesting carbohydrate) and protease (for digesting protein). Some also contain papain (from papaya) or bromelain (from pineapple). Eating these fruits fresh can also aid digestion. (See Resources, page 483.)

Also supplement a multivitamin and mineral containing 10mg of zinc because zinc is needed to make stomach acid. If you improve your eating habits you may well find that within a month, you can stop taking the digestive enzymes and still stay well.

If these steps don't work, you should see a nutritional therapist, who can assess other potential problems in your digestive system (such as dysbiosis or an imbalance in intestinal flora, or parasites).

Q *I thought beans and greens were good for you, but when I eat them I get bloated. Why?*

A Beans and greens *are* good for you: they contain a rich variety of nutrients including protein, minerals and vitamins. Yet beans, cabbage, Brussels sprouts, cauliflower, turnips, leeks, onions and garlic can all cause gas and bloating. The culprits are the indigestible carbohydrates they contain, such as galactosides.

While a small amount of gas from eating these foods is quite normal, excessive gas can be prevented by supplementing the enzyme alpha-galactosidase. This breaks down the indigestible carbohydrates and reduces flatulence. Some digestive enzyme formulas contain this enzyme as well as enzymes that digest protein, fat and carbohydrate. You can also help yourself by eating slowly and chewing well, plus making sure your digestion is working as well as it can be. If all else fails, charcoal tablets or capsules are effective absorbers of gas, helping to reduce flatulence and bloating.

Indigestion

Q *What can you recommend for acid reflux?*

A Acid reflux happens when stomach acid backs into the oesophagus, and is often accompanied by frequent heartburn. You may be experiencing excess acid reflux because you're eating foods that irritate the stomach lining, or cause an allergic reaction. To rule the latter out, it is well worth having a food intolerance test (see Resources, page 483).

Certain nutrients calm down the effects of excess acidity, such as vitamin A. Aloe vera is also excellent in this regard. You should also follow a digestion-friendly diet for a month, as outlined in my book *Improve Your Digestion* (Piatkus, 1999).

Basically, this means you need to cut out all gluten grains (barley, oats, rye and wheat), red meat, dairy products, eggs, refined foods, sugar, salt, hydrogenated fats, artificial sweeteners, food additives, alcohol, stimulants and fizzy drinks. Eat plenty of vegetables, although keep your intake of potatoes and avocado moderate; and plenty of fruit, especially apricots, berries, cantaloupe, kiwi fruits, papaya, peaches, mangoes, melons and red grapes. For the rest, choose brown rice, corn, millet or quinoa; three servings of oily fish a week; a modicum of extra-virgin olive oil; organic skinless chicken or turkey; and a handful of raw nuts and seeds a day. Drink 1.5 litres of water a day, as well as herbal teas.

Q *How can I tell whether I have too much stomach acid or too little?*

A The symptoms of low stomach acid include burping after eating; bad breath; indigestion, especially after eating protein-rich foods; upper abdominal pain and flatulence; bloating; diarrhoea; and/or constipation. Another indicator is feeling full shortly after eating or the sensation that food is slow to pass from the stomach.

One of the most common reasons for a lack of stomach acid is zinc deficiency because the production of hydrochloric acid in the stomach is dependent on a sufficient intake of zinc. Stress is also a suppressor of stomach acid production. This is because when we are in stress the body channels energy towards 'fight or flight' and away from digestion. So eating on the move or when you're under real pressure is definitely a bad idea. The nutritional solution is to take a digestive enzyme supplement containing betaine hydrochloride, plus at least 15mg of zinc in an easily absorbable form such as zinc citrate.

If you're producing too much stomach acid, the symptoms can be surprisingly similar, with one big difference: you may experience a burning sensation. If this is the case, supplementing betaine hydrochloride is likely to make matters worse rather than better. But you

may not know until you try. So start off with one capsule and monitor your reaction. If nothing happens,
then you're probably not producing enough stomach
acid (in which case follow the advice above). If you get
a warm feeling, you're probably over-producing it.

If this is this case, lay off alcohol, coffee, tea and
aspirin, which all irritate the gut wall, as does eating
too much wheat (in bread, pasta, crackers, biscuits
and so on). Very hot drinks and spicy foods, especially chilli, are also stomach-unfriendly. All meat,
fish, eggs and other concentrated proteins stimulate
acid production, which will further irritate an already
unhealthy and inflamed stomach lining, so avoid eating too much protein in any given meal.

Q *I get terrible indigestion and live on antacids. Is
there a natural solution?*

A There are several possible reasons for your indigestion. Are you eating too fast, drinking too much liquid with your meals, drinking more than three coffees
a day or eating hard-to-digest fatty, spicy or stodgy
foods? If not, your digestion may be below par, so
digestive aids are the next step.

Antacids aren't the answer, as they make your
stomach very alkaline, a condition that actually interferes with digestion (remember, it's stomach *acid* that
helps digest food). They may also contain aluminium,
which is toxic. So try a digestive enzyme supplement
with each main meal – one that contains amylase,

protease and lipase, which digest carbohydrate, protein and fat respectively. Ironically, indigestion is often caused by too little stomach acid (betaine hydrochloride). If you feel this might be so (for a list of symptoms, see 'How can I tell whether I have too much stomach acid or too little?', page 181), you can look for digestive enzyme supplements containing betaine hydrochloride. (See Resources, page 483.)

Q **I've been feeling nauseated ever since returning from holiday in India. Any suggestions?**

A There's a reasonable chance you've picked up a UFO (unidentified faecal organism). Given that there are 20 times more micro-organisms inside each of us than living cells, it isn't that difficult to pick up a pathogen on holiday in less hygienic parts of the world. Some of these, like Giardia, can make you seriously sick. Others, like *Blastocystis hominis*, can leave you with mild nausea and tiredness, sometimes worse after eating.

The first step is to get yourself tested. You can either do this by going to your doctor, or by seeing a nutritional therapist who can arrange a stool test (see Resources, page 483). If you do have a UFO, there are natural remedies that can help eliminate them. My favourites are olive leaf extract and grapefruit seed extract. However, some strong bugs need drugs to eliminate them; your doctor will advise. If you end up having to take a course of such drugs, I recommend supplementing both something like olive leaf or grapefruit seed extract for a month, and some probiotics to top up your beneficial gut bacteria. *Lactobacillus acidophilus* and *Bifidobacterium bifidum* are excellent. These two 'good guys' (think of A for acidophilus and B for bifidum) not only get wiped out by bugs and bug-killing drugs, but are also your first line of defence against getting infected in the first place. Next time you go to India, supplementing probiotics and taking some grapefruit seed extract every day will act as a preventive against infection, as will only eating peelable fruit, such as mangoes, and cooked vegetables, and drinking bottled water.

Dizziness

Q *I get feelings of dizziness and when I move my head I have the sensation that everything around me is moving at a different speed. What's going on?*

A There are a number of possibilities. One is low blood pressure, another sinus infections. However, I have often had patients who reported this symptom coming back, after following a good nutrition strategy, to tell me it had disappeared. So one possible reason for this strange sensation is a lack of key nutrients such as the B vitamins, magnesium and manganese, which may be required for the middle ear, which controls the sense of equilibrium, to function properly.

In any case, I'd recommend you first see a doctor to rule out any medical conditions. If all's well, you can treat yourself with a daily course of supplements, starting with a high-strength multivitamin and mineral containing 25 to 50mg of the B vitamins, 200mg of magnesium and 2 to 5mg of manganese.

Eczema

Q *I have chronic eczema, even on my eyelids. Can you help?*

A There are three main avenues you can explore. The first is allergies. Many eczema suffers are allergic to something they're eating, or putting on the skin. The most common foods in this context are dairy products and eggs, but citrus fruits, gluten (the protein found in wheat and also oats, barley and rye), nuts (including peanuts), soya, chocolate, tea and coffee are also common allergens. You could try eliminating these one at a time to see if you get any relief; do so for 10 days per type of food, since it takes a while for your skin to calm down. It is also well worth having a food intolerance test to pin down precisely what you are intolerant to, if anything. Allergies to chemicals can trigger eczema, so try changing to a neutral eco-washing powder and fabric softener (these are now available from healthfood shops and large supermarkets) and investigate allergy protection bed covering.

The second possibility is that you have a deficiency in essential fats, without which the skin will become dry and sensitive. It seems that eczema suffers have an especially high need for these essential fatty acids

(EFAs), found mainly in coldwater fish and pumpkin, sesame, sunflower, flax and other seeds, and their oils. Seeds and fish are both natural anti-inflammatories, too, which helps to explain their effect on eczema, which is an inflammatory condition. So it's a good idea to supplement EFAs – either GLA, found in evening primrose and borage or starflower oils (250mg daily), or EPA and DHA, found in most abundance in fish oils. You'll need 400mg of EPA and DHA both a day. I'd recommend taking a supplement that contains all three. I'd also recommend a good optimum nutrition multivitamin because B vitamins, zinc and magnesium all help the body use essential fats to keep skin healthy.

Finally, you may be low on antioxidants, some of which also have anti-inflammatory properties. Quercetin (300mg before meals) or grapeseed extract (50mg with meals), available from healthfood shops, may help. Certain foods, particularly berries, are also very high in flavonoids that have been shown to help eczema.

Meanwhile, there are certain drug-free creams worth trying. Try MSM (organic sulphur) cream or aloe vera gel, although be careful with these, as some people are sensitive to them, especially if the skin is broken.

Q *Are there any creams, other than cortisone, that help with eczema?*

A Yes, there are, and they're often more effective. While any serious eczema treatment regime must start from the inside (see 'I have chronic eczema', page 185), applying soothing creams to affected areas can dramatically reduce the irritating and painful symptoms of itching and inflammation. This can be especially important in children, as their constant unconscious scratching of affected areas can really exacerbate the condition.

The best creams contain anti-inflammatory herbs such as ginger, frankinsence, burdock or chickweed. MSM cream, which contains organic sulphur, can also help relieve soreness and itching. These are available in healthfood stores. These are both most suitable for small areas. For larger areas, try aloe vera gel, renowned for its soothing and cooling properties. Eczema suffers are usually highly sensitive, so all of these creams should be tested on small areas before liberal use, especially if the skin is broken.

DIG DEEPER: For more tips on treating eczema, see my book *Solve Your Skin Problems*, coauthored with Natalie Savona (Piatkus, 2001).

Emphysema

Q *What nutritional advice can you give for emphysema?*

A Emphysema is a chronic pulmonary condition where breathing becomes very difficult. It results essentially from an inflammation inside the lungs that may or may not be caused by exposure to the toxic mineral cadmium (found in cigarettes and some toxic emissions from factories).

You'll be pleased to hear that there are many nutritional ways of helping to reduce the symptoms of emphysema. An important mineral in the body, which also counteracts the harmful effects of cadmium, is zinc, so start by taking 15mg of that a day. To help reduce inflammation, it's best to take a good antioxidant blend that contains vitamins A, C and E, as well as other powerful nutrients such as lipoic acid or glutathione. A powerful natural anti-inflammatory is found in fish oils; look for the ones containing the omega-3 essential fatty acids EPA and DHA. Vitamin A plays an important role in the lungs, and is found abundantly in cod liver oil. So you can kill two birds with one stone by supplementing a cod liver oil supplement that is high in both the omega-3s and vitamin A. (See Resources, page 483.) Many people with congestion in the lungs find that avoiding dairy products can help, as this will reduce mucus production. Try giving up milk and milk products for three to four weeks and see if that makes any difference for you.

Exhaustion

 I feel tired a lot of the time. Are there any natural energy boosters?

A There are two common reasons for tiredness, apart from a lack of sleep. The first is blood sugar problems.

You can solve this by staying off sugar and stimulants, and eating 'slow-release' carbohydrates such as rye or oats as part of a balanced, wholefood diet. This means lots of fresh fruit and vegetables. Supplementing 200mcg of chromium, available in any healthfood shop, can also help.

The second reason is adrenal exhaustion, made worse by stimulants like caffeine and stress. If you supplement the amino acids tyrosine and/or phenylalanine (1 to 2g a day), from which the body can make adrenal hormones, this can give you a natural energy boost and more capacity to deal with stress. Also excellent are 'adaptogenic' herbs which keep adrenal hormones on an even keel, and increase your energy. The best are ginseng, both Asian and Siberian, rhodiola, reishi and ashwaganda. (See Resources, page 483.)

Q **I'm always tired and feel even worse if I exercise. Is this ME?**

A These are classic signs of ME, now known as chronic fatigue syndrome, and indicate that your body is having a problem detoxifying the normal toxins generated when it turns food into energy. This is why you feel excessively tired after exercise and probably feel bad if you eat too much, especially of less healthy food.

You need to improve your detox potential by following a liver cleansing diet for two weeks, as well as taking supplements that help to cleanse the system.

For the first week this means eating lots of fresh fruit, vegetables and wholefoods such as rice, beans, fish and the like, and staying completely off meat, dairy products, wheat, tea, coffee and alcohol. The best vegetables to eat are broccoli, Brussels sprouts, cabbage, kale and cauliflower, all of which contain substances called glucosinolates that help to support the liver. Also good are carrots, tomatoes, sweet potatoes and other orange-coloured foods that are rich in beta-carotene. Be sure, too, to supplement a good high-strength multivitamin and an antioxidant complex. (See Resources, page 483.)

Q *How can I stop myself from getting drowsy after lunch?*

A There are three reasons for feeling as if you're nodding off after lunch. You are eating too much; you are eating too much carbohydrate and drinking stimulants; or you are allergic to something you are eating.

The first is easy to rule out. Just eat lightly, and see how you feel. The second is much more common, so chances are you're overdosing on refined carbohydrates. If you're lunching on pasta, baked potatoes, sandwiches or wraps made with refined bread, sugary drinks, tea or coffee or snacks like chocolate, beware: all these can send your blood sugar through the roof. In too short a time it then comes crashing down and you end up feeling sleepy or exhausted. If this sounds like you, try eating something like a piece of fish or chicken with vegetables or salad only. If this makes a difference, make sure from now on that when you lunch, any serving of starchy carbohydrate such as rice, potatoes, bread or pasta is balanced out by a serving of protein (fish, meat, tofu, cottage cheese or hummus) of equal size. Drink water, herbal teas, coffee substitutes and diluted juices instead of tea or coffee, and snack on fresh fruit paired with nuts and seeds if you're hungry after lunch. The mineral chromium can also help stabilise your blood sugar; take 200mcg with lunch.

The most common reason for wanting to snooze after lunch, however, is a food allergy. Perhaps 1 in 10 people have minor reactions to certain foods, the most common being drowsiness. For some people it's yeast, for others wheat, milk, beef or soya. I thought I was allergic to wheat because I was drowsy after eating bread. I wasn't. After testing, I realised I was reacting to yeast, which is present in bread and beer, but not in pasta and champagne. It's worth investing in such a test to discover any food intolerance you may have.

Q *I get tired and low when I eat bread. Am I gluten sensitive?*

A You may well be. Tiredness, depression and digestive problems are the most common symptoms of gluten sensitivity. Also called coeliac disease, gluten sensitivity is far more common than most people realise. Recent research from Italy, where they have been randomly testing school children, show than 1 in 120 people are gluten sensitive.

Gluten is highest in wheat, although it is also present in rye, barley and oats. Some people, however, are sensitive to something in gluten called gliadin, which isn't present in oats. Of course, let's not jump to conclusions that you're gluten sensitive. You might be allergic to wheat only, or may even react to the yeast in bread, not the wheat. How are you with beer? Many people react to brewer's and bakers' yeast. The only sure way to find out is to get yourself tested. (See Resources, page 483.)

Q *When I go on holiday I feel exhausted and often get sick. Why?*

A You were probably adrenally exhausted before you went. When the adrenal glands are on their last legs, most people can keep going only by staying hyped up – for example, by working long hours, or keeping up a regular supply of stimulants such as tea, coffee, caffeinated drinks or cigarettes. Adrenal hormones also suppress infections and pain. But when the pressure is off and you get on that plane for your week's break, your adrenal glands go into retirement and your true state – utterly knackered – emerges. You can get headaches, nausea, body aches and flu-like symptoms, and feel chronically tired.

My advice is to eat very well, sleep long, do some mild exercise, and take 3g of vitamin C and a high dose B complex every day, plus some rhodiola, a herb that breathes life into flagging adrenal glands. Meanwhile, try and get some balance into your life so you're not living on the edge of exhaustion.

Q *In the winter it's dark when I wake up and I just can't get going. Why is this?*

A You are probably suffering from a lack of light. This is very common. An estimated 3 million people suffer from seasonal affective disorder (SAD), a form of depression that can happen when you don't get enough light, as during short winter days. Light has a direct effect on the brain, helping to control how you sleep and how you wake up. Of course, waking up in the dark, which is what we do in winter, is not natural and not ideal; but trying telling your boss that!

There is a solution that works remarkably well. It a 'dawn simulation' alarm. Basically, it's a bedside light with a built-in dimmer and alarm clock in one. When you set it to wake you up at, say, 6.30 a.m., it gradually turns up the light intensity, starting 20 minutes before your wake-up time, simulating what dawn does. If this doesn't wake you, the alarm goes off at your wake-up time. I've never heard the alarm because the light works so well. The extraordinary thing is you wake up seemingly of your own accord, with much more energy and natural alertness.

I'd also recommend taking a combination of amino acids, tyrosine and phenylalanine, and adaptogenic herbs such as Asian and Siberian ginseng and reishi. These are available in combined supplements (see Resources, page 483.) In the early winter mornings, this is what works for me.

Eye conditions

Q *Can nutrition help prevent eyestrain and shortsightedness?*

A The right nutrition can definitely prevent shortsightedness and protect against eyestrain and damage. The key nutrient is vitamin A, which is abundant in meat, and carrots and other red/orange foods, from sweet potatoes to tomatoes. I recommend supplementing 2,250mcg (7,500iu) a day. Also excellent is bilberry extract, lutein, and anthocyanidins, antioxidants that protect the eyes from radiation and pollution and improve the delivery of oxygen to the eyes. Another herb, gingko biloba, improves circulation to the eyes and hence helps nutrients get to the right place. The herb eyebright, which has been used as a natural remedy for centuries, is known to reduce eye inflammation and irritation, as well as helping prevent cataracts.

The simplest way to give your eyes nutritional support is to take a supplement that provides vitamin A and other antioxidants such as vitamin C, E and selenium, plus additional herbs and food extracts which also protect against radiation from computer screens. (See Resources, page 483.)

Q ***What can you recommend to protect against age-related macular degeneration and cataracts?***

A A recent study by the Florida International University found that people whose eyes contained higher amounts of a nutrient called lutein were up to 80 per cent less likely to be suffering from age-related macular degeneration (ARMD), a condition that includes cataracts. Lutein protects the eye by forming pigments in the macula – the part of the eye right behind the lens in the centre of the retina. These pigments help with vision by filtering out harmful blue light wavelengths that can damage the eye. The more pigments your eye contains, the less likely it is to fall prey to ARMD.

As the body does not naturally generate lutein, you need to make sure you are getting enough from other sources. The best are green leafy vegetables such as cabbage, spinach, broccoli, cauliflower and kale. A study in the *American Journal of Clinical Nutrition* found that eating a teaspoon of green leafy vegetables (with a small amount of fat) raised blood lutein levels by nearly 90 per cent. But you need to eat lutein-rich vegetables for several months before you'll see any benefits, so I'd advise taking a supplement.

This should include antioxidants, also found abundantly in green leafy vegetables. Vitamins A and C, plentiful in brightly coloured fruit and vegetables such as carrots, red peppers, sweet potatoes, kiwi fruits, plums and berries, are key.

I recommend supplementing at least 2g of vitamin C and 2,250mcg (7,500iu) of vitamin A a day, and including cherries, blueberries and blackberries in your diet. Bilberry extract, an antioxidant that boosts the supply of oxygen to the eyes, is also very good, and ginkgo biloba improves circulation to the eyes, which ensures a good delivery of nutrients. Astaxanthin is another very powerful antioxidant that can cross the blood-brain barrier to target the eye. (See Resources, page 483.) Finally, limiting sugar and saturated fats is important, as these can damage the eye if blood levels are too high.

Q *My eyes are very dry – I can't wear contact lenses any more. Are there any supplements that might help?*

A Dry eyes is a classic symptom of vitamin A deficiency. The best sources are cod liver oil, liver and eggs, while carrots and other dark green, red and yellow vegetables contain beta-carotene, which your body converts to vitamin A. In addition to a vitamin A and beta-carotene-rich diet, supplement 5,000mcg (17,000iu) of vitamin A or 18mg of beta-carotene daily if your eyes are dry. (Note, however, that if you're pregnant or likely to conceive you shouldn't take over 3,000mcg, or 10,000iu, of vitamin A.) Try this for two months, then reduce the amount to 3,000mcg.

Other possible causes of dry eyes are dehydration and a lack of essential fats, so drink at least 1.5 litres of filtered or bottled water daily and eat oily fish – sardines, mackerel, herring, trout, wild salmon and the occasional piece of fresh tuna – at least three times per week.

Q *Can nutrition help conjunctivitis?*

A Conjunctivitis is an inflammation causing pain, itching and redness on the surface of the eye. It can be caused by viruses, bacteria or an allergy, and is more often environmental than food related. Fortunately, optimum nutrition can dramatically improve the condition.

A sufficient intake of essential fats from oily fish and/or seeds and oils is a vital prerequisite for good eye health and to reduce allergic reactions, if that's what's causing the conjunctivitis. Vitamin A is well known to be a key nutrient for the eyes, and supplementing 5,000mcg (17,000iu) of vitamin A or 18mg of beta-carotene (and no more than 3,000mcg, or 10,000iu, of vitamin A if you're pregnant), plus 2g of vitamin C and 30mg of zinc daily while you have the infection, has been shown to boost the immune system and help clear conjunctivitis. Vitamin D is also known to be helpful for conjunctivitis, and the best source – cod liver oil – also provides essential fats and vitamin A (but remember to limit your overall vitamin A to the levels listed above). The herb euphrasia, often called eyebright, makes an excellent tea which can be drunk three times a day, as well as cooled and used as an eye rinse. Chamomile and fennel teas can be used in this way too. Colloidal silver solution spray is an effective remedy for conjunctivitis and can be sprayed directly around the closed eye. It's available from healthfood shops.

Fibromyalgia

Q *What do you recommend for fibromyalgia?*

A Fibromyalgia is a chronic condition accompanied by many symptoms, including widespread pain and fatigue. Research indicates that the painful muscles characteristic of fibromyalgia are due to lowered energy production and a reduction in the ability of muscles to relax.

Supplementing magnesium malate has been shown to reduce pain after as little as two days. Eat a healthy diet with plenty of magnesium-rich foods such as green vegetables, nuts and seeds. Supplement the key vitamins and minerals (the Bs, C, E, calcium and so on) in a good multivitamin, along with 600mg of magnesium malate. Reducing your stress levels, relearning how to relax and increasing exercise slowly are all important. Especially helpful are Psychocalisthenics exercises, which involve precise breathing patterns. By deepening breathing muscles work better (See Resources, page 483).

Gallbladder problems and gallstones

Q *I've had my gallbladder removed and have difficulty digesting fats. Any suggestions?*

A It's not surprising you have a problem digesting fats: the gallbladder stores bile, which is released into the intestines when we eat, and one of its jobs is to emulsify fats. During this process, bile breaks the fats up, giving them a bigger surface area on which enzymes can then get to work.

To help your body cope without a gallbladder, you'll need to give your digestion a hand. So eat less fatty food and avoid having a lot of fat in one go – limit or omit cream, butter and other spreads, and meat products such as sausages, salami or streaky bacon. It is vital to eat some fats, however; the omega-3 fatty acids from fish, nuts and seeds are essential for health.

To help digest fat, sprinkle a tablespoon of lecithin granules on food daily, or take a 1,200mg lecithin capsule with each meal. Also take a digestive enzyme supplement that contains lipase (the fat-digesting enzyme).

Q *Is there a natural way to get rid of gallstones?*

A There are two kinds of gallstone: calcified stones and fat deposits. The former need laser treatment to break them up. The latter respond to an increase in your intake of lecithin and a 'gallbladder flush' (see page 200). If you suspect you have a gallstone, you'll need to discover which type. Calcified gallstones will probably be more painful, as they can cause the gallbladder to become inflamed. If you lie down and press down under your ribcage you can normally detect whether this has happened, from the pain. A calcified stone will show up on an X-ray.

To ease the condition, increase fibre; this will stop bile being reabsorbed, which can contribute to gallstones. Take 3,000mcg (10,000iu) of vitamin A a day, as this will ensure a smooth lining to the gallbladder and thus prevent the bile from precipitating and forming stones. And sprinkle a tablespoon of lecithin granules, which help to emulsify fatty gallstones, on your cereal every morning, or have two 1,200mg lecithin capsules. It's also key to limit your intake of fat, so avoid fried or processed foods – but make sure you get enough good fats in the form of oily fish, fresh nuts and seeds.

If you don't have calcified stones, a nutritional therapist or naturopath may recommend a gallbladder flush. This involves drinking a lot of olive oil, swallowed down with lemon juice, a procedure that will probably leave you feeling quite nauseated. This acts to soften and remove fat-based gallbladder deposits. However, do not do this without professional guidance.

Genital herpes

Q *I suffer from genital herpes. Is there any alternative treatment that can help?*

A The herpes virus feeds off an amino acid called arginine. If you supplement lysine, an amino acid that looks like arginine, you fool the virus and effectively starve it.

I recommend supplementing 1,000mg of lysine every day, away from food, to keep the virus at bay. When you have an active infection, supplement 3,000mg of lysine a day and cut right back on foods rich in arginine, which include beans, lentils, nuts and chocolate. The more stressed you are, the weaker your immune system becomes and the more chances the virus has to become active. A good way to boost your immune system is to supplement 3g of vitamin C every day and 2g of the herb cat's claw, which is one of the most powerful immune-boosting herbs yet discovered.

Glandular fever

Q *What nutritional support to aid recovery from glandular fever do you recommend?*

A Glandular fever is a viral illness with symptoms very similar to those of flu. As well as feeling out of sorts, and possibly feverish or headachy, you might have swollen lymph glands. To recover from this nasty infection you'll need to support your immune system as much as possible.

Start by following an optimum diet rich in wholefoods such as wholegrains, good-quality proteins such as free-range chicken, fish and tofu, and plenty of organic fruit and vegetable, including carrots, beetroots and beet greens, sweet potatoes, tomatoes, garlic and beansprouts, and berries, watermelon, oranges and kiwi fruits. Investing in a juicer is a good idea, as every day you should include nutrient-rich juices made from these fruit and vegetable.

Also add in supplements to support the immune system – a multi, vitamin C and an antioxidant complex. Vitamins A, B1, B2, B6, B12, folic acid, C and E are all immune-boosters, as are zinc, magnesium and selenium. Try taking two multis and two antioxidants every day, plus 6g of vitamin C, taken in 2g increments with each meal. (See Resources, page 483.) I recommend that you see a nutritional therapist.

Gout

Q **Is there anything apart from prescribed drugs that can help with gout?**

A Gout can occur when proteins, usually from animal sources, are not being properly metabolised. The result is uric acid crystal deposits in fingers, toes and joints, which cause inflammation and pain.

Diets low in fat and moderate in protein alleviate this condition, so a vegetarian diet should help, so long as you don't eat too much cheese and other dairy products. Exercise is a real plus too. And it's essential to supplement the many nutrients involved in protein metabolism, especially B6 and zinc.

To combat gout or prevent a reoccurrence, cut out red meat and alcohol completely. Follow the optimum nutrition diet: avoid refined carbohydrates and eat wholefoods such as wholegrains; eat high-quality protein such as tofu and free-range chicken, beans and lentils; include plenty of vegetables, steamed or raw, and three pieces of fresh fruit a day. Go for organic. Be sure to drink 1 to 1.5 litres of pure water. And don't leave out the omega-3 essential fats from oily fish and seeds. For vegetarians, I recommend using cold-pressed seed oil blends, as these help to lubricate joints and reduce inflammation; ask in your local healthfood store. Non-vegetarians can top up their omega-3s by eating mackerel, trout or sardines three times a week or supplementing with an omega-3-rich fish oil. Other supplements should include a good multivitamin and mineral, 3g of vitamin C taken as 1g with each meal, 100mg of vitamin B6, 15mg of zinc and a bone mineral complex rich in alkaline-forming calcium and magnesium daily. (See Resources, page 483.)

Graves' disease

Q *What is Graves' disease and what can I do to treat it?*

A Graves' disease is a hyperthyroid condition caused by a basic defect in the immune system. People with Graves' suffer from an array of symptoms, including weight loss, fatigue, eye problems and muscle weakness. The condition may well be exacerbated by food sensitivities and has specifically been linked to gluten, the protein found in grains such as wheat, barley and rye. But there could be another underlying factor. People with autoimmune conditions often have raised homocysteine – a natural by-product of protein metabolism that should be converted to other substances, but can get 'stuck' without sufficient nutrients from the diet to do this.

I strongly recommend you see a nutritional therapist who can test you for potential food intolerances and check your homocysteine levels. (See Resources, page 483.)

If after testing you find your levels of homocysteine are above 10, supplementing with B12, B6 and folic acid has been shown to lower levels. And if you find you have intolerance to gluten, you can cut these grains out of your diet.

Haemorrhoids

Q *What do you recommend for haemorrhoids?*

A Haemorrhoids can develop after straining on defecation. The less compacted and softer the stools, the easier they are to pass and the less chance of developing haemorrhoids. The main symptom is anal itching (also sometimes a sign of candidiasis infection or inflammatory bowel disease), which in turn can lead to excessive scratching and aggravation of the condition. Diarrhoea and stress can also make the itching worse.

While frequent warm baths and anti-inflammatory creams can relieve symptoms, you can only achieve long-term relief through dietary changes. This means more fibre, but the often-recommended bran is not the way to go: as an insoluble and sometimes allergenic fibre, it can be harsh on the digestive system. A much better alternative is soluble fibre, such as is found in fruit and vegetables. Cabbage and prunes are rich in soluble fibre, as are psyllium husks and flax seeds, both widely available at healthfood stores. Celery has a lot of insoluble fibre, but doesn't tend to irritate the gut, so it's a good choice. As for the rest, choose wholegrains and wholefoods: try eating more beans, lentils, oats and rye. And be sure to drink 1 to 1.5 litres of water a day.

Halitosis

Q *I am really self-conscious over having bad breath, and breath fresheners don't work. Have you got any suggestions?*

A Unless you have rotten teeth or gums, bad breath rarely has anything to do with your mouth, which is why breath fresheners don't help. The most common underlying reason is that your stomach isn't digesting food properly. You may not, for instance, be producing enough hydrochloric acid (HCl), the substance that digests food in the stomach. Food will then be left fermenting in your stomach, which is what makes your breath smell.

You can buy HCl in capsules, usually in the form of betaine hydrochoride. Take 300mg with each meal. As stress interferes with the body's HCl production, chill out over meals: chew your food well, and relax when you sit down to eat.

Headache and migraine

Q *I keep getting headaches. Are there any natural remedies?*

A There are many causes of headaches and migraines, including a drop in blood sugar, dehydration, allergy, stress and tension, or a critical combination of some or all of these. Peaks and troughs in adrenalin and blood sugar can bring on a headache. Often they go away with optimum nutrition. Try eating small and often, and avoid long periods without food, especially if you are stressed or tense. Also, make sure you have a regular intake of fluid; drink 1 to 1.5 litres of water a day. Avoid sugar and stimulants like tea, coffee and chocolate. If the headaches persist, look carefully at the possibility of allergy. See if you can notice any patterns between the foods you eat and the incidence of headaches. It's well worth having a food intolerance test (see Resources, page 483).

Instead of taking an aspirin, or migraine drugs that constrict the blood vessels, try taking 100 to 200mg of vitamin B3 in the niacin form, which is a vasodilator. Start with the smaller dose. This will cause a 'blushing' sensation as well as a feeling of increased heat and can often stop or reduce a headache in the early stages. It's best to do this at home in a relaxed environment.

Q **When I'm exposed to a lot of exhaust fumes I get headaches. How can I stop this?**

A Obviously, the main aim is to reduce your exposure to the fumes in the first place. If you ride your bicycle to work through traffic-ridden areas, for instance, map out a less crowded route. That said, you can also improve the way your body processes these harmful chemicals, which contain lots of free radicals or oxidants. You'll need a good supply of antioxidant nutrients, so eat plenty of fresh fruit and vegetables, especially the red, orange and purple foods such as berries, apricots, sweet potatoes, peppers and carrots. Probably the best weapon against oxidants is a watermelon smoothie – just put chunks of it in a blender, seeds and all, and once it's whizzed up you've got a refreshing drink loaded with antioxidant nutrients. You can also supplement an antioxidant complex. (See Resources, page 483.) Also make sure you're drinking at least 1.5 litres of bottled or filtered water a day and avoiding things that burden your body, such as coffee and alcohol.

Q *I get headaches after I've used my mobile phone. Are there any natural remedies?*

A Nobody in the science community or the government seems to be able to make up their minds on the possible link between mobile phones and health problems. And no research has been done specifically on headaches caused by overexposure to mobile phone electromagnetic radiation. But while the research is variable, there is some evidence showing that antioxidants can minimise the effects of such overexposure. First, however, you need to reduce your mobile phone use as much as possible: just ruthlessly cut out all unnecessary calls. Note that hands-free phones also expose you to electromagnetic radiation, so make sure you don't have a base unit right by your bed, for example.

Then, to protect yourself, supplement an anti-oxidant complex. I would also supplement omega-3 fats and lecithin, high in phospholipids, because these substances help build the nerve and cell membranes that are particularly susceptible to damage by radiation. One tablespoon of lecithin granules a day and two 400mg omega-3 fish oil capsules should do it.

Q *I always seem to get headaches when I take multivitamin supplements. Any idea why this might be?*

A You are obviously reacting to something in your multivitamin. Try this experiment. Take 1g of vitamin C for four days, then add an antioxidant supplement. If you have no headaches, you've eliminated A, C, E and some other possibilities. (Reactions to sources of vitamin A, C and E are very rare.) Then try a B complex. If that triggers the headache, check that it's yeast-free. If it isn't, it may be prompting an allergic reaction. The supplements I recommend are yeast-free since studies show that as many as 20 per cent of people react to either brewer's or baker's yeast.

Some people are genetically pre-programmed to produce more of the neurotransmitter histamine. This condition can make them prone to headaches in the first place; but supplementing extra folic acid (as found in a B complex) can actually make them worse because folate promotes histamine production. So try cutting out folic acid and see how you feel.

Q *I often get migraines. Is there a nutrition connection?*

A The so-called 'classic' migraines are very severe recurring headaches that may involve a host of other symptoms, from vomiting to light sensitivity, speech difficulty and even loss of vision. Attacks can last as long as a day or two. Common migraines are less severe but not much fun to endure, either. The good news is that most migraine sufferers can get complete or substantial relief with optimum nutrition, although it's important to try to discover which factors are contributing to your migraines.

These could include too much sugar, stress or stimulants, going without food or not drinking enough water, and poor sleeping habits. A number of foods and additives have been found to trigger migraines, including aged cheese and other dairy products, alcohol, caffeine, MSG, citrus fruits and aspartame. A reliable food intolerance test (see Resources, page 483) can help you isolate any culprits. In the meantime, following an organic wholefood diet with good-quality proteins and carbohydrates, and plenty of fruit and vegetables, will help.

Generally, vitamins B1, B2 and B3 also reduce the incidence of migraines. Medical studies have shown substantial relief from migraines by supplementing either vitamin B2 or B3 (niacin). In a recent study, those taking high-dose vitamin B2 (try 100mg) for four months had fewer migraines. In another study, people who took 100mg of niacin a day halved their number of migraines. However, you can often stop a migraine in its tracks if you take 100mg of niacin at the first sign of an attack. Niacin is a vasodilator and you'll blush for about 20 minutes, so it's best to do this at home while relaxing.

Heart and circulatory conditions

Circulation

Q **What can I do to improve my circulation? I freeze in the winter.**

A You're spoilt for choice when it comes to ways of improving your circulation. First off, exercise regularly. Your best bet is to do some that raises your heart rate at least three times a week, such as a brisk walk or swim or session at the gym. But while exercise stimulates circulation, particularly to the extremities, that's not the whole story. Done rightly, it also helps build lean muscle mass, which means insultation. Sure, fat is good insulation too, but muscle is better. And since you want all-over insulation, don't forget to do exercises that strengthen your upper body as well as your legs – so don't restrict yourself just to walking or running. Psychocalisthenics is excellent.

Vitamins help too. Take 400mg of vitamin E and 50mg to 100mg of niacin (B3) a day, and you will see a difference. Vitamin E helps the body use oxygen, while niacin dilates blood vessels, so you get a real boost to your blood flow. You may also blush, possibly quite strongly for the first few days you take it. This is harmless, but you may feel hot during the flush, as your blood flow increases, and then cold afterwards.

So take niacin when you've got some time at home, possibly having a warm bath after the flush. One month of this and you may find your circulation is much improved, so you'll be able to stop taking the additional niacin.

The herb ginkgo biloba – a traditional remedy renowned for its ability to improve circulation – can help too. Take 40mg a day, making sure the supplement contains 24 per cent ginkgoflavonglycosides. Ginger and cayenne are other circulation boosters, so drink fresh ginger tea (pour boiling water over the chopped or grated root) and use cayenne pepper freely in your cooking. If you are also suffering from fatigue, low libido and dry skin, your thyroid gland may well be working below par, so ask your doctor to run tests to check that out.

Q *I get pins and needles all over my body during the day, but especially in my hands. What could I take to help this?*

A First, if you are anxious or stressed, muscle tension can interfere with your nerves, leaving a tingling sensation in your extremities. So calming tension with massage, exercise or osteopathy could help. If your pins and needles are due to a circulation problem, meaning that not enough oxygen is getting into the cells, vitamin B3 (niacin) gives it a good boost. Take 100mg.

Recurrent pins and needles, especially if accompanied by other symptoms such as fatigue and aching or inflamed joints, may be a sign of toxic overload. For this, you should work with a nutritionist to detoxify your system by following a very healthy diet and taking supplements such as a good antioxidant complex and liver support that includes the herb milk thistle. Generally, detox diets mean you'll need to cut out all gluten grains such as wheat, barley, oats and rye, and all refined foods, red meat, alcohol and stimulants; concentrate on fresh fruit such as watermelon, kiwi fruits, apricots, red grapes and berries, and fresh vegetables including sweet potatoes, carrots, peas, watercress, broccoli, peppers, spinach and tomatoes; drink 1 to 1.5 litres of pure water a day; and eat judicious amounts of wholegrains such as brown rice, along with oily fish and raw nuts and seeds.

Q *I wake up with pins and needles – what nutrients could help this?*

A Feeling pins and needles on waking is usually caused by lying on part of your body at an awkward angle, which cuts off the blood supply. If this is definitely not the case with you, other things to consider are physical tension and poor circulation. If your muscles do get tense, the mineral magnesium acts as a gentle, natural relaxant – take 300mg before you go to bed. Vitamin B3 (niacin) can also help relax tension and improve blood flow; take 50 to 100mg. Or you can take it as part of a high-strength mutlivitamin, which should provide up to 50mg in the non-blushing niacinamide form. The herb ginkgo is renowned for improving circulation: take 40mg (standardised to contain 24 per cent ginkgoflavonglycosides) three times daily.

Clotting, stroke and thrombosis

Q *What are the nutritional recommendations for someone prone to blood clots?*

A The nutritional approach to preventing blood clots involves thinning the blood with essential fats and vitamin E. Essential fats are found in oily fish such as wild salmon and mackerel, and seeds and their oils. Try having either 1,000mg of an omega-3 fish oil or a tablespoon of flax seed oil, or the equivalent in capsules every day, as well as supplementing 300mg vitamin E (400iu) a day. However, note that any food supplements that thin the blood must not be taken in conjunction with blood-thinning medications. So if you are on these drugs, just make sure you have an adequate dietary intake of E and the essential fats by eating avocados, wheatgerm, cashews, beans, oily fish and seeds (pumpkin, sunflower and flax). If you'd like to supplement anyway, only do so under professional guidance.

Garlic may also help. Eric Block, a professor of chemistry at the State University of New York, thinks it's all down to the chemical ajoene, found in the bulb. And vitamin C and vitamin B, or niacin, have been shown to be beneficial. Maintaining physical activity keeps the blood flowing and so less likely to clot, so exercise, in moderation, is important.

Another common cause of blood clots is excessively high levels of fibrinogen, a substance in blood plasma that causes coagulation. This is strongly linked to having high homocysteine, which is something I recommend anyone with cardiovascular symptoms having checked (see Resources, page 483). If your homocysteine is high there are specific supplements that help normalise it (see 'I've had a heart attack', page 215).

Q *What do you recommend to avoid deep vein thrombosis of the legs where the blood is referred to as 'sticky'?*

A 'Sticky' blood, due to either high levels of a sticky substance in the blood called fibrinogen or a high platelet adhesion index, can cause clots in different parts of the body – for example, behind the knees, calves or groin. So it can be quite a risky condition, but nutrition can help you control it. Essentially, the diet you'll need to follow is the one outlined in the answer to 'What are the nutritional recommendations for someone prone to blood clots?', page 213. Note that natural blood thinners such as the omega-3s and vitamin E should not be supplemented if you are already on blood-thinning medication.

Also check your homocysteine levels (see Resources, page 483). Two-thirds of people with thrombosis have raised levels. Homocysteine is strongly linked to fibrinogen, the sticky, fibrous substance in the blood that's the main mechanism for the formation of clots. When fibrinogen levels go up, the blood starts producing blood clots. You can normalise your homocysteine and fibrinogen levels with special supplements (see 'I've had a heart attack', below).

Heart attacks

Q *I've had a heart attack but my cholesterol levels are OK – what do you suggest I do?*

A It is a complete myth that cholesterol is the only baddie in heart disease. In fact, more than half of heart attack victims have normal cholesterol levels. Two rarely checked factors linked to heart attacks are lipoprotein(a) and homocysteine. Lipoprotein(a), a type of fat in the blood, increases the risk of heart disease if it builds up on artery walls. Homocysteine is an amino acid present in the blood and a normal by-product of body processes, but it is not detoxified well in people with low levels of vitamins B6, B12 and folic acid. Many studies showed that people with high blood levels of homocysteine have a substantially increased risk of a heart attack. In the US, cardiologists routinely measure homocysteine levels, but this is still a rarity in the UK. (See Resources, page 483.)

You can keep your homocysteine levels in check by taking vitamins B6, B12, folic acid and an amino acid called trimethylglycine (TMG). There are specific supplements that contain all of these. Other risk factors for high homocysteine include high-meat diets, too much coffee, tea or alcohol, smoking and lack of exercise, so a shift in lifestyle might be in order.

You can counteract lipoprotein(a) build-up by taking 3g of vitamin C daily and 1,000mg of the amino acid Lysine. In short, there's a lot you can do to minimise risk and maximise recovery from a heart attack.

Q ***Why do people have heart attacks – is it more than just too many fried breakfasts?***

A Heart attacks are caused by arterial blockages, which have three principal causes. Firstly, the artery itself can become narrower because of an accumulation of fatty deposits on its walls, a condition known as atherosclerosis. Secondly, if the blood is too sticky, a blood clot can get stuck in a narrower artery. Thirdly, the arteries can become narrower due to muscular contraction.

A diet high in fried fatty foods and sugar does lead to an accumulation of damaged fats in the arteries, hence atherosclerosis. But there are many other factors that could trigger one of the conditions leading to a heart attack. Stress, too much sodium or even smoking a cigarette can cause the muscular contractions that narrow arteries, especially in an unfit person. A lack of magnesium-rich green vegetables, beans and fruits can do the same, because magnesium deficiency makes it difficult for the muscles to relax. Green vegetables and beans are also high in B vitamins, especially folic acid, which keep the amino acid homocysteine, an arterial toxin, at bay. And if you don't have enough Bs, the homocysteine will be free to damage the arteries, causing atherosclerosis, and also makes the blood stickier. Finally, failing to eat enough essential fats, found in oily fish and seeds, can also harden your arteries – not all fats are villains, after all.

So a combination of all these factors – too much fried, damaged and saturated fats, sugar, stress, smoking and salt, and too little exercise, magnesium, fruit, vegetables, nuts, seeds, beans, B vitamins, minerals and essential fats – will really lay you open to the risk of having a heart attack.

Q *There is a history of heart attacks in my family. Can I do anything with my diet to lessen my risk?*

A By far the biggest contributor to heart disease is diet plus lifestyle factors, such as smoking and exercise. But it is certainly true that some people genetically inherit a predisposition to heart attacks. This is linked to the two arterial toxins that you don't want to have too much of – lipoprotein(a) and homocysteine.

Of these two, homocysteine is probably the most important. One in 10 people inherit a predisposition to having high levels of homocysteine because the enzyme (MTHFR) that clears homocysteine from the system doesn't work so well. The MTHFR enzyme depends on an intake of vitamins B6, B12 and folic acid, and another nutrient called TMG. (Of lesser importance are zinc, magnesium and vitamin B2.) People with this condition therefore need more B6, B12, folic acid and TMG to keep their homocysteine levels normal. Lipoprotein(a) can be lowered by taking vitamin C.

My advice, if you have a family history of heart attacks but no symptoms, is to have your homocysteine level measured (see Resources, page 483). If it is above 6 units then supplement more of these vitamins. The website www.thehfactor.com tells you how much to supplement depending on your level. If you have symptoms, I'd also recommend testing your cholesterol and lipoprotein(a) level and upping your vitamin C intake to 3g a day if high.

High blood pressure

Q *I've got high blood pressure. Should my doctor be checking my homocysteine level?*

A High levels of homocysteine, an amino acid in the blood, have been found to be more predictive of heart attack or stroke risk than cholesterol, so the answer is yes. In fact, it's vital for you to know your homocysteine level because this is a highly reversible risk factor for cardiovascular problems. The ideal level is below 6. A score of 15 means four times the risk of a heart attack.

Catherine is a case in point. She had high blood pressure of 220/130 and shortly after had a stroke. She then tested her H score, which was very high at 22 units. She followed my H factor diet, focusing on 'greens and beans' because dark green leafy vegetables and beans are very high in folic acid, which can vanquish high H levels over time. It has been shown that supplementing large amounts of B6, B12 and folic acid definitely helps lower homocysteine levels. This is what Catherine did and, two months later, her H score had dropped to 7.6, and her blood pressure has stabilised at 120/70 without medication. This means that her risk of a stroke or heart attack is less than a tenth of what it had been.

I believe anyone with cardiovascular problems including high blood pressure, or a family history of heart disease, should routinely test for homocysteine levels. If your doctor won't do it you can either get a home test kit or visit a private lab that will test you. (See Resources, page 483.)

Treatments

Q *My husband has been prescribed aspirin every day because he's got heart disease. Are there any alternatives?*

A Aspirin is widely prescribed to people who have heart disease because it thins the blood, but a study published in the *British Medical Journal* showed it could actually be dangerous. It found that men with high blood pressure are at risk of possible serious bleeding when they take aspirin.

The alternatives (not to be taken in conjunction with aspirin but instead of it) are vitamin E and omega-3 fish oils. Both have proven more effective than aspirin. A study at the University of Cambridge showed that 400mg of vitamin E cuts the risk of a heart attack by 75 per cent – that's four times better than aspirin, although not all other studies have confirmed this result. Omega-

3 fish oils lower cholesterol, thin the blood and reduce risk of a heart attack. I recommend taking 400mg(600iu) of vitamin E and omega-3-rich fish oil, giving the equivalent of 500mg of combined EPA, the highly beneficial omega-3 fatty acid. Diet-wise, make sure your husband is eating plenty of fish, nuts and seeds, all sources of essential fats; fresh fruits and vegetables; and garlic.

Q *What's your view on chelation therapy for preventing heart disease?*

A Chelation therapy is a non-surgical way to unblock arteries, thereby reducing the risk of a heart attack or stroke. It involves giving the synthetic amino acid ethylenediamine tetra-acetic acid, or EDTA, by a drip infusion into the vein, usually for a couple of hours once or twice a week. The EDTA attaches to toxic minerals and to calcium, all of which hold arterial deposits together, and removes them from the body. The net result is that blockages in the arteries start to clear. In addition to the EDTA, the drip contains large amount of nutrients, especially antioxidants, which help to heal and rebuild the arteries.

Chelation therapy has been well proven to reverse arterial disease. Of course, the first line of defence against heart disease is to prevent it in the first place with a healthy diet and lifestyle. But for people with advanced arterial disease who cannot or don't want surgery, chelation therapy is a valid option.

Q *What's your view on statin drugs for lowering high cholesterol?*

A Statin drugs are designed to lower LDL cholesterol, which is implicated in atherosclerosis or clogged arteries. Overall, statin medication can be expected to lower concentrations of LDL cholesterol by around 2 mmol/l if taken for several years, which reduces the risk of a heart attack by about 60 per cent and stroke by 17 per cent. The risk reduction in the first year is minimal.

The trouble with statins is that they do their job by blocking an enzyme that makes something called mevalonate, from which the body makes both cholesterol and Co-enzyme Q10. CoQ10 is a nutrient vital for the heart, and a deficiency in it is associated with fatigue, muscle weakness and soreness, and heart failure. So, as has been well established in trials with people, statins effectively cause a CoQ10 deficiency, and taking them long term is therefore itself risky. Women are particularly susceptible to CoQ10 deficiency, which suppresses immunity. But just how serious these problems are isn't known. The major trials of statin drugs excluded people with the most severe forms of heart failure, class 3 and 4, so any link between the drugs and death rates from congestive heart failure remains a mystery.

A number of symptoms have been linked to statins, ranging from dizziness, headache, extreme fatigue and swelling of the ankles to muscle aches. Statins can be dangerous if taken with high levels of long-acting (time-release) niacin, or vitamin B3. (Large amounts of niacin have been shown to lower cholesterol very effectively on its own, and often form a part of nutritional strategies for people with raised cholesterol levels.) Personally, I think statins should be taken as a last resort, used only if someone has undergone a complete nutritional strategy and failed to lower their raised cholesterol.

Q *My 78-year-old father is on warfarin, and since having a stroke is rapidly losing his memory and focus. I want to wean him off warfarin and wondered about supplements.*

A Our brains are made largely out of phospholipids and essential fats. Phospholipids, combinations of fatty acids and phosphate groups, are one of the building blocks of membranes; essential fats are the beneficial fatty acids found in seeds, nuts and oily fish as well as grey matter. The evidence is mounting that a person's intake of these has a direct effect on their mental health and emotional intelligence. So I would give your father phospholipids – particularly phosphatidyl serine and choline. You can find these in lecithin granules (available from healthfood shops); give him a dessertspoonful twice a day. Free-range organic eggs and organic organ meats such as kidneys are also excellent sources of phospholipids. I would also advise getting his homocysteine tested (see Resources, page 483), as this amino acid can affect brain function as well as cardiovascular health.

Essential fatty acids such as the omega-3s are trickier, as these thin the blood as well as benefit the brain. So he can't supplement significant amounts of them while he's on warfarin. Ensure, however, that he's eating oily fish, or flax or pumpkin seeds, as the omega-3s in these will boost his brain power safely. In terms of weaning him off warfarin, he'll have to do this under the guidance of his doctor. Once he is safely off it, he can supplement with omega-3s and vitamin E as alternative blood thinners. A table-spoon of flax seed oil and 300mg (approximately 400iu) of vitamin E will probably do it, but you really need to do this under the guidance of an informed doctor or a nutritional therapist.

Q **The hospital has advised my wife, who is 73, to come off garlic, CoQ10, glucosamine, high vitamin C, calcium and omega-3, as they conflict with the warfarin she is taking. What is your view?**

A Warfarin is a blood-thinning drug that interferes with the action of vitamin K, which the body synthesises in the gut, and controls normal blood clotting. It is also used to kill rats by overthinning their blood. I know of no reason why vitamin C, calcium or Co-enzyme Q10 would conflict with warfarin.

That leaves the omega-3s and garlic, and these are a somewhat different story. Omega-3 fats naturally reduce platelet adhesion, so they are an alternative blood-thinning agent. Garlic, too, has blood-thinning properties. But that doesn't mean these need be barred completely. Ideally, one would want to lower warfarin and increase omega-3s, which have numerous other positive effects on reducing risk of a heart attack or stroke. However, that is something your wife would need to discuss with her doctor or cardiologist. Since her doctor has not mentioned avoiding fish or seeds, both of which contain omega-3 fats, the question is also one of quantity and hence level of effect.

Eating garlic in, say, pasta sauces and stir-fries, shouldn't cause a problem. And I doubt that taking an omega-3 supplement every day providing 200mg of EPA and 150mg of DHA (adding up to 350mg of omega-3 fats), or eating fish three times a week and a spoonful of ground flax seeds a day on cereal, would have any harmful effect. I don't advise larger amounts, however. It would be wise for your wife to monitor her platelet adhesion index and if this goes too low, to lower the warfarin dose accordingly.

DIG DEEPER: To find out more about heart disease generally, see my books *Say No to Heart Disease* (Piatkus, 1998), and *The H Factor* (Piatkus, 2003), coauthored with Dr James Braly.

Hiatus hernia

Q *What sort of dietary advice would you recommend for someone suffering from hiatus hernia?*

A A hiatus hernia happens when the top part of the stomach moves up through the hole in the diaphragm through which the oesophagus runs. Severe heartburn and acid reflux from the stomach can result. So it's vital to minimise your intake of gastric irritants – aspirin, coffee, alcohol, very hot drinks and spicy food – and reduce the amount of concentrated, protein-rich and therefore acidic foods you eat, such as meat, fish and eggs, in favour of vegetable proteins such as beans or tofu. If muscle spasm is involved, capsules of peppermint oil, which is an anti-spasmodic, can be of benefit.

There are also physical techniques practised by naturopaths and some osteopaths and kinesiologists that can help correct this condition, so you may want to book an appointment with one, having checked they practise this therapy.

HIV and AIDS

Q *I'm on combination therapy for HIV. Are there any supplements that could help me?*

A Without a doubt. The main focus of current research is on antioxidant nutrients that strengthen the immune system. Leading researcher Dr Raxit Jariwalla from the Linus Pauling Institute in California has shown that vitamin C can suppress the HIV virus in laboratory cultures of infected cells. He found that with continuous exposure to ascorbic acid (vitamin C) in concentrations not harmful to cells, the growth of HIV in immune cells could be reduced by 99.5 per cent.

Dr Jariwalla suggests that in healthy humans a daily dose of at least 10g is needed for an anti-viral effect. N-acetyl cysteine (NAC), an altered form of the amino acid cysteine, which is a powerful antioxidant, has also been found to have anti-viral properties. When Dr Jariwalla added vitamin C to NAC, he found the mixture showed an eightfold increase in anti-HIV activity. I'd recommend supplementing 2 to 3g of NAC a day. Also follow an immune-boosting diet.

That means one that's as organic as possible, and rich in colourful fruit and vegetables (think carrots, broccoli, garlic, sweet potatoes, tomatoes, berries, kiwi, watermelon and the like), oily omega-3-rich fish, seeds, wholegrains, lentils and beans, free-range chicken and plenty of pure water. Cut out refined, sugary and fried foods and go for a proportion of raw food and steam-frying (a light stir-fry with minimal oil, then a short steaming with a small amount of water or a soy/lemon juice/water mixture). And in addition to C be sure to supplement the antioxidant vitamins A and E and take a B complex, plus zinc and magnesium.

DIG DEEPER: Also see my book *Boost Your Immune System* (Piatkus, 1998).

Hormonal conditions

Q *What causes high levels of the hormone DHEA and how can I lower it?*

A DHEA is a hormone produced in the adrenal glands. Levels of this hormone in the body fall steeply with age. DHEA is actually highly beneficial, known to improve mood, muscles and immunity while lowering your risk of heart disease. A high level of DHEA and a normal one of cortisol is a natural state, particularly when someone is recovering from prolonged and excessive stress.

The only possible negative symptoms from excessive DHEA that I'm aware of result from its being a precursor of testosterone and oestrogen. After it is transformed into these sex hormones, it may be a factor in symptoms of hormonal imbalance – cycle irregularities, aggression, acne, mood swings and so on. It has to be said, however, that these symptoms have only emerged in people who supplement high levels of DHEA (in the US, it is available over the counter as an anti-ageing and anti-stress hormone).

I don't know of any direct ways to keep DHEA on an even keel, other than generally supporting your adrenals. To do this, try to reduce your levels of stress by relaxing more; cut out stimulants such as coffee, tea, chocolate, cigarettes and sugary, refined foods that will send your blood sugar on a rollercoaster; and supplement with B vitamins and C, plus Siberian ginseng.

Human papilloma virus

Q *I've recently been diagnosed as having the human papilloma virus. Any suggestions?*

A The human papilloma virus (HPV) causes wart-like growths. The conventional medical treatment is burning or freezing them, then letting the body's immune system take over.

To support yourself nutritionally, either alone or alongside conventional medical treatment, I suggest you dramatically up your intake of vitamin C, as this is the most powerful antiviral agent and will make it very hard for any virus to survive. Over the next three months, I suggest you take 5g a day. The best form is pure ascorbic acid powder, which you can mix into a large bottle of juice mixed with water and drink throughout the day. If you get loose bowels, reduce the dose to a level where this doesn't occur. At the end of the three months, reduce the dose down to 3g a day, then 2 grams a day after a further three months. It is best to do this alongside a basic multivitamin and antioxidant complex supplement.

There are other ways of boosting your immune system, too – that is, eating a wholefood, nutrient-rich diet, drinking lots of water and limiting refined or processed foods and alcohol. Concentrate on fresh, organic vegetables, fruits such as watermelon, berries and kiwi, and be sure to include seeds, lentils, beans and fish. Avoid frying, which introduces free radicals, and steam your vegetables or eat a proportion of them raw. Salads, fresh diluted juices and lightly cooked soups are the way to go.

Injuries and accidents

Q *I was injured in a car accident. What can I do to help the healing process?*

A The most important nutrient immediately after an accident is an amino acid called glutamine. Glutamine helps the body to heal any injury and is now used by some surgeons after operations. You need 5g a day, best taken as a powder dissolved in water, away from food. Glutamine powder is much cheaper than capsules (see Resources, page 483).

Also important are zinc and vitamins A and E. A good multivitamin should provide 10mg, 1,500mcg and 100mg (150iu) respectively of these vital healing nutrients. I'd recommend eating seeds every day, which are rich in zinc and vitamin E. Provided you don't have an open wound, rubbing the content of a vitamin E capsule directly into the skin around a cut can help reduce scarring. Also eat plenty of fruit and vegetables and supplement 1g of vitamin C. This will help the body make collagen, which is essential in the repair of both cuts and bruises.

Q *I have just fractured my humerus and the bicep muscle keeps going into spasm. Can you recommend any supplements that will help?*

A Take 500mg of calcium and 300mg of magnesium to ease the muscle spasms. To get your humerus back to normal, you'll need to take bone-building nutrients. The key vitamins and minerals here are calcium, magnesium, boron and vitamins B, C, D and K. As you rarely get adequate quantities of these from a good multivitamin and mineral formula, you may want to supplement a bone-friendly mineral formula on top of your daily multi (see Resources, page 483). The naturally occurring plant chemicals isoflavones, found in soya beans and soya products such as tofu, also enhance bone-building after a fracture. Ipriflavone, a derivative of isoflavones, has been extensively tested and proven to increase bone density when given along with calcium and/or vitamin D. This too is available in supplements.

Q *What are the best nutrients to supplement if you're suffering from shock?*

A Shock, which can set in after accidents or assaults, causes a considerable release of adrenalin. Make sure you have the time and place to relax and ensure an intake of 3g of vitamin C, two B complex tablets and 300mg of magnesium over the following day. To really help you calm down, take a herbal supplement containing hops and passion flower. Valerian is also relaxing, but more soporific; it may be useful if you need a good night's sleep. The best herb of all for shock is kava kava. While no longer available in the UK, you can still buy it in the US.

Q *I'm a semi-professional tennis player and can't play any more because of tennis elbow. Can you help?*

A Tennis elbow, technically called epicondylitis, is caused by inflammation and possibly slight tearing to the tendons that connect to the elbow. It is slow to heal, but you can help this along considerably by taking the strain off the joint. I strongly recommend you get an EpiSport Arm Band (£17.51 by mail on 01457 860444) for the job.

There are several things you can do to reduce the inflammation. Apply an ice pack for 10 minutes once or twice a day. Rub in MSM (organic sulphur) cream, and take anti-inflammatory herbs such as boswellia and capsaicin. (See Resources, page 483.) Osteopaths can also help by reducing muscular tension and using heat treatments to de-stress the muscles and tendons.

Insect bites

Q *What's the best way to calm down an insect bite?*

A Insect bites cause a histamine reaction that isolates the poison, resulting in an itchy lump. Applying MSM (organic sulphur) cream or aloe vera gel as soon as possible cools the sting and helps reduce itchiness. Vitamin C is an antihistamine, so take 1g an hour for the first three hours after you were bitten.

And to help promote healing, cut open a vitamin E capsule and put the oil on the bite.

Irritable bowel syndrome

Q *What causes irritable bowel syndrome (IBS)?*

A Bloating, abdominal pain, flatulence, diarrhoea, cramps, depression, anxiety and constipation – these are some of the more common, and unpleasant, symptoms of IBS. In this disorder, the sufferer's bowel nerves and muscles are highly sensitive; their muscles may cramp up when they have a meal. It's thought that most cases are caused by food allergies, but it is not always easy to pinpoint the culprit.

To test this theory, researchers from the University of York tested 300 IBS suffers for allergies using a highly advanced blood test called IgG ELISA testing. They then gave the patients' doctors either real or faked results. The patients then avoided the alleged allergy-provoking food indicated in the test results for three months. At the end of three months, only those people on the real allergy-free diet showed a marked improvement in symptoms.

Wheat gluten is behind many cases of IBS. Gluten can also be found in rye, barley and oats, but oats are free of gliadin, a substance in gluten that is particularly allergenic. So if you've developed IBS, the first step is to avoid all gluten grains. If after 10 days, say, your condition improves, reintroduce oats and see what happens. If all is well you can keep on eating oats, a useful source of soluble fibre, vitamins and minerals and slow-release energy. But it is important to get yourself tested. We are all different, and you may be reacting to foods you've never suspected. (See Resources, page 483.)

Q *What's a good diet for IBS? Should I avoid starch?*

A Starch isn't the baddie here. In fact, the soluble fibres found in some starchy food are very helpful in alleviating the symptoms of IBS. Seeds, fruits and raw or lightly cooked vegetables can help provide the right kind of fibre too, and if you suffer from frequent diarrhoea, the pectin in apples and bananas can help. Brown rice is generally regarded as the best grain for IBS sufferers. It is the least allergenic choice – vital, as the key factors contributing to IBS are stress and food intolerances (see 'What causes irritable bowel syndrome (IBS)?', page 232). You can test for these either at home, with a 10-day elimination diet, or by sending blood samples off for testing.

Otherwise, eat plenty of fresh vegetables, simply cooked; drink 1 to 1.5 litres of pure water a day; and avoid sulphur-rich foods such as eggs and onions (they contribute to flatulence), sugar, wheat, refined foods, spicy foods, dairy products, alcohol and stimulants. Helpful supplements include a vitamin B complex, magnesium, alfalfa and peppermint oil – choose the enterically coated kind that isn't absorbed in the stomach.

> **DIG DEEPER:** For more advice, see my book *Improve Your Digestion* (Piatkus, 1999).

Kidney stones

Q *I've had kidney stones twice. What can I do to prevent it happening again?*

A Kidney stones are abnormal accumulations of mineral salts found in the kidneys, bladder or anywhere along the urinary tract, and can be anything from sand grain to fingertip sized. There are various kinds, but 80 per cent of kidney stones are calcium oxalate stones, which form when excessive calcium in too-alkaline urine crystallises.

By far the most important thing to do to prevent kidney stones is to drink plenty of filtered or bottled water – 2 litres a day – to flush the kidneys and urinary tract regularly. A lack of certain nutrients can also contribute, especially magnesium, vitamin B6, vitamin D and potassium, all of which are involved in calcium metabolism. So you should include green leafy vegetables, wholegrains, bananas, nuts and seeds in your diet on a regular basis. Vitamin A, abundant in carrots, red peppers, sweet potatoes and green leafy vegetables, also benefits the urinary tract and helps inhibit the formation of stones. Avoid antacids and minimise your consumption of animal protein, as it can cause the body to excrete calcium and uric acid, which can in turn contribute to the formation of the two most common forms of kidney stones.

ME

Q *I have ME. What is the best way to keep as fit as possible? I am also going through the menopause.*

A Chronic fatigue seems to be a sign of our times: some 30 per cent of visits to the doctor are from people complaining of it. But ME, now known as chronic fatigue syndrome (CFS), is much rarer, probably affecting fewer than 1 per cent of patients. It's characterised not just by severe, prolonged fatigue, but also by symptoms such as recurrent sore throat, painful lymph nodes, muscle weakness and pain, headaches and joint pain. Its cause remains a mystery, although a weakened immune system and problems with detoxifying the body have been suggested. When coupled with the menopause, the syndrome can be a huge drain on the body and mind.

First, you need to tackle the CFS to get your energy levels back again. This will involve a detox aimed at cleansing the liver. For the first week, cut out meat, dairy products, wheat and other gluten grains, tea, coffee and alcohol. Eat lots of fresh fruit and vegetables, particularly broccoli, Brussels sprouts, cabbage, kale and cauliflower for their liver-supporting glucosinolates; carrots, tomatoes, sweet potatoes and other orange-coloured foods, and spinach and watercress, for their beta-carotene; and fresh apricots, berries, melons, mango and papaya. Eat wholefoods such as brown rice and beans, high-quality protein such as oily fish and free-range chicken, and add in a large handful of raw, unsalted nuts and seeds a day, whole or ground in a fruit salad. Drink plenty of water, 1.5 litres a day.

Also supplement a good high-strength multivitamin and an antioxidant supplement (see Resources, page 483). Vitamins B2, B3, B6, B12, folic acid, glutathione, amino acids such as glutamine, and flavonoids, phospholipids, and antioxidants such as vitamins E and C are all important. Milk thistle, 100mg twice a day, helps with the detoxification process.

To answer your question about exercise, have you thought about yoga? Yoga can harmonise breath, movement and posture to remove physical blocks and tension in the body, and while gentle, can leave you feeling energised.

Motion sickness

 I suffer from motion sickness. Is there anything that can help?

A With travel sickness the best strategy is prevention, so make your anti-motion-sickness regime part of all your travel plans. One hour before you travel, take five charcoal tablets to help settle and cleanse your guts. Also take enough ginger capsules to give you the equivalent of 1,000mg before you go, and continue to take this amount every three hours. You could take fresh ginger tea in a flask – grate the fresh root and pour on boiling water. Dabbing a drop of peppermint oil on your tongue every now and then can also help stave off nausea.

It's also important to avoid spicy, fatty and junk foods before and during your journey, as they don't do your digestion any favours. The same goes for alcohol, which disrupts the balance mechanisms that are affected by motion. You may find that limiting any visual stimulation such as ocean waves or the views from a car window helps. That's why closing your eyes or lying down can stop you from feeling sick.

Muscular problems

Q *I keep getting muscle cramps after exercise. Are there any natural remedies?*

A First make sure you are warming up and cooling down properly before and after you exercise. Otherwise, you can help reduce cramping by addressing your body's mineral balance. Cramps are popularly believed to be the result of a salt deficiency, but this is actually very rare. The spasms are actually caused by the inability of muscles to relax, and this is likely to be due to low magnesium and potassium – which work with the sodium in salt and another mineral, calcium, to control muscle contraction and relaxation. You need to eat a diet rich in foods that have a lot of magnesium, such as green vegetables, nuts and seeds. Most fruits and vegetables are rich in potassium (bananas are a great source), so have at least five portions of fruit and vegetables a day. To absolutely ensure you're getting enough magnesium, you may want to try taking a supplement – 300mg twice a day.

Q *I've been getting muscle pains in my shoulders and neck and a lot of muscle cramps. Painkillers don't help.*

A You may well have a condition called fibromyalgia. This chronic condition is characterised by many symptoms, including widespread muscle pain, constant aches, general stiffness, fatigue, sleep disturbances and depression. The muscle pain in fibromyalgia is apparently due to reductions in energy production and in the ability of muscles to relax. Fibromylagia is not an inflammatory disease so anti-inflammatory painkillers don't help. So, if you've been prescribed cortisone, such as Prednisolene, or had a cortisone injection that didn't work, it is even more likely that you have fibromylagia.

Magnesium, stress reduction and breathing exercises will all help. For detailed suggestions on diet, supplements and exercise, see 'What do you recommend for fibromyalgia?', page 198.

Q *I get muscle spasms when sitting down for a while. What can I do to stop this?*

A Muscle spasms and cramping can be linked to nutritional deficiencies, particularly the important mineral magnesium. You could increase your intake of magnesium-rich foods such as nuts, seeds, beans and green vegetables, or take 200mg of magnesium twice a day. However, I would also take steps to have a more structural check-up. Visit an osteopath, who can discover whether you are trapping any nerves, cutting off circulation or somehow interfering with the muscles involved.

You may find it useful to get up regularly during the day to have a good stretch and walk around. Also look into the way you are sitting, and your chair itself, to make sure you are maintaining good posture. An ergonomic chair, designed to align the body properly, could be a good investment if yours is broken down or poorly designed. If you habitually breathe shallowly, this can also make your muscles go into spasm because they are not getting enough oxygen. So do daily breathing exercises such as taking 10 deep breaths, holding them in and slowly exhaling.

Nervous system conditions

Q *Can nutrition help with motor neurone disease?*

A In motor neurone disease, motor cells in the brain and spinal cord progressively degenerate, hindering the sufferer's ability to move, breathe, speak and swallow. There may be paralysis and muscle weakness. It is a serious condition, but it can almost certainly be helped by nutritional support.

Start with a hair mineral analysis to check for heavy metal toxicity – especially mercury – as this can destroy the myelin sheath around nerves that helps in the transmission of nerve impulses. It's important to rule out this possibility, or detoxify if any are found to be present. (See Resources, page 483.)

Otherwise, you'll need to follow a diet that supports your nerves. Antioxidants disarm damaging free radicals in the body and may help, as they do with most degenerative diseases, so supplement an all-round antioxidant complex including A, C, E, beta-carotene, glutathione and anthocyanidins. Cut down on saturated, animal, fried and hydrogenated fats, and boost your intake of essential fats from seeds and their oils, and oily fish. These last are essential for brain and nerve health. They help rebuild the myelin sheath, which is composed largely of the same fatty acids, and so protect the nerves and boost brain cell communication. Another nutrient that sometimes produces excellent results is niacin (vitamin B3). However, you need 500mg twice a day and, at this amount, you'll experience considerable blushing for 30 minutes afterwards. There are other important nutritional considerations, too; it is best to see a nutritional therapist to have a full health evaluation, for specific dietary and nutritional recommendations.

Q *A friend is suffering from multiple sclerosis. Can optimum nutrition help?*

A Multiple sclerosis is a condition affecting the central nervous system – the brain, spinal cord and optic nerves. In MS, the fatty tissue surrounding nerve fibres, known as the myelin sheath, is lost in many places, causing symptoms that range from extreme fatigue to difficulties with walking or vision. While MS is thought to be an autoimmune disease, its cause is still unknown. People with the condition, particularly in the early stages, often respond well to nutritional support.

Start with a look at your friend's diet and lifestyle. As a high intake of animal fats is linked to MS, they should cut out cheese, milk and meat and eat plenty of fish, nuts and seeds that are rich in omega-3 fatty acids. Omega-3 fats have been found to be vital in the formation of myelin. I recommend you supplement a combination of the essential fats GLA, DHA and EPA. Myelin has been found to be very susceptible to oxidation, so avoid smoking, smoky atmospheres and fried or burnt food, and take a good antioxidant complex.

Mercury toxicity may also contribute to the condition, either through mercury fillings, vaccinations, heavy pollution or a lack of other minerals in the body to counteract mercury accumulation. B vitamins (in particular B12) are key. So in addition to eating and supplementing with omega-3s, the ideal nutritional support strategy would be a wholefood, low-toxin diet supported by a high-strength multivitamin and mineral formula and a B complex. A hair mineral analysis would give an indication of any toxicity in the body. Some think MS may be linked to food allergies, particularly to gluten (in wheat, oats, rye and barley) and milk. It's worth cutting these out to see if it helps and getting yourself tested for allergies. There's also a link between high homocysteine and MS so this is worth testing too. (See Resources, page 483.) Finally, research has shown digestive enzymes may help.

Nosebleeds

Q *Is there anything you can recommend to stop me from getting nosebleeds?*

A Nosebleeds are usually a sign of weak blood capillaries (the small blood vessels) in the lining of the nose. This could just be due to temporary pressure, say from blowing your nose a lot because of a cold; or it could be a sign that the capillaries throughout your body are not as strong as they should be.

To strengthen fragile capillaries, make sure you are getting plenty of bioflavonoids. These remarkable nutrients are found most abundantly in citrus fruits, berries, broccoli, cherries, red grapes, rosehips, papaya and tomatoes as well as tea and red wine. Bioflavonoids work best with vitamin C and are usually found in a blend, so go for a good complex. See (Resources, page 483.)

Oral and dental problems

Q *What can I do for a tooth abscess?*

A Increase vitamin C intake to 1g up to five times a day, and take 2,500mcg of vitamin A or 6mg beta-carotene four times day. Also take 15mg of zinc twice a day for no more than two weeks, plus 200mcg of selenium. This will help strengthen your immune system. Vitamin B6 at 100mg twice a day helps to localise the infection and acts as a mild analgesic. And if you're on antibiotics, take a B complex and a probiotic supplement for the duration of the course. (See Resources, page 483, for supplement suppliers.)

Q *I'm prone to cold sores. Are there any natural remedies that work?*

A Cold sores are caused by the herpes virus, which feeds off an amino acid called arginine. If you supplement lysine, an amino acid that looks like arginine, you fool the virus and effectively starve it. I recommend supplementing 1,000mg of lysine every day, away from food, to keep the virus at bay. When you have an active infection, supplement 3,000mg of lysine a day and cut right back on foods rich in arginine, which include beans, lentils, nuts and chocolate. The more stressed you are, the weaker your immune system becomes, and this allows the virus to become active – which is why many people succumb to cold sores when they're run down. A powerful immune-boosting combination is 3g of vitamin C every day; take it with your lysine.

Some people are now getting great results staving off cold sores with a special form of sulphur, MSM. This is an anti-viral and appears to strip away the protective coating of a virus. You can get MSM in supplement and cream form. Start by taking 3g a day, and work up until you find the dose that keeps your cold sores away; for some people this is 10g.

Q *My gums bleed a lot. Can diet help?*

A Bleeding gums can be caused by many factors, but the classic reason is a deficiency in vitamin C, the extreme version of which is scurvy. Start by eating a healthy diet of fresh, unprocessed foods, minimising things that deplete your body of nutrients (such as smoking, sugar and alcohol) and taking 1g of vitamin C three times a day. Vitamin C works best in conjunction with substances called bioflavonoids, which are abundant in berry extracts and particularly important in strengthening capillaries, or small blood vessels. So look for a C/bioflavonoid blend. Some dentists also suggest 30mg of the naturally occurring compound CoQ10 to improve oxygen and nutrient supply to the gums. I also recommend a daily mouthwash to minimise any risk of infection. Make it up by diluting a few drops of tea tree oil (available from healthfood shops and chemists) in a glass of water and gargling with this.

Q *Why do I get mouth ulcers when I'm stressed?*

A There are several factors that can trigger mouth ulcers, including nutrient deficiencies and food sensitivities. The link with stress appears to be that stress increases your need for vitamin C, and a deficiency in vitamin C is a factor in ulcers. When you are stressed, vitamin C is needed in higher quantities by the adrenal glands, which provide the body's main stress response. So if you are under a lot of pressure, the adrenals are likely to be getting the lion's share of your vitamin C supplies, leaving other areas low.

Obviously, the first thing to do is tackle the way you deal with stress so it's not so much of a burden. When you are under pressure, take 1g of vitamin C three times a day. It's best to take a less acidic form such as magnesium ascorbate, rather than ascorbic acid. You may also need more vitamin A, which strengthens the 'inside skin'. Try supplementing 250mcg (7,500iu) of vitamin A a day, as well as 15mg of zinc, which helps ulcers to heal.

Food allergies, to wheat in particular, can also trigger mouth ulcers; eating foods you're sensitive to only every fourth day can help keep the allergic reaction at bay. Also, check your toothbrush. Splayed-out bristles, especially if you brush too hard, often cause the initial damage that leads to a mouth ulcer.

Osteoporosis and other bone conditions

Q *What's the best way to avoid getting osteoporosis? I'm only 30, but I'd like to start now.*

A With osteoporosis, the bones get thinner due to loss of calcium; but the cause of this disease is much more complex than simply not getting enough of this mineral. There are many diet and lifestyle factors that adversely affect the body's calcium balance, including prolonged stress, blood sugar problems, too much protein, excess stimulants (such as tea, coffee, alcohol or chocolate), or a lack of exercise, sunlight or key bone-building vitamins and minerals including magnesium, boron, zinc and silica and vitamins B, C, D and K. For these reasons a good diet, plus all-round multivitamin and mineral supplementation, is far more protective than just supplementing calcium.

The best foods for all the bone-building minerals are seeds. If you eat a daily heaped tablespoon of pumpkin, sesame, sunflower or flax seeds, perhaps ground on cereal or nibbled as a snack throughout the day, you'll get all the minerals you need. Peppers, cabbage, broccoli, tomatoes, strawberries and oranges are rich in vitamin C, while boron can be found in most fruit and vegetables, including peaches, lettuce, cabbage, peas and leafy vegetables. Vitamin D is abundant in eggs and fish.

Eating too much animal protein, such as meat two or three times a day, can be bad for bones. The reason is that excess protein makes the bloodstream more acidic, which in turn causes the body to release calcium from bone to reduce the acidity. So excessive amounts of milk and cheese, both high in protein and calcium but low in magnesium, are not necessarily the best bone food.

Soya products such as tofu or soya milk, on the other hand, are very beneficial for the bones. They contain phytoestrogens called isoflavones, which enhance bone-building and prevent the breakdown of bone. Ipriflavone, a derivative of these naturally occurring isoflavones, has been extensively tested and proven to increase bone density when given along with calcium and/or vitamin D and is now available in supplements. Later, when you reach the menopause, you might like to think about natural progesterone (see 'I'm a 53-year-old woman diagnosed with osteoporosis', below).

Exercise is another excellent preventative against osteoporosis. Because the action of muscles pulling on bone builds bone, weight-bearing exercise can really help. Brisk walking, running, climbing stairs and yoga are all good for keeping your bones strong.

Q *I'm a 53-year-old woman diagnosed with osteoporosis. My doctor wants to put me on HRT. What would you recommend?*

A Given that HRT increases your risk of breast cancer and that its bone-protecting benefits disappear as soon as you stop taking it, you may wish to opt instead for the safer alternatives offered by natural remedies.

A recent American study showed that menopausal symptoms in 83 per cent of women using natural progesterone creams were significantly better or disappeared. As osteoporosis has been linked to hormonal imbalance, it's likely that natural progesterone will prove more effective than oestrogen HRT in protecting against it.

Other studies have had great results alleviating menopausal symptoms with extracts from soya and red clover, which contain naturally occurring hormone-like substances called isoflavones. Isoflavones, a type of phytoestrogen, or oestrogen-like plant compound, also enhance bone building and prevent the breakdown of bone. Ipriflavone, a derivative of these naturally occurring isoflavones, has been extensively tested and proven to increase bone density when given along with calcium and/or vitamin D. Combine this with a good multivitamin and mineral supplement each day.

If you do decide to pursue the HRT option, you should first have your oestrogen and progesterone levels tested to determine if you really need it. The only effective way to do this is with a saliva test (see Resources, page 483). Far safer and equally, if not more, effective than oestrogen HRT is natural progesterone. It's called natural because it is exactly the same as the body's own progesterone and is given in amounts akin to what the body should produce every day, as a transdermal skin cream. This is available on prescription.

DIG DEEPER: For details on natural progesterone, contact the Natural Progesterone Information Service on 07000 784849, and read my book, *Balancing Hormones Naturally*, coauthored by Kate Neil (Piatkus, 1999).

 I have been diagnosed with osteopenia. I'm on the Pill. How can I reduce my risk of bone fractures?

A Osteopenia simply means that your bone density is less than normal; it can be a precursor to osteoporosis, but there is much that you can do to increase your bone density.

And there is so much more to bone density than calcium. In fact, combining calcium with magnesium, vitamin D, boron and silica is much more effective than taking calcium alone. Dietwise, the best and simplest way to get these vital minerals is to eat a lot of ground pumpkin, sesame, sunflower and flax seeds: try a tablespoon or two on your cereal in the morning, or a handful of raw pumpkin or sunflower seeds as a snack. You would also be wise to supplement a bone-friendly multimineral formula containing the above nutrients. You'll also need to consider your protein consumption. Too much protein may also lead to loss of bone density, so you'll need to look carefully at how much meat and dairy products you're eating, and keep them to a sensible minimum: avoid them two or three times a day when you ordinarily would have eaten them. Tofu and other soya products are a better option for bone strength, although you don't want to overdose on them either; as with many foods, it's possible to develop an allergy to soya if you eat too much of it.

Also, if you are progesterone deficient and hence oestrogen dominant, which can be checked with a saliva hormone test (see Resources, page 483), this definitely leads to loss of bone mass. It is highly likely that being on the Pill is disrupting your hormonal balance. You will need to consult your doctor about your hormonal health.

DIG DEEPER: Contact the Natural Progesterone Information Service on 07000 784849 for a list of natural hormone-friendly doctors. I also strongly recommend that you read the late Dr John Lee's book *What Your Doctor May Not Tell You about the Menopause* (Time Warner, 1996). You'll find a lot of applicable information in this.

Q *I'm a vegan. How can I get enough calcium to prevent osteoporosis?*

A The dairy industry has done a very good job of convincing us that we must consume dairy foods to get enough calcium in our diets, and many people drink milk for just this reason. But it doesn't agree with quite a few of us. Dairy foods are a common allergen, can cause mucus and sinus problems and can exacerbate asthma, hay fever and digestive problems. Some also think it can up your risk of getting osteoporosis by providing too much acidic protein and not enough magnesium and other nutrients needed to get calcium into the bones.

The thing I always ask those who assert we can't get enough calcium without dairy foods is 'Where do cows get their calcium?' The answer, of course, is green leafy vegetables. But you don't have to eat grass – spinach, kale, broccoli, watercress, parsley and green cabbage are great sources of calcium as well as the magnesium needed to use it properly. Seeds and nuts are also rich in both calcium and magnesium. Finally, many products, like tofu, breakfast cereals and soya milk, are now fortified with calcium, so getting enough shouldn't be a problem on a sensible vegan diet.

Pain (see also Fibromyalgia)

Q *My partner had a micro-decompression operation on his back earlier this year. Despite regular physiotherapy, he still has a lot of pain with minimal movement. Any suggestions?*

A By following a simple, healthy diet with absolutely no additives or processed foods, he may be able to reduce the nerve inflammation and kickstart his recovery. Start by removing all sugars, milk and dairy foods, farmed meat, refined foods like white pasta and white rice, and gluten grains, especially wheat (although you may be able to introduce oats, barley and rye once the pain has subsided, but note his responses to these).

Get him to focus on eating oily fish like sardines, mackerel, wild salmon, herring and trout, organic lean chicken and game, nuts, seeds (especially flax seeds or linseed, which should be ground to aid digestion), brown rice, quinoa, millet, lots of organic fruit and vegetables of all sorts, and organic eggs. He must not smoke or drink alcohol, tea or coffee, as these rob valuable minerals from the bone and make the body acidic. He should drink up to 2 litres of filtered or bottled water a day to cleanse the cells and assist repair.

Good and bad prostaglandins (hormone-like substances) that govern pain responses are produced from the breakdown of fats from digestion. The essential fatty acids he'll be getting from flax seeds and oily fish are a step towards producing more of these good anti-inflammatory prostaglandins, but supplementing alongside is even better. I recommend supplementing the essential omega-3 and 6 fatty acids – GLA, EPA and DHA – together with a good quality multivitamin and mineral.

Your partner should keep up the changes in his diet for as long as possible, although it may take some weeks to become pain-free.

Q *The soles of my feet are excruciatingly painful to walk on first thing in the morning. What is this?*

A Very tender and burning feet or heels are a sign of a deficiency in vitamin B5, or pantothenic acid. Other signs of deficiency in this vitamin can include anxiety, teeth grinding, muscle tremors, exhaustion and sleep problems. You could certainly try supplementing 500mg of pantothenic acid to check the burning in your feet. B5 is also found in brewer's yeast, peas, beans, organ meat, chicken, fish and wholegrains.

If this doesn't help, it is possible you have a circulation problem. See your doctor to rule out that possibility.

Q *Which painkiller is worse for you – aspirin or paracetamol – and is there a healthy alternative?*

A The bottom line is that neither is great for you, especially over a long time. Aspirin is harsh on your stomach and digestive tract because it irritates and causes bleeding. The longest recorded intestinal bleeding from one aspirin was three days! Frequent use of aspirin causes gastrointestinal problems, ulceration and occasional death.

Paracetamol puts a strain on the liver. It is detoxified using the same pathway in the body as alcohol, and combining the two is particularly lethal. Most liver transplants and cases of liver failure are the result of people taking both. You can reduce the toxic effects of paracetamol by taking glutathione, which helps detoxify it in the liver. Either take a good antioxidant complex, which should include it, or eat onions and garlic, which contain cysteine from which glutathione is made in the body.

Ultimately, however, you need to ask yourself why you're using either of them. It is always best to tackle the cause of the pain, rather than numbing it constantly. So if, for example, you have tender joints, you can reduce the inflammation with anti-inflammatories such as omega-3 fish oils or a blend of the herbs boswellia and curcumin.

And if you get headaches regularly, you should look into the possible causes: are you drinking enough water, stressed and living off stimulants, or sensitive to something you're eating? For ways of treating headaches naturally, see 'I keep getting headaches', page 205.

Q *I have terrible pain in my wrists from repetitive strain injury (RSI). Is there anything I can do nutritionally for it?*

A RSI is a complex condition that occurs, as the name suggests, from overworking the wrist and fingers, although there are usually underlying weaknesses that enable it to develop in the first place. With so many of us using computer keyboards for hours every day, RSI is a real risk.

Nutrition can definitely help reduce the typical symptoms of pain, tingling and stiffness. First, as the nerves and tissues are often internally inflamed, limit the inflammation-promoting foods in your diet. The real baddies are red meat and dairy products. Some people also find that cutting out vegetables from the 'nightshade' family – potatoes, tomatoes, aubergines and peppers – really helps. Next, boost your intake of anti-inflammatories containing omega-3 fats, such as oily fish (sardines, organic or wild salmon, mackerel or herring) and seeds. Seeds are a delicious and nutritious addition to your diet – either snack on whole seeds or, to really ensure you release the essential oils, grind a mixture (ideally, half flax and half pumpkin, sunflower and sesame) in a coffee grinder and sprinkle a tablespoon fresh on cereals, soups or salads each day.

Antioxidants also help to reduce inflammation and

you can increase your intake by eating a multicoloured array of fruits and vegetables – carrots, beetroot, avocado, green leafy vegetables, berries, kiwi fruits, apricots, sweet potatoes, plums and so on. Have as many as you can, but no less than five portions a day. And take a good antioxidant supplement twice a day. (See Resources, page 483.) Also supplement B vitamins, as these are essential for healthy nerve responses. Choose a supplement that provides at least 25mg of B1, B2, B3, B5 and B6, 10mg of B12 and 100mg of folic acid.

When you're sitting at the computer, ensure that your posture when typing is good and that your forearms are supported on a table of the right height for your chair. An ergonomic chair can be a good idea. Make sure, too, that you take frequent breaks from this and other repetitive tasks, relaxing and stretching your arms and shoulders. Reducing your stress levels is important, say through yoga or complimentary therapies such as osteopathy, acupuncture and the Alexander Technique.

Finally, try some homegrown hydrotherapy. Every evening before bed, fill two large bowls or sinks side by side – one with water as hot as you can stand; the other with ice-cold water (add ice cubes to make it really cold). Immerse your lower arms up to the elbows in the hot water and keep them there for 30 seconds; do the same in the cold water for 30 seconds. Repeat this alternative immersion 16 times in total – 8 times in the hot and 8 in the cold, making sure you finish with cold. This exercise will help to drain the lymph fluid and boost circulation in your arms and fingers.

Parkinson's disease

Q Can nutrition help Parkinson's?

A Although Parkinson's needs close medical supervision, sufferers can benefit enormously from nutritional therapy. Research has shown they are often deficient in certain nutrients, so supplements can be helpful. Digestive difficulties are also common, so identifying food sensitivities, taking enzymes and healing the gut lining are important. Many people with Parkinson's also suffer from chronic constipation, which can be alleviated by drinking 1.5 litres of water daily, taking aloe vera juice, eating foods such as prunes, cabbage and celery, and exercising (with the help of a physiotherapist).

The known cause of Parkinson's is a difficulty with converting amino acids into dopamine, adrenalin and noradrenalin. So a nutritional approach demands a very specific type of diet that controls the amounts of the amino acids tyrosine and phenylalanine in the diet, and ensures an optimal intake of vitamin B6 and zinc, among other nutrients, that help to convert them into dopamine, adrenalin and noradrenalin. Many people with Parkinson's also have high levels of the amino acid homocysteine, which indicates an inability to balance the brain's chemistry and which can be substantially helped by taking vitamins B12, B6 and folic acid. Keeping all these nutrients in balance is quite complicated, however, and for this reason I strongly recommend you see a nutritional therapist who has experience in treating people with Parkinson's. (See Resources, page 483.)

DIG DEEPER: See my book *Optimum Nutrition for the Mind* (Piatkus, 2003) for more on Parkinson's. An excellent book on the role of nutrition in this condition is *The Parkinson's Disease Workbook – Optimising Function and Wellbeing* by the nutritionist Lucille Leader and her husband Dr Geoffrey Leader.

Raynaud's disease

Q *Do you have any nutritional recommendations for Raynaud's disease?*

A Raynaud's disease is a circulation problem made worse by stress. Capillaries in the fingers, toes, hands and feet contract and deprive the area of blood, causing painful chilblains and itching, and in extreme cases, ulcers.

There's plenty you can do to help control Raynaud's. Start by keeping your extremities warm, avoiding fatty and fried foods, caffeine and cigarettes, and reducing your stress levels. Gingko biloba can be very effective in counteracting Raynaud's. Recent research at the University of Dundee showed that people with Raynaud's taking ginkgo had half as many attacks during which their extremities went white. Ginkgo is usually taken in capsule form and you should look for a brand with a flavonoid concentration of 24 per cent: two to three doses of 120mg a day. Often it takes a month or two before you begin to see results. Note that ginkgo is a blood-thinning agent so you must use caution if you're taking other blood thinners such as coumadin, heparin or even aspirin. Side-effects of headaches, nausea or nosebleeds have been reported, but only rarely and at high doses.

Vitamin E (start with 100mg/200iu daily and build to 400mg/600iu daily) also improves circulation, and taking 100mg of a B complex daily, plus an extra 100mg of niacin (B3), can boost circulation too; be aware that niacin often triggers harmless blushing, which lasts about half an hour. Try this for a month. Also useful are 100 to 200mg of Coenzyme-Q10 a day, as this improves tissue oxygenation.

Moderate exercise is key for promoting circulation. If you're low in magnesium, however, your muscles won't be working optimally, and that will affect your capillaries, which explains why excessive exercise can worsen Raynaud's. So it's a good idea to take 450mg of magnesium a day. Lastly, I'd check yourself out for allergies. One woman cured her Raynaud's by giving up gluten grains such as wheat. (See information on tests in Resources, page 483.)

Restless legs

Q *What do you recommend for restless legs?*

A Restless legs are a common stress-related sleep problem; the affected person will jerk their legs about while asleep. They can also feel an urge to move their legs while sitting or resting. The condition is thought to be linked either to drinking coffee at night or to a deficiency in certain minerals important for muscle relaxation.

The B vitamins are important for stress-related nerve function, and iron has been suggested as important in this condition. Calcium, magnesium, potassium and zinc can all help. I'd recommend taking a high-strength multivitamin in the morning and a multimineral giving at least 250mg of magnesium in the evening. Meanwhile, avoid stimulants and alcohol in the evening. Regular exercise can also really help – try taking a walk after dinner. It's advisable to see a nutritional therapist, who can run a hair mineral analysis to pinpoint which minerals are low or imbalanced.

Rheumatic disorders

Q *My mother suffers from polymyalgia rheumatica and whenever she reduces her steroid treatment, it gets worse. Can you help?*

A Polymyalgia rheumatica mainly affects older adults. It's an inflammatory disorder that causes muscular aches and stiffness, especially in the neck, shoulders and hips. The condition is often brought on when the body's detoxification systems are overloaded, and the liver, kidneys, brain and all the cells, including muscle cells, fail to deal with the toxic by-products of digestion and daily living. Different systems of the body can be affected: in your mother's case, it's her joints and immune system.

She can boost her detox ability by taking a good antioxidant supplement and 1g of vitamin C twice a day, drinking more water and eating healthy, unprocessed (and preferably organic) foods with the emphasis on fresh fruit, vegetables, organic chicken and, for those valuable anti-inflammatories, oily fish, nuts and seeds. She may also benefit from taking a digestive enzyme to improve digestion. Folic acid, as part of a B complex supplement, can help too. This is probably because some sufferers have high levels of the amino acid homocysteine in their blood, which is associated with pain. I recommend testing your mother and if her level is high then giving her a supplement of nutrients designed to help maintain healthy homocysteine levels. This will contain folic acid. (See Resources, page 483.)

Shingles

Q *What nutritional supplements do you recommend for shingles?*

A Shingles – an unpleasant illness characterised by tingling or pain followed by small blisters on the body or face – is caused by the chickenpox virus varicella-zoster, itself a variant of the herpes virus. It usually affects older people; in young adults it may mean a weakened immune system.

To treat shingles, supplement 3g of the amino acid

lysine away from food and 3g of vitamin C; also take two 2,500mcg vitamin A (retinol) supplements two times a day. This is slightly higher than what's recommended in pregnancy so, if there's any chance of your being or getting pregnant, do this for one month only. While you have the infection, it's a good idea to limit foods rich in arginine, the amino acid that feeds the virus. These include beans, lentils, nuts and chocolate.

Side effects of drugs

Q *Antibiotics give me an upset stomach. Is there anything I can do to stop this?*

A Antibiotics have a kind of 'throw the baby out with the bathwater' effect, stripping out the healthy bacteria in your gut along with the baddies. This can lead to stomach and other digestive upsets. Taking a probiotic supplement will help to repopulate your gut with healthy bacteria, the two most prevalent strains of which are *Lactobacillus acidophilus* and *Bifidobacterium bifidum*. Some fermented products, such as the cultured milk drink *kefir*, contain these bacteria, but a more direct way to boost levels is to take a supplement. (See Resources, page 483.)

It's best to take probiotics on an empty stomach – one tablet first thing in the morning and again before you go to bed. Start when you begin the antibiotics and continue for one week after you finish the course. Don't take probiotics and antibiotics at the same time of day. If it's a one-day antibiotic, for instance, and you take it at night, then take the probiotic in the morning.

Q *I'm having my wisdom teeth out. Can you recommend something that will help me deal with the effects of the general anaesthetic?*

A Vitamin C helps detoxify the body from the effects of anaesthetic, either local or general. Take 5g spread over the day, for two days after, then 3g a day for a week. This vitamin also helps the body to heal and has been shown to speed recovery from surgery, as does the amino acid glutamine: take 5g a day on an empty stomach until your mouth is healed. An additional 3,300mcg (10,000iu) of vitamin A (retinol) per day is also helpful, as is zinc. You should get enough of both by taking a high strength multivitamin twice a day on an ongoing basis.

Right before surgery, you can keep taking your supplements, except for omega-3s, vitamin E and - garlic, as these can thin the blood and cause clotting problems. I would also avoid taking very large amounts (above 2g) of vitamin C, since this might make the anaesthetic a little less effective. As for eating well after surgery, there are plenty of no-chew options. Try smoothies made with fruit, ground nuts and seeds and yoghurt, or Get Up & Go! whizzed up in the blender with dairy or soya milk and fruit. Soups blended with silken tofu are good too. (See Resources for where to buy Get Up & Go!, page 483.)

Skin, hair and nails

Skin

Q *What's the solution for acne? I'm an otherwise healthy adult.*

A Given that your skin is a major organ of elimination and good barometer of your internal health, I would start by looking at your internal detoxification capacity and elimination processes – that is, your liver and your gut. I usually find a remarkable improvement in people's skin from cleansing these.

Diet-wise, avoid alcohol, coffee, tea, fried foods, excess animal fats and sugar. Increase your intake of water, fruit, vegetables, wholegrains and proteins from fish, chicken, soya and lean meat. Keep your digestive tract moving with a good intake of fibre from wholegrains, vegetables, beans and lentils. If you get constipated, soak a dessertspoon of organic golden flax seeds overnight in a glass of water and drink the mixture. I recommend a good colon and liver cleansing programme involving herbs and fibres (see Resources, page 483). Supplementing 20mg of zinc and up to 5,000mcg of vitamin A can help, although you need to limit your vitamin A intake to 3,000mcg (or 10,000iu) if you're pregnant.

Q *Do you recommend the Pill for hormone-related acne?*

A While the Pill can help in the short term, it clearly doesn't address the underlying problems causing acne. I would encourage you to look for those, rather than just masking the problem, especially given the health concerns regarding long-term Pill use. Even with today's lower-dose Pills, women taking them have a higher chance of getting a blood clot, and may also experience nausea.

Hormonal changes, usually in teenagers, generate more oily secretions that block up skin pores. These then become infected. A diet high in saturated fat and fried food will have a similar effect. Vitamin A and zinc deficiency leads to a lowered ability to fight infection. So it's sensible to eat a healthy diet of wholefoods; avoid fatty meats, too much cheese and fried foods; and have plenty of fruit and vegetables, as well as 1.5 litres of pure water a day.

Supplementing 20mg of zinc and up to 5,000mcg of vitamin A can help, but limit the A to 3,000mcg if you're pregnant.

Q *I'm a woman with acne on the jaw and neck (the 'beard' area). What causes this and what should I do?*

A This can be caused by low oestrogen. High oestrogen affects your sebaceous glands by making them smaller and reducing sebum production, making your skin less oily. Low oestrogen has the opposite effect, making your skin oilier and more susceptible to blockage and infection of the pores. Low levels of oestrogen leave the very small amount of testosterone in women unopposed, so it is able to exert its effects, which may include aggressive behaviour, facial hair and even spots in the 'beard' region – testosterone controls beard growth in men.

Oestrogen also increases the rate at which the cells of the epidermis divide and reproduce, so as it declines, the reproduction of new cells does too, and this ends up thinning the skin. Oestrogen also stimulates the production of substances (such as hyaluronic acid), which keep the skin well hydrated, supple and smooth, so low levels can make the skin become dull-looking.

Natural progesterone cream may help, as your body can make oestrogen out of it. Ask your doctor to prescribe it, or contact the Natural Progesterone Information Service (see below). Excess sebum production can also result from a vitamin B6 deficiency, so you may benefit from taking B6 in addition to a high-strength multi, up to 100mg. In the meantime, it would be a good idea to get your hormone levels checked by either your doctor or a nutritional therapist.

DIG DEEPER: For details on natural progesterone, contact the Natural Progesterone Information Service on 07000 784849.

Q *I suffer from acne but am 30! What can I do about it?*

A Sadly, adult onset acne is becoming more common. There are many potential causes, from stress to gut bacteria imbalance.

I'd start by looking at your diet and boosting levels of fresh fruit, vegetables and wholegrains (brown rice, rye bread and wholemeal pasta, for instance). Eat oily fish (such as organically farmed or wild salmon, sardines, mackerel and occasionally fresh but not tinned tuna), as the omega-3 fats they contain, far from exacerbating oily skin, keep the skin smooth and your hormones in balance. Cut back on refined or processed foods and sugar, fizzy drinks and alcohol, coffee and fried or fatty foods, and drink 1.5 to 2 litres of pure water each day.

Take regular exercise and think about ways of managing your stress if you feel overburdened: yoga and other calming exercise, meditation or simply chilling out are all useful. Also, supplement your diet with a good multivitamin and mineral and take a course of probiotics that help to restore a healthy balance of bacteria in your gut. (See Resources, page 483.) Topically, tea tree oil, an extract from the Australian plant *Melaleuca alternifolia*, has remarkable antibacterial properties, so try dabbing this on any spots.

Q *What natural products can I use for my acne, which seems to be worse in winter?*

A Aside from improving your diet (see 'What's the solution for acne?', page 263), take a look at what you're putting on your face. If your acne is worse in winter, it may be worth changing your moisturiser – many contain substances that block the pores. Dermalogica make an excellent range of products for cleansing and protecting your skin – call 01372 363600 to find your nearest stockist. The best topical substance I know of for acne is tea tree oil. Studies have shown it to be as effective as the usual spot cream ingredient benzoyl peroxide, and it is widely available in chemists and healthfood shops. Only use it directly on the spots, as it can dry out the skin, or dab it on with a piece of wet cotton wool. Another useful cream is MSM, which contains sulphur, an old, effective remedy for skin complaints. Check out your local healthfood store for this.

Q *My skin looks like I'm blushing and I get little red spots. My doctor confirmed this is acne rosacea. Can you help?*

A Acne rosacea is a rather mysterious but quite common condition which usually affects people between the ages of 30 and 50. Acne-like eruptions of red spots appear on the face, and particularly the cheeks. The cheeks then become very red as the capillaries there fill with blood.

To strengthen fragile capillaries, make sure you're taking in plenty of bioflavonoids: eat lots of red and purple fruits and vegetables, especially berries, and take a 1g vitamin C supplement containing at least 250mg of bioflavonoids or an equivalent amount of berry extracts. Inadequate digestive enzymes and low stomach acid (hydrochloric acid, or HCl) have also been linked to acne rosacea, as has a lack of the fat-digesting enzyme lipase. Many sufferers find supplementing these enzymes with their main meals helps. (See Resources, page 483.) As the condition has been linked to B vitamin deficiency, take a high strength B complex providing 100mg of the full range of Bs. It's also a good idea to avoid too many alcoholic or hot drinks and spicy foods, as these can all aggravate the condition. And as alcohol-based skincare products can do the same, choose the purest, simplest facial creams you can find.

Q *How can I treat the red spots with yellow heads on the end of my nose?*

A Acne is often called diabetes of the skin – so although the spots you describe aren't classic acne, following a blood sugar balancing regime may help. Supplementing 200mcg of chromium a day is a good start, but you need to back this up with a diet high in fibre, fresh fruit and vegetables, and low in sugars, saturated fat and refined carbohydrates. Also eat regular meals that include protein, which further helps to regulate blood sugar.

In terms of supplements, zinc, vitamin A and antioxidants are all essential for skin health. Supplementing 20mg of zinc and up to 5,000mcg of vitamin A can help. (Limit your A to 3,000mcg a day if you're pregnant.) The best topical substance I know of for spots is tea tree oil, which has remarkable antibacterial properties. Use it directly on the spots, not the surrounding skin, as it has a drying effect, or dab it on with a piece of wet cotton wool. Another useful cream is MSM, which contains sulphur and is available in healthfood shops.

Q *I have brown spots on the backs of my hands and my body. What causes them and can I get rid of them?*

A The spots you are describing, popularly called liver spots, are pigmentary changes associated with older skin due to oxidant damage to tissue. These are extremely common in those over 40. They can be brought on by ageing, exposure to sun or other forms of ultraviolet light. Antioxidant supplements can help to stop new ones from appearing, and applying vitamin E oil (cut open a capsule and smear the oil on the spot) can help to fade them, but will not eliminate them completely.

Your liver could also do with some support, as these spots can be a sign that it's not coping with its detoxification load. The liver is the primary organ in the body for disarming harmful oxidants. So eat plenty of fresh fruit and vegetables, organic if possible (especially broccoli, cabbage, onions, garlic and kale), drink at least 1.5 litres of water daily, have fibre-rich foods such as beans and wholegrains such as brown rice, oats and rye bread. Vitamin C (2g a day) and the herbs milk thistle and artichoke also give your liver a boost.

Q *I suffer from facial blushing – what can I take for this?*

A This can either be physiological or psychological. If the former, it can be caused by an allergic reaction – for example, to caffeine, alcohol or spicy food. So you need to figure out if there's a trigger. If it's acne rosacea (see 'My skin looks like I'm blushing', page 267), a lack of digestive enzymes can also contribute indirectly, so if you feel full or heavy after eating, or have difficulty digesting fatty foods, consider taking a betaine hydrochloride (stomach acid) supplement, or a digestive enzyme formula that contains betaine with food. As for other supplements, taking a high-quality multivitamin and mineral formula with extra vitamin C is a good daily programme to follow to ensure you're getting all the nutrients you need. Bioflavonoids help to strengthen the integrity of blood capillaries, and so may have an indirect effect on the blushing. Take 1 to 2g of vitamin C containing bioflavanoids or berry extracts. (See Resources, page 483.)

Q *I bruise really easily, especially on my thighs. What can I do about this?*

A Easy bruising is a classic sign of vitamin C or E deficiency. If you get bruises and don't know where they came from, you need to up your intake of these antioxidant vitamins that help to keep skin and blood vessels strong and healthy. The best food sources of vitamin C are carrots, cabbage, watercress, broccoli, cauliflower, green peppers, tomatoes, kiwi fruits, lemons, oranges and strawberries. The best food sources of vitamin E are nuts and seeds, such as pumpkin seeds, or their cold-pressed oils; avocados are good too, as is wheatgerm, as long as you're not allergic to wheat. Also helpful are bioflavonoids, which are found in blue/purple foods such as blueberries, blackcurrants, red grapes and beetroot. As well as eating these foods, try supplementing 1g of vitamin C and 300mg/400iuof vitamin E a day. The best vitamin C supplements, called C complex, also provide around 250mg of bioflavonoids.

Q *How can I get rid of dark circles under my eyes?*

A Dark circles under the eyes are usually linked to some sort of allergy or sensitivity to a particular food, which causes inflammation in the tiny blood vessels under them. Wheat and milk products are the two biggest culprits, although different people react to different foods, including alcohol. The easiest way to find out if a food is triggering reactions is to avoid it for 10 days and see if there is any difference and then, when you start eating it again, to take note of any changes. Wheat is in most bread (choose 100 per cent rye instead), most cereals (choose corn or oat-based types), pasta, pizza, biscuits and so on. Instead of milk, have soya or rice milk.

There can be other reasons for those dark circles, however. Apart from needing more sleep, they could indicate poorly functioning kidneys. Follow a kidney-friendly diet by drinking at least 2 litres of bottled or filtered water every day, eating more raw foods (aim for 75 per cent) and reducing your intake of animal proteins, as too much can put stress on the kidneys. Alternative protein sources include peas, beans, lentils, nuts, seeds, millet, quinoa, soya and whole-grains. Foods that support the kidneys include garlic, potatoes, asparagus, parsley, watercress, celery, cucumbers and papaya, plus lentils, seeds and soya, which contain kidney-friendly arginine. It's also important to reduce your intake of potassium and phosphates. Avoid salt and potassium chloride (a salt substitute), beet greens, chocolate, cocoa, eggs, fish, meat, spinach, rhubarb, Swiss chard and tea, and limit your consumption of bananas to no more than three a week.

Additional considerations include checking for heavy metal toxicity, as heavy metals are very harmful to the kidneys and need to be eliminated if present. A nutritionist can arrange a hair mineral analysis to check this. Note that if you have severe back pain, this could indicate kidney stones or other problems with your kidneys; you should see a doctor immediately to check for these. However, by far the most common cause of dark circles is an allergy.

Q **I suffer from dermatitis. Is there a diet connection?**

A The word dermatitis literally means skin inflammation. It's a condition similar to eczema, where the skin can be irritated, swollen, red and itchy. Usually the term dermatitis is used when the primary cause appears to be a contact allergy – that is, you've touched or worn something you're allergic to. Consider all possibilities, such as metals in jewellery, watches, perfumes, cosmetics, detergents in washing-up liquid, soaps, shampoos or washing powders.

Where there is a contact allergy, there's often a food allergy too, the most common being to dairy products and wheat. Sometimes only a combination of eating an allergy-provoking food and contact with an external allergen will trigger the symptoms. It's a good idea to do elimination tests on all these allergens, both edible and nonedible. Cut out each one for 10 days and see what happens. Even better is to test yourself for food intolerances (see Resources, page 483).

Another predisposing factor is a lack of essential fatty acids from seeds and their oils, and oily fish, which control inflammation in the body. Try supplementing starflower or borage oil; 1,000mg provides roughly 250mg of the essential fat GLA, which is what you are looking for. GLA has been proven to help reduce skin inflammation and is widely available in healthfood stores.

Q *How can I stop my skin from being dry and rough?*

A There are two underlying causes of dry, rough skin. The first is deficiency in essential fats. If you don't eat seeds or nuts and the only oil you use in dressings is olive oil, the chances are you're not getting enough essential fats. Go to a healthfood shop and buy a bottle of flax seed oil. Have a tablespoon a day, on cereal or salads, in soups – or straight down the hatch. If this is your problem you'll see a difference in a week.

The other possibility is you're not getting enough vitamin A – a common cause of dried-out, roughened skin. Arch your fingers and look at the underlying colour on the palm side of your fingers. They should have a yellowish hue. If you're all white/grey there, you're not getting enough vitamin A. Eat a carrot every day, preferably organic, as there's twice as much vitamin A in an organic carrot. In a couple of weeks you should notice a slight yellow underlying skin colour when you do the 'palm test'.

Q *How can I keep my skin from drying out on my summer holiday?*

A Although avoiding the sun is a good prescription for keeping your skin supple, let's face it: you're likely to ignore that at least some of the time. And anyway, moderate sunlight on your skin is actually good for you. So apart from being sensible about when and how long you are in the sun, give your skin all the protection you can with nutrients.

Antioxidants such as vitamins A, C and E are essential for protecting against the harmful effects of the sun – so eat plenty of fruit, vegetables, nuts and seeds. I also recommend you take a good antioxidant formula. Apart from using a good sun cream, you should moisturise your skin from the inside with essential fatty acids. Oily fish, nuts, and seeds such as pumpkin and sunflower are particularly rich in these important nutrients, so eat mackerel, organic or wild salmon, herring or sardines three times a week and have a handful of nuts and seeds every day.

Q *Every winter I get itchy red patches on my legs and arms. Can you help?*

A Redness and itching is more often than not a sign of skin inflammation. This tendency can be aggravated by temperature changes and cold weather as well as a diet low in antioxidant-rich fresh fruit and vegetables, which may be why you get it only in the winter. You can reduce your tendency to inflammation by increasing your intake of essential fatty acids from foods such as oily fish, nuts, pumpkin, flax and sunflower seeds or their oils. Supplementing 1,000mg of flax seed oil capsules three times daily usually helps. Vitamin C (1g three times a day) can also help reduce inflammation. Many people find relief from all sorts of skin irritations by applying MSM cream, which contains sulphur compounds; just be aware it can sting on sensitive skin at first.

Q *What can you do to stop oily skin?*

A Your skin normally produces a substance called sebum. Some people, however, produce an excess, which usually causes very oily skin. Although this can be hereditary, it's also affected by diet and hormone balance.

Diet-wise, reduce saturated fats, mainly from meat and milk products. These fats can interfere with the body's processing of the important essential fats found in oily fish, fresh nuts and seeds such as pumpkin and sunflower. I also recommend supplementing flax seed oil – 1,000mg, twice a day. And it's important to reduce your intake of sugary foods such as sweets, chocolate, desserts and biscuits, and sugar in drinks such as coffee, tea or fizzy drinks, because sugar feeds infections.

People with oily skin can also be tempted to overclean their skin, but this only stimulates more oil production. It's best to get the advice of a skincare professional about what is best for your skin.

Q *Are there any natural remedies that can help psoriasis?*

A Psoriasis is a chronic disease in which cells in the outer layers of skin reproduce too fast, causing the skin to scale. There is also usually inflammation, and can be pain, itching and restricted movement in some joints. Some natural health therapists say that psoriasis can be linked to stress and psychological issues, so it's important to address this aspect of your life. There is a link between a build-up of toxins in the bowel and psoriasis, because the toxins can increase the speed of skin cell regeneration.

First, make sure you're digesting well, to avoid leaving toxins in the gut. Taking a digestive enzyme supplement with each meal will help. It's important to cleanse the bowel by following a high-fibre, high-water diet. But rather than wheat bran, take a spoonful of flax seeds soaked in water and drink this daily alongside colon-cleansing herbs such as Oregon grape or oregano. Eating foods rich in essential fatty acids such as oily fish, nuts and pumpkin or sunflower seeds, and taking an omega-3 fish oil supplement (1 or 2 1g fish oil capsules a day) can help reduce the inflammation and moisturise the skin.

Q *What can I do to remove or diminish stretch marks and prevent more from appearing?*

A You need to supplement 15mg of zinc every day and ensure a good intake of essential fats. Both are needed to help skin and muscle cells strengthen and repair. The best way is to buy a glass jar, fill it half with flax seeds, half with sesame/sunflower/pumpkin seeds and keep it in the fridge. Every day grind some in a coffee grinder and have a tablespoon on your cereal, or sprinkle them on soups or salads or add to fruit smoothies. I'd also recommend taking a supplement providing the essential omegas GLA, EPA and DHA Ideally take 300mg of EPA, 200mg of DHA and 100mg of GLA a day.

Q *I keep getting warts. What can you suggest?*

A Warts are caused by a virus, and any recurrent infection may be a sign that you have a beleaguered immune system. Common warts, however, are notoriously difficult to get rid of. In order to strengthen your immunity, make sure you're eating a healthy diet of fresh, unprocessed foods and avoiding sugar and alcohol. Deficiencies in vitamins A and C and zinc reduce the immune system's strength, so take a good antioxidant or multivitamin. There are various recommendations for topical applications of natural substances: a thin slice of garlic, aloe vera gel and vitamin C cream (or a paste made from vitamin C powder). You can buy the latter two from your healthfood shop. Viruses have a hard time surviving in a vitamin C-rich environment, so I'd start with that one.

Q *What causes varicose veins?*

A A varicose vein is a vein that has become enlarged and swollen through poor circulation; they usually show up on the legs, where circulation is most difficult. It is unlikely that optimum nutrition can do much for veins that are already varicose. However, getting adequate amounts of vitamin C (1g twice a day – get a formula with bioflavanoids or berry extracts) and vitamin E (400mg/600iu once a day), as well as other antioxidants, can help to prevent further occurrences.

There is some evidence that a high-fibre diet can help to prevent varicose veins. That means plenty of fruit, vegetables and wholegrains such as oats, brown rice and rye bread. Regular exercise, especially swimming, will also improve circulation, and putting your feet up and gently massaging your legs may help too. Application of vitamin E cream to the vein area, or using the oil in a capsule, can also be beneficial.

Q *My hands and feet have a yellow tinge. Is this a problem?*

A Yellowish hands and feet are most likely to be the result of one of two things, one good, and the other not so healthy.

First, you may just be consuming particularly high levels of beta-carotene, the plant version of vitamin A, from foods such as carrots, sweet potatoes, pumpkin, watercress and mangoes. It's well known, after all, that people who drink large amounts of carrot juice get a yellowy tinge all over. This is not really unhealthy, but you should reduce your intake slightly. The other possible cause is that your liver is not detoxifying properly. If the whites of your eyes are yellow too, ask your doctor to do a liver function test. Otherwise, a nutritional therapist could advise you on a liver detoxification programme to lessen the burden on this vital organ and get it going properly.

Q **Do vitamins in skin creams really do any good?**

A Your skin is quite capable of absorbing substances from the outside in (think of hormone or nicotine patches), although the form of the vitamin used is key to how well this happens and whether it actually helps. Certain forms of vitamins are susceptible to damage when put on your skin and exposed to oxygen; for example, vitamin C as ascorbic acid is much less stable than ascorbyl palmitate. Most reputable companies formulate the vitamins so that they are in a stable form.

DIG DEEPER: Dermalogica's Multivitamin Power range includes Multivitamin Power Concentrate, which is excellent for sun-damaged or prematurely ageing skin. See www.dermalogica.com.

Q **What are parabens in cosmetic creams?**

A Parabens are synthetic preservatives that are used not just in cosmetic creams, but also in shampoos, conditioners, hair styling gels, make-up and deodorants. They may cause skin irritation, dermatitis or allergic skin reactions. Some research suggests that long-term exposure from leave-on products (make-up and skin lotions) enables migration via the skin into the bloodstream, and this can have oestrogenic effects that can interfere with hormone balance. Look out for good alternatives – naturally produced skin care products such as Dr Hauschka

(www.drhauschka.com), Jurlique (www.jurlique.com)
or Energys (www.highernature.co.uk).

DIG DEEPER: For more on caring for your skin
generally, read my book *Solve Your Skin Problems*,
coauthored with Natalie Savona (Piatkus, 2001).

Hair and scalp

Q *I suffer from dandruff. Can you help?*

A The first thing to check is whether any hair products
– shampoo, mousse, gel – are irritating your scalp.
Many contain alcohol and harsh chemicals that can
dry out your skin, making it itchy and flaky. So switch
to a different type to see if that makes any difference,
especially if you've recently changed brands. Some
people find that rubbing pure aloe vera gel into their
scalp when their hair is still wet after shampooing
helps.

Otherwise, there's the inside-out approach.
Omega-3 and omega-6 essential fatty acids are key
when it comes to skin, as they form part of each skin
cell and help keep it from drying out and flaking. Oily
fish, nuts and seeds such as pumpkin and sunflower are
particularly rich in these important nutrients. Try to
eat wild or organically farmed salmon, herring, sardines or mackerel three times a week, grind up a tablespoon of seeds to sprinkle over your cereal in the
morning, and snack on a handful of nuts for your
elevenses. Or you can supplement with fish oil

capsules (1g a day) or a tablespoon of flax seed oil each day. You may also be low in vitamin A, which is important for skin health. So eat eggs, yellow and orange fruits (mangoes, apricots) and vegetables (peppers, sweet potatoes) and take a multivitamin that contains at least 2,500mcg of A (and no more than 3,000mcg if you're pregnant). Many people find MSM, a type of sulphur, helps all sorts of skin problems. Take 3g a day. MSM also comes in a topical cream form.

Q *My hair is always dry. Can this be linked to my diet?*

A Your body is smart – it prioritises the distribution of essential nutrients to the vital organs, leaving the parts of the body that are least important for survival until last. Your hair may be vital to your appearance, but it actually comes way down on your body's list, so if your hair is dull and lifeless this usually means you're taking in so few nutrients there's little left over for it. A lack of essential fats – important oils found in oily fish and seeds (such as pumpkin and sunflower) – is the most common cause of dry hair. So have oily fish such as sardines or trout three times a week and a handful of seeds each day as snacks, on salads or cereal. To ensure you're getting enough, supplement an omega-3-rich-fish oil. Cod liver oil is a very good source. To safeguard against any other nutrient shortfalls, supplement a good diet with a high strength multivitamin and mineral too.

Q *I am losing a lot of hair. Am I missing something in my diet?*

A Hair loss is connected to many different factors, from stress to a general nutrient deficiency. Nutrients particularly linked to falling hair are iron, vitamin B1, vitamin C and the amino acid lysine. Some hair supplements contain all of these. To optimise hair growth, make sure you are getting adequate protein from fish, lean chicken and soya products like tofu, as well as the mineral zinc, which is essential for growth. Meat, shellfish, eggs, wholegrains such as oats, nuts, and seeds such as pumpkin and sunflower are all rich in zinc. Vitamin B5 (pantothenic acid) has also been shown to help stimulate hair growth. Take a good multivitamin which contains at least 15mg of zinc and 50mg of vitamin B5. (See Resources, page 483.) If you have other symptoms, such as fatigue, dry skin and low libido, you may have low thyroid function, so ask your doctor to run a test.

Q *My hair is starting to thin on top and I don't want to end up a monk! Any help?*

A Premature hair loss in men is linked to three things: hormones, circulation and nutrition. The body makes the sex hormone testosterone and stress hormones from the same raw material. Too much stress can upset the balance and encourage hair loss.

Women's hair loss is most often linked primarily to low iron levels. The ability to absorb and use iron is helped by the amino acid lysine, plus vitamin C and vitamin B12. Some hair formula supplements contain all of these, which are good for both men and women. (See Resources, page 483.)

DIG DEEPER: Hair Tomorrow (call 01628 776587 for details) have a proven approach that tests and corrects hormonal and nutritional deficiencies and then prescribes diet, plus supplements to 'feed' the scalp and exercises that stimulate circulation to the hair bed such as vigorous scalp massage or hanging upside down! Strange as it sounds, it works. I've seen 'monks' grow back a full head of hair.

Q *My hair grows very slowly. Any suggestions?*

A You may well just have a natural tendency to slower hair growth than most people. There are also other, external factors that affect the speed at which hair grows. One is sunlight, which revs up cellular division. This means that in the relatively gloomy winter, your hair tends to grow more slowly anyway (unless you head off to the Caribbean). Otherwise, you may be deficient in protein, zinc or B5, all of which affect hair growth. Make sure you're getting enough high-quality protein (two servings a day), in the form of fish, lean chicken or soya. Zinc is found in meat, shellfish, eggs, wholegrains such as oats or rye, and nuts and seeds such as pumpkin and sunflower. And take a good multivitamin containing at least 15mg of zinc and 50mg of vitamin B5, plus other B vitamins.

Nails

Q *My nails keep cracking. Is there anything I can do to stop this?*

A Brittle, cracking nails are often a signal of nutrient deficiency. The body prioritises the distribution of nutrients, and while vital organs are first on the list, skin and nails are pretty much the last. You could be low in vitamin A, B vitamins, calcium or iron, but rather than supplementing these individually, take a high-strength multivitamin and mineral.

Another key factor is how well you are digesting and absorbing nutrients from your food. Low levels of stomach acid, which prepares minerals for absorption, and digestive enzymes, are a common problem. A supplement containing both of these can really boost the condition of your nails, although note that you shouldn't take it if you've had stomach ulcers or other stomach problems. And don't forget to protect your nails from external damage, such as harsh detergents and hot water.

Q *What causes pronounced vertical ridges in both fingernails and toenails?*

A The vertical ridges in your nails can indicate a deficiency of B vitamins. Many foods are rich in the Bs, but these vitamins can be removed by processing and refining (of grains, for example), and are depleted in the body by stress and alcohol. Consequently many people today are not getting enough. In addition to a good multivitamin and mineral, I'd recommend a B complex supplement of 50mg with breakfast and dinner. Also reduce your alcohol intake and stress levels (yoga, walking and just chilling out will help, as well as laying off stimulants such as coffee), and eat plenty of vitamin B-rich foods (wholegrains, brewer's yeast, lentils, and most vegetables – watercress, broccoli, cauliflower, cabbage and tomatoes are good sources).

Q *What do white marks on your fingernails mean?*

A This is a classic sign of zinc deficiency, as are ridges that run across the nail. If you've got white marks or stripes on three or more nails, this is a clear sign that you are not getting enough zinc. Zinc is rapidly depleted by stress and in men, by excessive sex – semen is zinc-rich! So supplement with 15mg of zinc a day, and eat foods rich in the mineral. Luckily, it's a delicious array. If you like oysters, these are far and away the best source, but you have plenty of other options: fresh ginger, lamb, pecan nuts, fresh green peas, dried split peas, haddock, shrimp, turnips, Brazil nuts, eggs, wholegrains such as rye and oats, and peanuts and almonds.

Stress

Q *My work is totally stressful. What's the best way to chill out?*

A Anything that relaxes you, from alcohol to valium, affects the brain's natural peacemaker – the nutrient and neurotransmitter GABA. Supplementing this amino acid helps you to unwind, but without the after-effects associated with alcohol or tranquillisers. So too do the herbs kava kava, used by Pacific Islanders, hops, passion flower and valerian. Combinations of these are most effective. In fact, a recent study found that kava and valerian together were as effective as tranquillisers, but completely non-addictive. Unfortunately, neither kava nor GABA are available in the UK, although they are in the US. It's useful to note, however, that GABA is made in the body from the amino acid glutamine or glutamic acid, which is sometimes combined with herbs in supplements. (See Resources, page 483.)

On the non-chemical front, blue light, the scent of lavender and the right 'chill' music all relax you, as do yoga, t'ai chi, meditation, exercise and sex. Try one of these after work, together with some relaxing nutrients and herbs, for a natural chill out.

DIG DEEPER: For more information on how the brain works and how to chill out effectively, see my book *Natural Highs Chill* (Piatkus, 2003).

Q **Stress from work caused me to suffer an energy burnout a year ago. Can you help?**

A I recommend you take charge of your energy now by doing the following:

- Give up all alcohol for 10 days to gauge the effect it's having on your energy levels.
- Take a day to learn how to meditate, to become master of your mind.
- Take a supplement that contains a combination of the amino acids tyrosine and phenylalanine and the herbs ginseng and reishi or rhodiola to support your adrenals and boost your energy.
- Track down some DHEA (a hormone that supports the adrenals) from the US; you'll have to do an Internet search. Take 25mg a day for one month.
- If you're not already, take 2g of vitamin C plus a good multivitamin and mineral every day.
- If you're not feeling sufficiently energised by your gym sessions, I suggest you learn an exercise and breathing system called Psychocalisthenics (or Pcals for short), which you can then do each day at home in 20 minutes. It exercises all the main muscle groups, and tones and energises the body. See Resources, page 483, for details on both the exercises and the supplements.

> **DIG DEEPER:** For more information on stress generally, see my book *Beat Stress and Fatigue* (Piatkus, 1999). You may also find *Natural Highs Energy* (Piatkus, 2003) useful as a guide to how the brain works and how to give your energy levels a big boost through diet and exercise.

Superbugs

Q *My mother has the methicillin-resistant staphylococcus aureus (MRSA) virus, which is highly resistant to treatment. Can you recommend a supplement?*

A To create an environment in which this virus would find survival difficult, I suggest you buy some vitamin C in powdered form and mix 10g in 2 litres of half water, half diluted juice for her to drink throughout the day. She may experience loose bowels with this amount; if this is a problem, reduce the amount she drinks until this stops. She should also take a good high-strength multivitamin and mineral plus an antioxidant containing at least 2,250mcg (7,500iu) of vitamin A, 200mg (300iu) of vitamin E, 100mg of B6, 20mg of zinc and 100mcg of selenium. Cat's claw tea and echinacea (10 drops three times a day) are also good immune boosters. She should do all this until she is better.

Sweating

Q *My hands and feet sweat a lot. Any suggestions?*

A The first thing I'd recommend for excessive sweating is to balance your blood sugar levels. If they are going up and down you're also likely to have see-sawing energy, mood and concentration levels; and irritation and anxiety can cause you to perspire more than is normal.

To even out your blood sugar, eat regularly, have some protein (fish, yoghurt, lean meat or soya) and fibre (vegetables, fruit or wholegrains) at each meal, cut out sugar, processed foods, coffee, tea and alcohol, and take 200mcg of the mineral chromium each day. Excessive sweating can also be caused by stress, which can in turn play havoc with your blood sugar levels, so take control of that by meditating, doing yoga, walking or just chilling out regularly to soothing music.

Many people find that they perspire less if they have a good intake of the omega-3 and 6 essential fatty acids (EFAs), which act as a kind of two-way waterproofing in the skin. EFA-rich foods include oily fish, nuts and seeds. Eat these as well as taking a good fish oil supplement (1g), or flax seed oil (a tablespoon a day) if you are vegetarian.

Q *I suffer from body odour, as I sweat a lot. What can I do to stop this?*

A Heavy sweating is often down to stress and problems with keeping your blood sugar on an even keel, while body odour could be the result of a need to detoxify your body. There are three things you have to do to balance your blood sugar and reduce stress: cut right back on sugar and stimulants such as tea and coffee; eat foods that release their sugar content slowly, such as oat-based bread or cereal, wholegrains, vegetables and fruit; and supplement 1g of vitamin C, a B complex and 200mcg of chromium daily. If you feel a detox is definitely in order, you'll need to follow a two-week detox diet.

Here's how. Cut all red meat and dairy products right out, and concentrate on fruit, vegetables and lots of water (1.5 to 2 litres a day). Choose organic whenever possible. Fresh apricots, berries, cantaloupe, kiwi fruits, peaches, red grapes and mangoes, among other fruits, are the best; while peppers, beetroot, Brussels sprouts, broccoli and other cruciferous vegetables, as well as cucumber, carrots, tomatoes, sweet potatoes, kale, spinach and watercress are excellent vegetable detoxifiers, as are beansprouts. Up to a third of your detox diet should be made up of grains such as millet, quinoa and brown rice, oily fish such as mackerel and sardines, and organic chicken or tofu. Every day, eat a handful of whole or ground raw nuts and seeds, either as a snack or in cereal, fruit-and-juice smoothies or soup.

Systemic lupus erythamatosis

Q *I suffer from systemic lupus erythamatosis. What's your dietary advice?*

A Systemic lupus erythamatosis (SLE) is an auto-immune disease in which the immune system, our internal police force, becomes too belligerent and begins to attack the body itself. The best thing you can do is support the immune system with good nutrition. This means plenty of antioxidant-rich foods such as fresh fruit, especially berries, and vegetables, plus enough protein from fish, beans, lentils and a small amount of organic meat. People with SLE often have hidden allergies, with gluten sensitivity the most common. For this reason it is vital that you get yourself checked out by having an IgG food intolerance test (see Resources, page 483, for details on where to take the test).

Sometimes the immune system 'cross-reacts' to a protein in a food and a protein in you. If you do find you are food sensitive avoiding the offending item can make a big difference.

I'd also recommend supplementing 3g of vitamin C a day, as well as a high strength multivitamin and antioxidant formula.

Thrush

Q *How can you get rid of thrush naturally?*

A Thrush is an infection caused by the yeast *Candida albicans*. Yeasts feed off sugar and are more likely to multiply when your defences are down. Factors that trigger thrush are taking a course of antibiotics, being on the Pill, smoking, a high sugar or alcohol diet and wearing tights.

If you've been on antibiotics, take a supplement

of the beneficial bacterium *Lactobacillus acidophilus* and *Bifidobacterium bifidus* for two months. Otherwise, clean up your diet by eating lots of vegetables, whole-foods and a clove of garlic every day, while cutting right back on sugar and alcohol. Douching is generally not a good idea, as you need to re-establish your natural vaginal flora, not wash it away. There are various vaginal creams and pessaries available in health-food shops that contain beneficial bacteria and/or substances like tea tree oil that fight candida. Finally, many women swear by the soothing ability of live natural yoghurt in the vagina, which of course also contains the beneficial bacteria to help restore the natural flora to the area.

Q *I have candida, and some anti-candida diets recommend avoiding gluten grains. Why is this?*

A Gluten is a protein in certain grains such as wheat, and one of the reasons for avoiding them on a candida regime is because they are often allergenic, and so compromise the immune system. Some practitioners also believe that, like sugar (but to a much lesser extent), gluten grains feed the candida by causing a rise in blood sugar. Finally, candida can damage the integrity of the gut lining, making it more susceptible to irritation by these grains.

If avoiding them altogether seems too extreme, a compromise would be to balance your intake of grains and other carbohydrates with protein, so that you don't flood your blood with glucose (the break-down product of carbohydrates). In practice, this means eating meat, fish or vegetable protein with brown rice, pasta, oatcakes, baked potatoes and so on in equal portion size, and non-starchy vegetables in unlimited quantities.

But ultimately, a candida diet is hard to follow, so you have to find a way to manage it that is workable. And if this means eating grains, then it's not going to undermine your good work; it may just take longer to clear the candida.

Q *I keep getting thrush and have been prescribed the drug Nystatin. Is there a natural alternative?*

A Nystatin works as an anti-fungal drug, which kills the fungus *Candida albicans* that triggers thrush and other symptoms such as fatigue, bad skin and digestive problems. Several natural substances have powerful anti-fungal properties and are good alternatives. The best ones are caprylic acid, oregano extract, grape-fruit seed extract and garlic. Otherwise, see 'How can you get rid of thrush naturally?', page 292.

Thyroid conditions (see also Graves' disease)

Q *How do I know if my thyroid is underactive?*

A Low blood pressure plus cold hands/feet and feeling tired or sluggish are all symptoms of an underactive thyroid. Test yourself at home like this: shake out a thermometer and keep it by your bed. When you wake up in the morning, and before getting up, put a thermometer under your arm and lie there for 10 minutes. Your basal temperature should be 36.5 to 36.7 degrees Celsius. Do this for at least two days. (Women should do this test on days 2 and 3 of their period, as body temperature fluctuates during the cycle.) If your temperature is below 36.5, take it again regularly over a longer period, say a week, to see if it is low on a fairly regular basis. If it is lower than 36.5 you are probably hypothyroid – that is, your thyroid gland is underfunctioning.

In many cases, a low temperature will not necessarily indicate a condition which would be medically diagnosed as an underactive thyroid, but nevertheless, you could benefit from supporting your thyroid nutritionally (see 'I have an underactive thyroid . . .', below).

Q *I have an underactive thyroid and don't want to be on thyroxine medication for the rest of my life. Any suggestions?*

A A sluggish thyroid can mean you'll have symptoms ranging from fatigue, low energy and cold hands and feet to a slow metabolism. Your doctor may have given you thyroxine to compensate for your symptoms, but you can boost your thyroid gland nutritionally so it can make its own thyroxine.

The key duo is iodine and tyrosine. Seaweeds such as dulse or kelp are very rich in iodine, as are sea vegetables (such as nori and arame), mushrooms, Swiss chard, butterbeans and sesame seeds. Tyrosine, an amino acid, can also be found in butterbeans, as well as fish, almonds, bananas, avocados and pumpkin seeds. To supplement, take 200mcg of iodine a day, and 500mg of L-tyrosine twice a day. Essential fatty acids are vital for proper thyroid function, so include oily fish, seeds and cold-pressed oils in your regular diet. As a range of other nutrients, such as zinc and selenium, is also needed for full thyroid support, you may be better off taking a special thyroid blend. (See Resources, page 483.) If you are on medication, you should have your needs monitored by your doctor once you start to support your thyroid nutritionally, as these may change.

It is also worth looking at the state of your adrenals. Excessive adrenal function hinders thyroid function, and if your adrenals are low too, it may be because they were being overworked for too long (as a result of stress) and have put the brakes on your thyroid. Consider ways of reducing your stress load: meditation, yoga, walking and just giving yourself time to chill out.

Q *I have a hypothyroid condition caused by an autoimmune reaction. What can I do?*

A Some people produce 'anti-thyroid antibodies' which destroy thryroid tissue. This can be due to a 'cross-reaction' in which your body reacts to a food and mistakenly attacks the thyroid. Gluten grains such as wheat, rye, oats and barley are strongly associated with many autoimmune disorders, so you could try eliminating these from your diet and see how you feel. Even better is to test yourself for food intolerance. It also would be wise to consult a nutritional therapist to investigate what is causing your immune system to overreact in this way. (See Resources, page 483.)

Tinnitus

Q *I suffer from tinnitus and have a constant ringing in my ears. Can you help?*

A Tinnitus is said to affect as many as 4 million people in Britain, and is caused and exacerbated by a number of factors. Many prescribed medications list it as a side effect, for example. It can also be triggered by a loud noise, either a single blast or exposure over a long period of time. Inflammation in the ear can be a cause, either from infection or allergy. So can restricted blood flow, which can happen with a blood sugar imbalance; low blood sugar boosts adrenalin levels and constricts blood vessels.

To handle the inflammation, a diet low in saturated fat and high in essential fats can help, as omega-3s from oily fish, nuts and seeds are natural anti-inflammatories. The herbs boswellia and curcumin are good for inflammation, too. Ensure your blood sugar is balanced by following a sensible organic wholefood diet, restricting carbohydrates to slow-release kinds such as whole rye or brown rice, eating protein when you eat carbs and avoiding stimulants and sugary foods. It's also a good idea to check out your food allergies (see Resources, page 483) and include 2g of vitamin C in your daily supplement programme.

Sometimes physical imbalances in your neck or skull can result in tinnitus. A cranial osteopath can correct these.

DIG DEEPER: To find a cranial osteopath near you, contact the International Cranial Association on 020 8367 5561 or 020 8202 6242.

Ulcers

Q *I have stomach ulcers and take Zantac every day. What can I do?*

A There is plenty you can do nutritionally to prevent stomach ulcers, rather than simply relieving the symptoms. First get your doctor to check you for the bacterium *Helicobacter pylori*, which is the cause of many ulcers. If this is ruled out, think about what you're eating. It's largely a myth that stomach ulcers are caused by too much acid – the body is well designed to protect itself from its own digestive juices. The problem arises from eating and drinking foods that irritate the digestive tract, a condition which is then aggravated by stomach acid. So start by cutting back on likely irritants – alcohol, coffee, spicy foods or wheat. Reduce the amount of protein-rich foods (such as meat and cheese) you eat, as these are acidic. Vitamin A and glutamine are important for healing ulcers and omega-3-rich fish oils help reduce any inflammation. Chewing deglycyrrhirised liquorice tablets 20 minutes before a meal can also help to soothe ulcers.

Urinary problems

Q *I get thirsty and I pee a lot. What does this mean?*

A Both of these are classic signs of a deficiency in essential fats. No doubt you've heard that the human body is 66 per cent water. But, you might wonder, why don't we slurp around? The answer is that we keep our water inside our cells via a fatty 'waterproof' membrane, partly made of the essential fats also found in seeds and oily fish. If you don't eat enough of these fats, you lose the ability to control your water balance and you might find you are retaining water, are very thirsty, urinate excessively and have dry skin, dry hair or dandruff.

If you find yourself with several of these symptoms, I recommend three things: 1. eat seeds every day, as a tablespoon of ground seeds (half flax, and half sesame, sunflower and pumpkin seeds) on your cereal or in a smoothie; 2. eat oily fish such as wild salmon, herring, mackerel or sardines (and the occasional piece of fresh tuna) three times a week. 3. take an omega-3 fish oil supplement. (See Resources, page 483.)

Be aware, however, that excessive thirst can be a classic sign of a blood sugar problem, even diabetes. Ask your doctor to do a blood test to rule this out. If you find you have an imbalance, you'll need to even out your levels through your diet. Although it's best to consult your doctor or a nutrition practitioner if you have diabetes, such a diet generally involves eating little and often; choosing slow-release carbohydrates which also have protein, such as wholegrains, peas, beans and lentils, and fruit as long as they are eaten with nuts or seeds; and avoiding all forms of concentrated sweetness, from dried fruit to fruit juice, as well as stimulants like coffee and tea. Supplementing 200mcg of chromium can help.

Q *I have been diagnosed with an irritable bladder and suffer from incontinence. I have no infection, prolapse, muscle problems or pain and have tried excluding alcohol, tea, coffee and sugar. Is there anything else you can possibly recommend?*

A Have you been tested for food sensitivities? These are often a factor in bladder problems, so if you haven't been tested, I'd recommend you get an IgG allergy test. (See Resources, page 483.) I'd also boost levels of magnesium because this mineral is vital for muscle function. Take 200 to 300mg a day, and eat seeds (pumpkin, sunflower and sesame), rich in both magnesium and calcium, which control muscle function.

If you've been very stressed lately, your adrenal glands may be under pressure. A sudden release of adrenal hormones can affect the bladder. If this is the case, I'd suggest you see a nutritional therapist. In the meantime, supplementing an 'adaptogen' such as the herbs ginseng, rhodiola or reishi can help to support your adrenal function.

Q **I've started getting cystitis since starting a relationship. Why is this?**

A Cystitis is more likely to happen when you are having a lot of sex. The condition is an irritation or inflammation of the bladder or urethra, the tube that connects up to the bladder. It can progress into an infection of the bladder, at which point I'd recommend you see your doctor. If you have any blood in your urine this points towards an infection.

Whether you have an infection or not, the bladder can be aggravated by acidic urine, which can cause pain when you pee. To reduce the acidity of your urine, drink half a pint of water as soon as you feel the symptoms, and every 20 minutes for the following three hours. Then start drinking unsweetened cranberry juice every day, or take a cranberry juice extract, which is available in healthfood stores.

Drinking a pint of water containing 1 heaped teaspoon of sodium bicarbonate can also help by alkalising the urine. This can have a mild purgative effect.

I'd also recommend boosting your immune system with probiotics, echinacea and/or garlic. Probiotics are beneficial bacteria, for example found in yoghurt. You can also buy probiotic capsules, powder and vaginal creams. These are especially useful if you are prone to thrush. Gentle exercise, and avoiding alcohol, coffee, spicy foods and high acid foods such as meat and cheese can also help. So too can a warm bath or a hot water bottle on your back or tummy, or wrapped in a towel between your legs. You don't have to stop having sex, although a break for a couple of days may help, but do wash after sex and generally keep yourself clean.

Urticaria

Q *My daughter has developed urticaria. What could be causing this?*

A Urticaria – or hives – is almost certainly an allergic reaction. I'd therefore suggest your daughter eliminates suspect foods, the most common being wheat, gluten (the protein found in wheat and also barley, rye and to a lesser extent oats), dairy foods, eggs, citrus fruits, tea, coffee, chocolate and soya. Start with one food group at a time, eliminate completely for 10 days, then reintroduce and monitor the results. If all is OK, repeat the process with the next food group. Chemicals, pharmaceutical drugs or household products (washing powder, detergents and so on) can also cause an allergic reaction, so think if there's something in these groups that may be aggravating her too.

Water retention

Q *What do you recommend to prevent water retention?*

A Food allergies or intolerances, often to wheat and dairy foods, are a common cause of water retention. Other foods can also be involved; check out those you eat a lot of. Water retention can also be a symptom of essential fatty acid deficiency (see also 'I get thirsty and I pee a lot', page 299). Ensure a high intake of seeds and their oils and oily fish. Although it seems counter-intuitive, water retention can also mean you're not drinking enough water, and are forcing your body to store what it's got. Be sure you take in 1.5 litres of pure water a day and eat water-rich foods like fruit and vegetables. Supplements worth looking into include fish oil or flax seed oil, vitamin B6, biotin, zinc and magnesium.

ENVIRONMENTAL HEALTH

As far as nutrition is concerned, there are two sides of the coin: your intake of nutrients, and your exposure to 'anti-nutrients'. These can include all sorts of elements that work against the health of the body, such as the wrong kind of food, or polluted water or air. Some, like mercury or exhaust fumes, use up nutrients, increasing your need for them and taxing the body's natural detoxification systems accordingly. Others, from microwaves to mobile phones, affect the body in ways we haven't yet pinned down. Staying 100 per cent healthy means minimising the bad guys, the anti-nutrients, and optimising the good guys, the nutrients. And as it's wise to know your enemy, in this section I answer questions about anti-nutrients and issues of environmental concern.

Q *I feel worse in the city. Is this the pollution?*

A Maybe. Urban life in the 21st century places enormous stresses and strains on both mind and body.

Although city life can be stimulating and exciting, it also exposes us to air pollution, noise pollution, unhealthy working and travelling environments, and even toxins from other people such as infectious bacteria or cigarette smoke. These toxins work against our bodies, affecting our immune systems, stress levels and thought processes.

If you're an urbanite, there are plenty of ways to deal with the pressure. Make sure you have nutritious snacks like fruits and nuts with you to keep your energy up instead of the ubiquitous teas and coffees, avoid busy roads where you can, drink 2 litres of filtered or bottled water throughout the day, avoid junk and fast foods (on almost every corner in many cities), and instead eat nutritious and antioxidant-rich foods like green leafy vegetables, berries, fresh fruits, red, yellow and orange vegetables, garlic and onions. By protecting your body from the stresses and pollution that city life brings, you can be free to enjoy all that cities have to offer, whether you seek work or pleasure.

Q *What's your view on clingfilm and aluminium foil – are these harmful?*

A As long as they don't touch your food, they're fine, especially the 'non-PVC' types. Clingfilm, like some other plastics, may release hormone-mimicking chemicals into your food, especially oily food (see 'Is it a bad idea to use plastic dishes when heating things up in the microwave?', page 310). This process and the potential risks are far from fully understood, but while uncertainty persists, it's better to be cautious. The effects of plastics on our reproductive health are the cause of some concern in research circles at present. This isn't an issue if the film doesn't touch your food, and if you use it to keep food such as salads fresh in storage, it's very useful. It's also less likely to be a problem if you wrap non-oily foods such as sandwiches in clingfilm.

Aluminium foil is a similar case. If you use it to cover something you're baking in the oven but it doesn't touch the food, I can't see it would cause a problem. Aluminium foil (or cookware or utensils, for that matter) in contact with food will leach small amounts of aluminium into your food. I wouldn't recommend grilling pieces of meat directly on aluminium foil. If you're deficient in zinc or calcium, for instance, you're more likely to absorb the aluminium. It's toxic to the nervous system and has been linked to various problems from hyperactivity in children to Alzheimer's in the elderly.

Q *What's your view on fluoride?*

A The debate as to whether fluoride is beneficial or outright dangerous has been raging since it was first put into British water supplies in 1964, in Birmingham. The theory is that by drinking water containing fluoride (a waste product from the petrochemical and fertiliser industries), you are less likely to need fillings because it re-mineralises tooth enamel and prevents bacteria in the mouth from producing the acid that causes tooth decay. In fact, many factors contribute to tooth decay: poor nutrition, high sugar intake, poor dental hygiene, a predisposition to the condition and so on. So fluoride plays a small role in protecting teeth, and some would say a harmful one in other ways: scientific reports increasingly link an accumulation of fluoride in the body to a higher risk of mottled teeth, hip fracture, and poor mental development in children. So I recommend that while putting fluoride on the surface of your teeth via toothpaste may reduce tooth decay, taking it into the body may be bad for you.

Q *Are mercury fillings dangerous?*

A Mercury is one of the most toxic elements known to us, and is being banned from virtually all uses. In some countries you can no longer buy mercury thermometers. Yet an equivalent amount of mercury is found in an amalgam or silver filling. These fillings are composed of roughly half mercury and they are only inches away from your brain! Quite rightly, a growing number of dentists are alarmed at their potential danger and no longer recommend amalgam fillings.

The question of whether or not those with mercury fillings should have them removed is a bit trickier. The truth is that many people do not appear to suffer at all from mercury fillings, while others find huge relief from symptoms such as depression, low immunity, fatigue and headaches when their fillings are removed. I even know of one man, Tom Warren, who had Alzheimer's disease, proven by brain scans, and who has made an almost complete recovery within one month of having his 26 mercury fillings removed (see 'Can Alzheimer's ever be reversed?', page 354)!

If you do have any unexplained health problems that your doctor cannot explain, from memory loss to multiple sclerosis, it is worth checking whether your fillings might be part of the cause. If you decide to have your fillings out, how they are taken out is very important. Make sure your dentist is up on the procedure for minimising your accumulation of mercury when the filling is extracted. If in doubt contact the British Society for Mercury-free Dentistry (see below). There are many good composite materials, for which you can be compatibility tested, that can be used instead.

As well as having the amalgam fillings removed and replaced by non-toxic materials, it's important to detoxify the body with a good intake of fibre (especially pectin in apples and pears), sulphur-containing amino acids such as cysteine and glutathione (found in eggs, onions, garlic and good antioxidant supplements), and extra supplemental vitamin C, zinc and selenium (also present in seafood, seeds and wholegrains).

DIG DEEPER: For more information and advice on alternatives to mercury fillings, contact the British Society for Mercury-free Dentistry on 0171 370 0055.

Q *I've heard fish is high in mercury. Should one avoid eating it?*

A Mercury, sadly, is a common pollutant in the world's oceans. It bio-accumulates up the food chain, starting in plankton, which is then eaten by small fish, who are eaten by medium fish, who are eaten by large fish. These larger fish, which include shark, tuna and swordfish, live a long time and eat a lot of smaller fish, thus accumulating sometimes unhealthy levels of mercury in their tissues. As a result, government agencies around the world advise that such fish should now be avoided by pregnant women and eaten no more than once per week by everyone else.

Similar surveys have found that while most fish contain some mercury, the levels are low in smaller fish and are unlikely to pose a significant health risk. Fish provides quality protein in your diet without the saturated fat, and oily fish such as sardines, mackerel, herring and trout contain health-promoting levels of omega-3 essential fats. These fish should be eaten at least three times per week.

Q *What's your view on microwaving foods?*

A This question has been bandied about for decades now, and microwave ovens are actually banned in Russia. I'm going to go out on a limb here and say 'Get rid of it.'

Microwaving works via non-ionising radiation, which vibrates food particles, particularly water particles, and thus heats them up. Conventional cooking does the same thing. The potential advantage of microwaving is that the food cooks in its own water, which minimises the leaching of nutrients, and it's true that overall, microwaving is better than most cooking methods for preserving the water-soluble vitamins B and C. The temperatures reached in fat particles, however, are very high and therefore it would not be a good idea to microwave fish as this will damage the essential fats it contains, as well as vitamin E.

There are also other reasons to be cautious. In one trial eight participants all strictly followed the same diet for eight weeks. Those who had all their food microwaved had worse health results upon blood testing at the end of the trial. Another study, published in the October 2003 *Journal of the Science of Food and Agriculture* by a team of Spanish researchers, may show why. After broccoli was cooked by various methods and the effect of these on its antioxidant content was measured, the results showed microwaving as the clear loser: microwaved broccoli had lost between 74 and 97 per cent of three major antioxidant phytonutrients, while steamed broccoli lost less than 11 per cent of the same antioxidants. As science learns more about nutrition and health, I imagine the only place you'll see microwave ovens is in museums and junkyards.

Q **Is it a bad idea to use plastic dishes when heating things up in the microwave?**

A We are surrounded by plastic, and it's almost impossible to buy foods that aren't wrapped in the stuff.

But the effects this can have on our health remain largely unknown. Certain chemicals are added to plastics during their manufacture to make them more stable, more pliable or less breakable, such as nonylphenol and bisphenol-A. These chemicals are similar in structure to the hormone oestrogen, and have been found both to leach out of the plastics into foods and liquids they come into contact with, and cause hormone disruption in animals and humans due to their oestrogen-mimicking action. This phenomenon is thought to have contributed to observed reproductive problems in humans and wild animals.

The plastics industry is moving away from using proven hormone-disrupting chemicals, but I'd still recommend using glass or ceramic containers rather than plastic when heating foods in a microwave. (I'd also recommend not using a microwave – see 'What's your view on microwaving foods?', page 309.) Oils/fats and plastics are generally not a good combination in any circumstance, being chemically similar and conducive to the transfer of chemicals from one to another. Heating increases the rate of any chemical reaction, and may make it more likely that hormone-disrupting chemicals are leached into your food. These concerns may not apply to all plastics – manufacturers are developing safer, more inert types all the time. In the meantime, it's probably best to err on the side of caution, and minimise your exposure to plastics as much as possible.

Q *Is there a link between mobile phones and brain cancer?*

A Without a doubt. Mobile phones, as well as hands-free home or office phones, microwaves, electric pylons, mobile phone masts and any wireless devices such as 'bluetooth' technology all give off electronic magnetic frequency radiation, called EMF, or microwaves. We are unwittingly bombarded with these microwaves on a fairly constant basis, yet they have been clearly demonstrated in animals to increase the incidence of cancer as well as Alzheimer's-like changes in brain cells. And the dramatic increase in brain cancer of 45 per cent over the last 30 years makes it highly likely that microwave radiation, including that from mobile phones, is contributing to the problem.

The critical issue is how much exposure at what intensity equates to risk? Microwave radiation is measured in units known as microtesla (μT). In some countries, exposure is strictly limited by enforcing phone companies to use low-frequency phones. For example, in Switzerland phones emit only 4μT, compared to UK phones which emit sometimes over 5,000μT! Many countries have buffer zones around mobile phone masts. With clusters of leukaemia occurring around electricity pylons, there's little doubt that being close to devices emitting EMF is a health hazard.

But while there is a clear pattern of risk emerging, much research is being suppressed and much research is still to be done, so at this point it's hard to quantify the risk. My advice is not to use mobile phones, and if you do, use them as little as possible and don't keep them on your body. Keep them in a bag so your exposure is less. Also, don't use hands-free phones at home, especially next to the bed, because the base station is permanently transmitting.

Q **What's your view on farmed salmon?**

A No all farmed salmon is equal. While fish farming is generally a good idea, as it provides a way of avoiding the continual depletion of already struggling fish stocks in the world's oceans, commercial pressures can lead to poor practices and corner-cutting. Farmed fish in general can be quite an unhealthy option compared to wild fish. Stocking rates in sea cages can be too high – the fish are too close together and sea lice and fish diseases are rampant. So chemicals, antibiotics and biocides are then used to keep the fish alive, and this regimen isn't conducive to breeding healthy fish. As recent news stories report, farmed salmon can also be highly contaminated with industrial chemicals and pesticides.

Another key consideration is what the fish eat. The fishmeal-based feed is often lacking in the essential fats the fish would naturally get in the wild from plankton and so on, and farmed salmon may thus have a much lower content of omega-3 essential fats than their wild cousins. Farms also often add colourants to the feed to make the flesh pinker, and while some are simply natural red pigments, I imagine others are not. If you can't get wild salmon, I recommend organically farmed salmon, where at least there are some controls on the stocking densities, the cleanliness of the waters, the types of feed used, and whether artificial colourants are prohibited.

Q **I wake up all blocked up. Could it be something in my bed?**

A Maybe. Sinus problems can result from sensitivities to something in your environment or your diet. You may have an allergy to house dust mites, which live in your mattress by the million feeding on your dead skin cells. Nice, huh? Try getting a new mattress or at the very least a mattress protector. This will prevent the mites from flourishing in your mattress as well as keeping them away from you as you sleep.

You should also have yourself checked for food intolerances, and regardless of the outcome eliminate dairy and wheat from your diet for 10 days to see if it helps. Dairy and wheat are both known to be mucus forming and are often the key cause of the sinus problem you're experiencing. A deficiency of essential fats will also make you more sensitive to allergens, so eat oily fish – sardines, mackerel, herring, trout or organic or wild salmon – three times a week, add pumpkin seeds, sunflower seeds and flax seeds to your breakfast every day, and supplement 1,000mg of fish oil or an omega-3/omega-6 blend twice daily.

FIRST AID
AND TRAVEL

The travel bug has bitten millions, but our love for exotic – or just plain hot – destinations can lay us open to bugs of a very different type. In fact, holidays can be a big strain on your health, exposing you to bites and bacteria your immune system has never had to cope with before, not to mention all kinds of injuries – whether you're jungle trekking in Java or scaling peaks in Peru. This section provides first aid tips designed to keep you healthy while on the go.

Q *If you're having an allergic reaction, how can you stop it quickly?*

A A sudden allergic reaction can set in when you have eaten or been exposed to an allergen. Whether you've got allergies or not, it's a good idea to take along the necessary treatment anyway, particularly if you'll be in remote regions far from medical clinics.

Alkalising your body with a combination of calcium and magnesium bicarbonate can shorten the duration of an allergic attack, and a number of supplements provide these minerals as a powder, available in health food shops. Follow the instructions on the label. If you can't get hold of these have a teaspoon of sodium bicarbonate (baking powder) in half a pint of water. You can also take 5g of vitamin C, ideally in the form of calcium ascorbate, and drink plenty of water. This will help you to return to normal.

Q **Can you deter mosquitoes and other biting insects through nutrition?**

A Some recommend 500mg of vitamin B1 taken every day for two weeks before you go and during your trip. My understanding is that 100mg per day is enough, but I have to say that B vitamins have never stopped the critters from biting me! Garlic supplements may be more effective – start taking a high-strength garlic supplement, or two cloves of garlic a day, a few days before you go. I'd also recommend using a good-quality natural insect repellent based on citronella, or citronella essential oil in a carrier oil applied liberally and frequently. Lavender oil works, but not as well as citronella. Although it's rare, some people are allergic to citronella, so it's a good idea to apply a bit before you go to see whether it provokes a reaction.

Q *What's the best way to heal a bruise, a burn and a cut?*

A To handle bruises, scrapes, burns and cuts while on the move, you'll need to tuck a few extra items in your first aid kit – selected vitamins, MSM supplements and cream (containing organic sulphur, which has renowned healing properties), aloe vera gel and tea tree oil among them.

Bruising occurs when the tissues under the skin are injured, which leads to an accumulation of blood. Apply MSM cream to the bruised area to speed healing and reduce pain. Vitamin C and bioflavonoids are essential for strengthening capillary walls so they are less susceptible to damage, and also supply oxygen to the area to help it heal. You can get vitamin C cream as ascorbyl palmitate. Both MSM and vitamin C can also be taken orally to speed recovery: I recommend 3g of each a day to recover from any major injury.

Burns need to be treated instantly. Apply aloe vera gel or MSM cream to help healing, soothe inflammation and minimise scarring. Never put a plaster on a burn till the heat is out of it. To promote healing supplement 5,000mcg of vitamin A per day (don't take more than 3,000mcg if you're pregnant), or 18mg of beta-carotene, and 30mg of zinc for one week or less, depending on the burn. Vitamin E oil (just cut open a capsule) can be applied when the burn is not an open wound. Drink plenty of fluids, and take 3g of MSM daily for a month and then reduce to 1g a day.

From a nutritional point of view, the treatment of cuts is similar to that for burns. Apply aloe vera gel and MSM cream alternately around the wound several times a day until it has healed – these two facilitate the healing process and reduce scarring. Continue this regime to prevent scarring, plus vitamin C, vitamin E and MSM taken orally. Scars from cuts heal up spectacularly well when you apply vitamin E oil to the injury site (but don't do this with big open wounds), which you can do by piercing a vitamin E capsule. Cleansing with diluted tea tree oil, a highly effective antibacterial, helps prevent infection.

Q *I often get constipated when I fly. How can I prevent this?*

A Flying is not only severely dehydrating, it also disturbs the normal balance of gut bacteria. That is why it is essential to drink a lot of water when you are flying, even if that means you pee a lot. I recommend a glass of water every hour, and complete avoidance of alcohol, which will simply amplify the dehydration you're already exposed to. I always take a few pieces of fruit along when I travel, too. Fruit provides a lot of water, plus many other nutrients, thus making it a healthy alternative to the usually sub-standard airline food.

It also helps to up your intake of vitamin C to 3g a day for the day of travel and a day after. When you land, take half a teaspoon of probiotics (acidophilus and bifidus bacteria), and make sure you eat a lot of water-rich foods. This means more fruit, and vegetables (taking into account local hygiene – you may need to stick to peelable types), and drinking enough water. Also, get some exercise. Sitting for a day is in itself constipating.

Q *What's the best prevention, and cure, for holiday diarrhoea?*

A If you're off to an exotic location, start taking a good probiotic supplement containing *Lactobacillus acidophilus* and *Bifidobacterium bifidum* for one week before you go, and continue while you're out there. Make sure to take one that doesn't need refrigeration. This helps build up the good bacteria in the intestines so the bad guys are less likely to take hold.

If you do get a bout of diarrhoea, take grapefruit seed extract, 15 drops three times a day, and drink plenty of water or diluted fruit juice. Don't eat for 24 hours, then start back on food with boiled rice and grated apple, which contains pectin that is binding. Take the probiotics for another two weeks when you get home. Combining them with glutamine powder speeds up recovery. I recommend half a teaspoon of probiotic powder containing acidophilus and bifidum with a heaped teaspoon (5g) of glutamine powder in water, away from food. (See Resources, page 483.)

Vitamin A is essential for maintaining strong

cellular membranes throughout the body, including the gut. The richest source of vitamin A is meat – but this, along with unpeeled vegetables and fruit, is the most likely source of holiday diarrhoea, so eat with caution if at all. If you do stay largely vegetarian I'd supplement 2,250mcg (7,500iu) of vitamin A a day, preferably in a good multivitamin. Essential fats are also crucial for cell repair. You can get them from seeds and oily fish, but if these are in short supply it's a good idea to take supplements along.

Q *What's the best way to recover quickly from jet lag?*

A During jet lag, your body clock effectively gets out of sync with the earth. Taking the neurotransmitter melatonin can be very helpful, but it needs to be used cautiously. It cannot be bought over the counter in Britain, but can be bought for your own personal use by mail order from the US or from American websites, as restrictions don't apply there.

Note that supplementing too much melatonin can have undesirable side effects such as diarrhoea, constipation, nausea, dizziness, reduced libido, headaches, depression and nightmares. However, none of this is likely with short-term use.

The best way to bring yourself back into balance is to start with 1mg of melatonin for every one-hour time difference, just before your new bedtime. Take this the first night, then halve the dose each subsequent night. So, if you fly from London to Los Angeles, which is eight hours behind, you take 8mg of melatonin on the first night, then halve it to 4mg for the second night, 2mg for the third, then 1mg, then stop.

Q *I often get sinus infections after long flights. How can I prevent this?*

A Air travel exposes you to a lot of potential infections. The first tip for avoiding sinus infections is to avoid eating any foods you may be allergic to for 24 hours before travelling, and also while you are travelling. As a rule of thumb, I'd avoid all dairy products, as these can cause excessive mucus production and thus contribute to sinus problems.

Secondly, I'd travel armed with a saline solution nasal spray, available in larger pharmacies. Spray each nostril once, then blow your nose, then spray again. Do this every hour or so. It not only keeps your sinuses clean, but also keeps them hydrated. Be sure to drink lots of water during the flight – at least a glass an hour.

The other method worth trying is to buy a face mask. These are available from the Aviation Health Institute and not only minimise the risk of infection, but cleanse the air you are breathing. Also, get a seat near the front: conditioned air circulates from the front to the back.

Finally, when you land, bump up your intake of

vitamin C and have a meal with some garlic and spices to clear your sinus passages and give your immune system a boost. Wasabe (Japanese horse-radish paste) is excellent for this.

DIG DEEPER: For details on face masks and useful advice, see the Aviation Health Institute's very informative website, www.aviation-health.org.

HERBAL AND OTHER NATURAL REMEDIES

Quite apart from vitamins, minerals and other essential nutrients, there are plant and food extracts that contain substances that can heal, energise and soothe us – herbal remedies. These have been with us since time immemorial, but we're now entering a new era for this ancient store of folk wisdom. First off, we're now able to pick and choose the best remedies from around the world. And secondly, research is revealing wonderful, sometimes unexpected properties in many of them. Here I answer questions about when and how to use them.

Herbal supplements A-Z

Q *Are there any herbs that shouldn't be taken alongside medications?*

A There are all sorts of possible reactions between herbs and drugs, nutrients and drugs and between medications themselves. Key ones to look out for are herbs and drugs that have similar aims. For example, garlic, which helps thin the blood, may exaggerate the effect of the drug warfarin, making blood dangerously thin so that it does not clot properly. Ginseng and garlic can have a similar interaction. Another combination to watch out for is ginkgo biloba and aspirin – taking these together has been linked to the eruption of blood vessels in the eye. Another popular herbal remedy, St John's wort, widely used to help depression, shouldn't be taken at the same time as anti-depressant drugs such as Prozac.

A viable alternative to taking herbs with medication is to concentrate on finding effective herbal remedies alone. But if you are on medication, do check with your doctor before stopping it – or in fact starting any herbal remedies.

Q *What other natural antihistamines are there apart from vitamin C?*

A Vitamin C is the best antihistamine, but if you're looking for alternatives, the antioxidant quercetin is also effective (take 500mg per day away from food), as is curcumin, which is a natural anti-inflammatory compound found in turmeric and mustard (take 500mg one to three times a day). As an antihistamine for hay fever or similar symptoms, bee propolis and royal jelly are also helpful. All these are available from your healthfood store.

Q **What is your view on aloe vera?**

A Aloe vera is a cactus-like member of the lily family. Extracts of the plant first became popular as a proven skin healer: it is known to actually improve collagen repair, helping to heal burns and prevent wrinkles.

But recent research shows this ancient remedy does much more. It is a powerful detoxifier, antiseptic and tonic for the nervous system. It also has immune-boosting and anti-viral properties. Research has proven that adding aloe vera to one's daily diet improves digestion, and it can also be taken as a general daily health tonic. Exactly what the 'active ingredient' is remains a bit of a mystery, however. Aloe vera is rich in mucopolysaccharides, one of which is called acemannan, but also contains enzymes, vitamins, minerals, essential fats and amino acids. Note that concentration can vary greatly from one product to another (see Resources, page 483).

Q *What's your view on black cohosh?*

A Native Americans have used the remarkable herb black cohosh for centuries to combat female hormone problems – earning it the nickname 'squaw root'. More recently, research has proven that it helps relieve menopausal symptoms arising from declining oestrogen levels in the body, such as hot flushes, night sweats, depression, anxiety, insomnia and a reduced sex drive. In Germany, in fact, it is widely prescribed for this as a safer alternative to hormone replacement therapy (HRT). An ideal dose is 4mg of the active ingredient, 27-deoxyactein, every day.

Q *What's your view on cat's claw?*

A The Peruvian rainforest herb *Uncaria tomentosa*, or cat's claw, is one of the most powerful immune-boosting, detoxifying and anti-cancer herbs yet discovered. It also has anti-inflammatory effects and so it can be helpful for people with arthritis, asthma and eczema. Some people find it helps soothe their digestion too. People who live in the rainforests make a tea from the thorny bark of this plant, which looks like cat's claws, as a daily tonic. In Peru it is best known for its anti-cancer properties, and has been well proven to stimulate phagocytosis, the process by which the body's immune system destroys misbehaving cells and unwanted organisms such as bacteria or viruses.

If you're fighting an infection, are run down or on the verge of a cold, taking 2g of cat's claw a day can really revive you fast. Make sure you buy a brand that is made from the bark of the tree, not the roots, as digging up the roots kills the plant and so is not a sustainable method of harvesting it.

Q *What's your view on cranberry?*

A Cranberries are much more than a garnish for the Christmas turkey. They have long been used as a traditional remedy for any bladder infections, especially by women suffering from cystitis. Now scientists have pinpointed a substance in cranberries called hippuric acid, which acidifies urine, making it more difficult for bacteria to survive, and also tougher for stones to form in the bladder or kidneys. Other substances in cranberries, proanthocyanidins, prevent bacteria from sticking to the urinary tract. So cranberries are great news, but not in just any form: most cranberry juices are laden with sugar, which isn't good for the immune system. So go for a pure powder extract of cranberry, which you can add to filtered water.

Q *What's your view on elderberry extract?*

A If you feel even the slightest hint of a sniffle, get some elderberry extract. Long hailed as a useful remedy for colds, it has now been shown in research to have a remarkable ability to fight off viruses in a number of ways. In fact, tests have shown that 90 per cent of people with flu felt completely better within three days after taking elderberry extract.

The cold virus is covered in tiny spikes that, aided by a special substance, puncture your cells, get inside them and ultimately make you feel ill. Elderberry works against the virus on various fronts. First, it can smother the spikes and destroy their special coating. It can also boost your immune system so that it is more able to fight off any infection in the first place, and it is rich in flavonoids, which work with vitamin C, another powerful cold-fighter. Elderberry extract comes in delicious syrups which are good for children and adults alike. Have a teaspoon or dessertspoon of this three times a day when you are fighting an infection (see Resources, page 483).

Q **How is ginger good for you?**

A Delicious as it is in stir-fries and gingerbread, there's a lot more to ginger root than just that distinctive flavour. It has been used medicinally for thousands of years in its native China, and even in the West, its healing properties have been exploited for at least 150 years. Its main uses are for soothing the digestive tract – it can help reduce nausea and vomiting, especially if you suffer from motion sickness. It's even been shown to help severe cases of morning sickness in pregnancy. Ginger also has powerful anti-inflammatory properties which people have found useful in soothing arthritic pain. This effect, combined with its ability to reduce blood stickiness, have made it helpful in combating migraine headaches.

For nausea, the best dosage appears to be 1 to 2g of dried root daily, or about a quarter-inch slice of the fresh root. For arthritis, you should take twice this. You can make your own ginger tea by putting fine slices in a thermos flask with the juice of half a lemon and a spoonful of honey – great for sore throats.

Q **What's your view on ginseng?**

A *Panax ginseng*, also known as Chinese or Korean ginseng, is an adaptogen – so-called because it can help you adapt to stress. American ginseng is another variant of *Panax*, but 'Siberian' ginseng is a completely different plant. Research has proven that *Panax ginseng* can boost energy, and improve resistance to and recovery from stress. It helps to balance your blood sugar and has proven helpful for diabetics, as well as having a mild effect on increasing libido. In short, ginseng helps you adapt to many of the health hurdles of 21st-century living, largely by regulating adrenal hormones. *Panax ginseng* may also reduce the side effects of corticosteroid drugs, which are taken for inflammatory conditions such as arthritis, asthma and eczema.

With its long history of use in the East, ginseng has proven to be non-toxic. You need 1 to 2g a day to experience the beneficial effects. Pick a packet that states the level of the active ingredients, called ginsenosides: a good ginseng product will contain 4 to 7 per cent of these.

Q *What's your view on grapefruit seed extract?*

A An essential item in your natural medicine chest, grapefruit seed extract is a powerful anti-viral, anti-fungal and anti-bacterial agent without anything like the damaging effect on beneficial gut bacteria that conventional antibiotics have. I never go travelling without it, and have often seen it sort out stomach bugs in hours. The extract can be used to treat many kinds of infection, from earaches to stomach bugs, and even athlete's foot.

It comes in drops, capsules, eardrops and a nasal spray. To fight an infection you need 10 drops, two or three times a day. It doesn't taste great, so either have it with some fruit juice or opt for capsules. Gargle with it if you have a sore throat. You can even use it to worm your pets!

Q *Is hemp seed oil good for you?*

A Hemp seeds are one of nature's superfoods. Better known as marijuana, this plant has seeds rich in essential fats that are important for countless uses in the body, not least your heart, your brain and your skin.

(The seeds won't make you high, and are treated so that they cannot be grown for other, better-known uses.) Hemp seeds are one of the richest plant sources of omega-3 fats, which make up a healthy brain and nervous system; keep your blood from getting too sticky and clotting too much; and are natural painkillers in conditions such as arthritis because of their anti-inflammatory properties. But the beauty of hemp oil is that it also contains an excellent balance of the important omega-6 fats. In fact, it is the only common seed oil that meets all your essential fat needs.

Q *I've heard kava described as 'Hawaii in a bottle'. What's your view?*

A Kava is probably why Pacific islanders are so chilled out: it can help relax both muscles and emotions, reduce excessive mind chatter, increase mental focus and expand overall awareness, all without causing addiction. Research shows that kava works just as well as well as Valium, but you don't need to keep increasing the dose to get the same effect, and there are no withdrawal problems when you stop taking it. It is great for specific anxiety-producing situations such as a job interview, or a final exam, where you want to be both calm and alert.

Note that at the moment, kava is banned in the UK due to a very small number of people with compromised livers or alcohol problems, or who were on liver-toxic medication, who also took kava and developed symptoms related to liver problems (see also 'Can kava damage your liver', below). Kava is not banned in the US.

The active ingredients in kava are called kavalactones. The taste is quite strong, and causes a brief numbing of the mouth and tongue. The recommended daily adult dose is 60 to 75 mg of kavalactones, taken two to three times daily – equivalent to 200 to 250 mg of standardised extract containing 30 per cent kavalactones. For sleep, getting high or an instant chill out, try double this amount. Don't combine with alcohol.

Q *Can kava damage your liver?*

A The South Pacific herb kava, which promotes relaxation and helps reduce anxiety and sleeping problems, has been banned in all EU countries following some cases in Germany where kava was associated with liver problems. Personally, I think this is likely to be a storm in a teacup since the majority of cases reported were of people who were either on prescribed drugs known to cause liver problems, or who had problems with alcohol. There were only two cases involving the kind of kava you could buy in the UK, and the outcome for these cases was far from clear. Clinical trials involving over 10,000 people on high amounts of kava have not discovered any liver problems in the people tested.

I hope the ban is rescinded in due course. Kava is

certainly a lot safer than tranquillisers, to which 1.5 million people in Britain are now addicted. Just ensure that you do not supplement kava along with prescribed drugs known to be taxing on the liver, or alcohol.

Q **What is your view on liquorice?**

A Even if you're not a fan of the Allsort, liquorice may well be what you need if you suffer from stress, infections, menstrual problems or ulcers. Liquorice has been used for thousands of years as a natural remedy and is one of the most popular components of Chinese medicines. It is also a common ingredient in natural cough remedies.

For people under long-term stress, liquorice supports the adrenal glands that provide the body's stress response. It also appears to help balance the hormones oestrogen and progesterone, thereby helping relieve premenstrual symptoms, especially if taken for two weeks before menstruation. Liquorice with one of the main ingredients removed, which is known as deglycyrrhizinated liquorice, or DGL, has been shown to be more effective at treating peptic ulcers than some of the most popular drugs for the condition.

Q **What's your view on milk thistle?**

A If you are a bit of a party animal, or become one around Christmas time, you'll be doing your liver a huge favour by getting hold of some milk thistle. This herb contains silymarin, one of the most powerful liver-protective substances known, which keeps toxins and oxidants – the reactive, destructive molecules also known as free radicals – at bay. Research has shown that silymarin is highly effective at protecting your liver against all sorts of poisons, from alcohol to toadstools, as well as pollution. It also encourages the growth of new liver cells to replace the old and damaged ones.

Be aware that taking milk thistle isn't a licence to abuse your liver, but you will certainly be better off for having some around during the party season. When you buy it, check that it contains at least 80 per cent silymarin.

Q *I've heard that certain mushrooms are very good for you. Which ones are they?*

A We're only just catching on now to the wonders of mushrooms that have been used in Japan and China medicinally for millennia. In addition to providing a great balance of nutrients such as proteins, minerals and vitamins, certain mushrooms have been investigated for their medicinal properties in preventing and treating some of the deadliest and most insidious diseases of our day, such as cancer and AIDS. Compounds in such mushrooms as maitake, shiitake, reishi and ganoderma have been isolated, and shown by research to fundamentally boost immunity and to be strongly anti-bacterial and anti-viral. Shiitake mushrooms, for example, contain something called lentinan, which has been proven to boost your immune system.

You can buy extracts of these mushrooms in tablet or liquid form, but it's probably best to eat the whole mushroom – that way, you'll benefit from the natural synergy of all the compounds. Luckily, they're as delicious as they are healthful. You can get fresh shiitake in most supermarkets. Otherwise, use dried ones from healthfood shops. Soak these in boiling water for 10 minutes and add (along with the strained soaking water) to soups, stir-fries, stews or risottos.

Q *What's your view on red clover?*

A Red clover, which is part of the legume family along with lentils and beans such as soya, is a rich source of the plant oestrogens known as isoflavones. Women with high levels of isoflavones in their diets not only lower their risk of developing breast cancer (and it also lowers the risk of developing prostate cancer in men), but also suffer from fewer symptoms of the menopause. In a study at Tufts University School of Medicine in the US, menopausal women given a concentrated supplement of red clover had half the incidence of hot flushes.

Isoflavones protect against breast cancer by blocking the receptor sites of oestrogen and hormone-disrupting chemicals, thereby preventing the oestrogen overload that stimulates excessive cell growth in both breast and womb. People whose diets include plenty of beans or lentils, especially soya or chickpeas, are much less likely to suffer such hormonal health problems. Alternatively, you can take a concentrated red clover supplement. Choose one that contains 40mg of isoflavones, equivalent to that consumed in a traditional Asian diet.

Q *What's your view on rhodiola?*

A Sometimes known as 'Arctic root' and a favourite with Chinese emperors, rhodiola isn't just the stuff of legend: it's clearly a herb for 21st-century living. The beneficial properties of this remarkable herb, first studied in Russia, are only just coming to light in the West.

Rhodiola's key properties centre around its ability to increase energy, boost endurance and increase alertness. It contains active ingredients which act as adaptogens in the body, improving how it deals with mental, physical and environmental stress. It stabilises the adrenal hormones and promotes the production of the 'happy' neurotransmitter serotonin. As a result, rhodiola also has a significant antidepressant effect. One study of 128 people taking rhodiola showed 64 per cent of them showed an improvement or a complete disappearance of symptoms such as fatigue, loss of strength, irritability, headache and decreased work capacity. Try taking 200 to 300mg of a standardised extract with meals.

Q *What's your view on sceletium?*

A Sceletium is one of the most ancient of mind-altering herbs. Hunter-gatherer tribes have used this native South African creeper, also called kou-goed, since prehistoric times. It lessens anxiety, stress and tension, raises spirits and enhances the sense of connection. Four hundred years of documented use by Dutch settlers have revealed no adverse effects, either. Psychiatrists have reported a wide range of positive uses for sceletium, from treating anxiety and depression to alleviating alcohol, cocaine and nicotine addiction. Sceletium has also been reported to enhance the experience of nature, increase the sensitivity of the skin and boost sexual arousal.

How does it work? Apart from being very rich in amino acids and minerals, the active constituents of the plant are alkaloids, including mesembrine, which enhances the activity of serotonin, the 'happy' neurotransmitter. It also appears to have a harmonising and balancing effect on the other feel-good neurotransmitters. It has no reported toxicity, but should not be taken with antidepressants, and as it has not been studied in pregnant women, it would be wise to avoid it during pregnancy. There are no reported cases, but it's theoretically possible that if taken with large amounts of tryptophan or 5-HTP, 'serotonin syndrome' – the symptoms of which are headache, higher body temperature and heavy sweating – could result.

Q **What's your view on sulphur?**

A Sulphur is a key mineral, one of the most crucial to life. A naturally occurring organic form of sulphur known as MSM has been found to have remarkable health benefits, promoting better hair, nails and skin, allergy relief and pain control. MSM helps the body build and repair, as well as calming down inflammation.

If you are prone to allergic or inflammatory health problems such as eczema, asthma or hay fever, MSM may provide substantial relief. People with chronic pain, perhaps frequent headaches, back or muscle pain, are reporting major improvement after supplementing 1 to 3g a day. Start with 1g for a week, then double the dose. However, don't expect results overnight. It often takes a week or two to work, and a few people have reported a flare-up of symptoms for a couple of days as sulphur helps the body detoxify and repair old injuries.

Other natural remedies

Q **Do anti-cellulite supplements really work?**

A Cellulite, one of the bugbears of the beauty industry, is simply hardened fat cells that make the skin look corrugated. This happens when fat cells become loaded with saturated (hard) fat, and when the body's ability to detoxify itself diminishes, at which point it dumps toxins out of the way in fat cells.

So the key to banishing cellulite is to cut right

back on saturated fat, which means less meat and dairy produce, and increase your intake of polyunsaturated oils from seeds, nuts, coldwater fish and their oils. Then, to boost your detox potential, you have to clean up your diet by eating lots of fresh fruit and vegetables, organic if possible, and staying away from junk food. Drink 1.5 litres of water every day and cut out alcohol and coffee, or decrease your intake of them drastically. The liver uses a whole host of vitamins to detoxify, so a good high-strength multi-vitamin plus 2g of vitamin C will make a difference. Anything to improve circulation is also good news, such as swimming, massage and skin brushing.

Most anti-cellulite supplements contain small amounts of some of these nutrients. However, I doubt very much that they will make any real difference unless you also change your diet.

Q *Do pills that claim to boost breast size work?*

A Pills claiming to increase breast size contain food sources of plant oestrogens, and while it is true that oestrogen stimulates breast growth, too much oestrogen is associated with increased risk for breast cancer. The advantage of plant oestrogens is that they are very weak compared to the real thing and can block oestrogen receptor sites, hence lowering the body's oestrogen load, not raising it. There is no evidence that people whose diet is high is plant oestrogens, such as the Japanese, have larger breasts, nor have the manufacturers been able to supply any clinical trials to back up the claims being made.

Q *How does light affect your health?*

A Ever wondered why a holiday in the sun leaves you feeling so good? Light is an often forgotten nutrient that tones up your immune system and boosts your mood. Quite apart from the positive associations we have with a sunny day, light is now known to stimulate the pineal gland, a tiny organ in the brain also known as the 'third eye'. The pineal gland produces certain types of important chemical called tryptamines that keep us feeling happy and 'connected' with nature. Melatonin, one type of tryptamine, keeps us tuned in to night and day and the seasons.

All this is to do with natural light. Artificial light is a very different proposition. Natural sunlight contains the full spectrum of different wavelengths that creates a 'white' light. Rainbows show the different wavelengths, broken up as bands of colour, which collectively make what we perceive as white light. Ordinary light bulbs do not produce the same kind of light. They contain a narrower band of wavelengths, and the light is yellower as a result. Fluorescent lighting is closer to natural, but the best indoor lighting is called 'full-spectrum' lighting, and it aims to mimic the wavelengths of natural light, including its benefits.

If you work indoors with little exposure to natural light, or if you're prone to the winter blues, it's certainly worth investing in full-spectrum light bulbs. Although they cost more, they last up to 100 times longer and use a quarter of the electricity of a normal bulb. (See Resources, page 483.)

Q *Can supplements help you tan?*

A Supplements containing carotenoids such as beta-carotene do have the effect of slightly colouring the skin as if you had a mild tan. You need about 20mg of beta-carotene a day for this effect, or just quaff a glass of carrot juice. The other way to get a fake tan is to use a skin cream containing dihydroxyacetone. This reacts with amino acids in the skin to provide an orange-brown shade after about three hours. It also provides some protection from harmful UVA rays. The best products also moisturise the skin and provide a guaranteed sun protection factor (try Dermalogica's Protective Self Tan SPF 15, for example – see www.dermalogica.com).

Either method is preferable to getting a suntan. Tanning ages the skin rapidly and increases the risk for skin cancer, especially if you have pale skin, red hair or a lot of moles. The worst combination is to drink alcohol and then get sunburnt, because alcohol suppresses the immune system's ability to repair DNA damage caused by intense sunlight. Supplementing a good antioxidant formula (see Resources, page 483) not only protects you from the damaging effects of sunlight but also gives you some beta-carotene for that natural glow.

MEN'S HEALTH

It seems strange that only a few decades ago, information on many issues to do with men's health were confined to chapters in medical textbooks. Some conditions, such as the male menopause, were virtually unheard of. Now all that has changed. The male menopause is undeniably real, and recognised as a common cause of decreased motivation, mood and sexual performance in middle-aged and older men. Prostate health is a widespread concern, too, and discussed here – although for information on prostate cancer, see the section on cancer, page 150.

Q **I'm 45 and have difficulty maintaining an erection. What can I do?**

A There are a number of potential biological reasons for this, and a range of natural solutions you can explore. A look at how Viagra works can help. Viagra promotes a key chemical involved in erections called nitric oxide, which is produced by the amino acid arginine. So supplementing arginine may help you. I'd recommend 2g a day. Another common cause is low levels of the hormone testosterone. This is quite common in men above the age of 40. I'd recommend you get your level checked: it should be above 12nmol/l.

Also worth a good look are a handful of natural aphrodisiacs that, at least anecdotally, have been reported to help sustain erections. These are ginseng, damiana, muira puama and maca. Ginseng is widely regarded as a 'sexual rejuvenator' and animal studies have shown it to increase testosterone levels, help the body adapt to stress and boost energy. You need about 1g a day of either *Panax ginseng* (standardised to 10 per cent ginsenosides) or Siberian ginseng (standardised to 1 per cent eleutherosides).

Damiana is a central American shrub that is said to stimulate production of testosterone, although the exact mechanism is not known. Try 400 to 800mg twice daily.

Muira puama is native to the Brazilian Amazon, and its workings, too, are shrouded in mystery. In a study in France, 62 per cent of men who took it claimed it had changed their lives. Try 1g a day.

Maca (*Lepidium meyenii*) is native to Peru's central highlands, where it has been used in traditional Andean culture to awaken healthy passion. Experiments on animals showed increased sexual performance and improved erectile function even in rats with their testes removed! Try 3 to 5g of ground

maca. You can find herbal remedies containing combinations of these herbs.

Q *When I hit 50 my weight went up and my energy
and sex drive went down dramatically. Is this the
male menopause, and what can I do about it?*

A Around a third of men in the 40 to 69 age group com-
plain of a range of symptoms that commonly include
loss of libido, erectile dysfunction (inability to get or
maintain an erection), depression, and worsening
memory and concentration. These are the classic
symptoms of the andropause – otherwise known as
the 'male menopause'.

Despite years of research – pioneered in Britain
by Dr Malcolm Carruthers, author of *The Testosterone
Revolution* – many doctors still deny the existence of
the male menopause. However, these symptoms, and
especially depression, should be taken seriously.
Depression in men is harder to diagnose since men
tend to get angry rather than sad. They are also more
likely to commit suicide. Luckily, there are many
ways of combating the andropause.

First off, if the symptoms above sound like
yours, it is well worth having your testosterone levels measured. If low, meaning below 12 nmol/l,
then you may benefit from testosterone replacement
therapy. However, symptoms are as important, if
not more so, than testosterone levels in the blood.
This is because most testosterone in the blood is

not 'free', but bound and consequently unavailable. If your doctor also measures your Sex Hormone Binding Globulin (SHBG) it is possible to estimate your level of 'free' testosterone. Salivary testosterone levels may be a better indicator, backed up by symptoms. You can both test your symptoms and get a salivary testosterone test by visiting www.andropause.com. The salivary test also measures your DHEA levels. These tests are also available through clinical nutritionists.

If you do have low testosterone, supplementing extra can really help. Dr Elizabeth Barrett-Connor studied 680 men aged between 50 and 89 and found a direct relationship between testosterone levels and mood. In the UK, Dr Carruthers has treated 1,500 men and found a consistent elevation in mood once testosterone levels become normal. Testosterone is only available on prescription from doctors.

From a nutritional point of view, make sure you are eating adequate protein and slow-releasing carbohydrates. Essential fats are required for healthy sperm and prostate function, antioxidant nutrients protect testosterone from being destroyed and zinc helps everything to do with male sexual health and hormonal balance.

DIG DEEPER: You might want to read Dr Carruther's *The Testosterone Revolution* (Thorsons, 1998) for more information on this essential hormone.

Q *I've been diagnosed with an enlarged prostate.
Can nutrition help?*

A An enlarged prostate is, at least in part, linked to hormonal imbalances, including oestrogen dominance and testosterone deficiency. These can leave the prostate inflamed.

The good news is that there are quite a few substances around that can help with this condition. Zinc (15mg a day) and vitamin E (400mg a day) regulate hormonal balance in the body. Essential fatty acids from fish or flax seed oil act as a natural anti-inflammatory. The herb saw palmetto is well known as a treatment for prostate problems, as are juniper berries and another herb, *Pygeum africanum*. Some herbal supplements contain a combination of these. An enlarged prostate has also been linked to exposure to oestrogen-like chemicals such as those in some pesticides and plastics. So try to eat organic whenever possible, and avoid plastic packaging, microwaving in plastic dishes and allowing clingfilm to touch the surface of stored foods. Natural plant substances found in lentils and soya can help counteract these oestrogen-like chemicals, so be sure to add these to your menus.

Otherwise, go for a sensible overall diet: avoid meat and milk, due to their hormone content; keep saturated fats very low; and eat wholegrains such as rye, good proteins such as tofu and other soya products, and plenty of fruit and vegetables which are high in the antioxidant vitamins A and C – sweet potatoes, carrots, watercress, broccoli, melon, pumpkin, tomatoes, cabbage, courgettes, apricots, cauliflower, lemons, mangoes, peppers, strawberries, oranges, grapefruit and kiwi fruit, among a host of others.

Q *My skin gets really irritated when I shave. Any suggestions?*

A Supersensitive skin is a very common problem among men. Generally speaking, the better your nutrition, the smoother your skin is likely to be, and the less likely it is to become inflamed. Eating a lot of fried food, or drinking a lot of alcohol and smoking, will all leave your skin ultrasensitive and prone to becoming sore and raw when you shave.

That's the inside-out story. You'll also need to look at the way you shave. When preparing for a shave, don't use very hot water on the skin as this will just irritate it before you've even begun. Most shaving foams are alkaline, stripping the skin of its acid mantle – use a shaving oil instead. The one I recommend is Dermalogica's Professional Shave, which contains essential oils that help to calm down the skin after shaving, too.

Another common mistake is to shave against the direction of hair growth. While this does give a closer shave, it further irritates the skin. It's better to shave in the direction of hair growth with a very sharp razor. Shaving effectively removes the top layer of skin cells, leaving the skin prone to inflammation, so after shaving, use a good moisturiser or apply some aloe vera gel.

Q *I keep getting thrush on my penis. What can I do to stop this?*

A Thrush, which is overgrowth of the *Candida albicans* fungus, is common. We all carry some *Candida albicans* in our large intestine, but if you eat the wrong kind of diet the fungus can get out of control. If your immune system is run down, or if your sexual partner has a low-grade infection, you are more likely to pick up thrush.

So, what should you do about it? I recommend a two-part strategy. Approach the problem from the outside by washing both before and after sex. Use a cream containing nystatin, which is an anti-fungal drug, locally. Three days of this should clear up the active infection. Then, be sure to keep yourself well aired. Fungi love warm, wet places, so wear cotton boxer shorts rather than tight pants. At the same time, aim to control candida from the inside out. Boost your immune system by taking vitamin C (try 2g a day), zinc, cats's claw and berry extracts. Control candida in the gut by supplementing a probiotic supplement providing both *Lactobacillus acidophilus* and *Bifidobacterium bifidum*. And maintain a candida-unfriendly diet, which means no sugar, yeast, alcohol and other fermented products.

MENTAL
HEALTH

Emotional wellbeing and clear thinking are as vital to health as a fit, well-nourished body. Yet according to the World Health Organization, mental health problems are fast becoming the number one health issue for the 21st century. One in 10 people is suffering from conditions such as depression at any point in time, and one in four is diagnosed with a mental health problem at some point in their life.

The statistics may be grim, but current research shows this story could have a very different ending – that the right nutrition can vanquish much of this misery, and even overturn serious psychosis. It has been found by some researchers, for instance, that supplementing large amounts of certain nutrients can alleviate the symptoms of schizophrenia. But optimum nutrition is also enormously effective at staving off depression, anxiety, poor concentration and all the other bugbears of our hectic lives. Here I deal with questions and concerns about a wide range of mental health issues relevant to all of us.

Alzheimer's and other forms of dementia (see also Memory)

Q *My mother has Alzheimer's. Is this hereditary?*

A The genetic predisposition to Alzheimer's is probably less than 10 per cent of the cause: this form of dementia is, like cancer and heart disease, largely preventable. We do, however, inherit bad habits! In fact, much of the same diet and lifestyle factors linked to heart disease apply to Alzheimer's as well. So, cut back on saturated fat, fried foods, alcohol, sugar and stress (see 'Can you prevent Alzheimer's', below, for full dietary guidelines on prevention).

One of the best predictors of Alzheimer's risk is your blood level of the amino acid homocysteine. If you are 65 and have a high level, this doubles your risk. This sounds like bad news, but isn't: you can lower your homocysteine in as little as two months by taking large daily amounts of B6 (100mg), B12 (100mcg) and folic acid (800mcg). Everyone would do well to supplement either a B complex or a multivitamin. Pick one that has the highest levels of these vitamins. Of course, the best thing is to know if you do have high homocysteine (see Resources, page 483).

Q *Can you prevent Alzheimer's?*

A Like many degenerative diseases, Alzheimer's stems primarily from not looking after your diet and lifestyle. The actual damage in the brain is caused by inflammation linked to too many oxidants – toxins generated from burning, whether from cigarettes, exhaust fumes, or fried or browned food.

Supplements are vital in treating dementia. High levels of the amino acid homocysteine in the blood can be an indicator of Alzheimer's, so taking the vitamins that lower homocysteine levels is crucial – that means B1, B3, B5, B6, folic acid and B12. The antioxidant nutrients such as vitamins A and C and particularly E are other important preventatives, helping to prevent oxidative damage from pollution and toxins. Eat plenty of fresh fruit and vegetables (aim for a mix of all colours, ranging from blueberries, beetroot, carrots and yellow peppers to green vegetables), and supplement with an all-round antioxidant supplement. The minerals zinc (15mg) and selenium (200mcg) are also important antioxidants; ensure your supplement has these as well as lipoic acid, NAC, glutathione, co-enzyme Q10 and anthocyanidins. A diet rich in vitamin E, found in seeds and fish, cuts risk by over 60 per cent. Supplementing vitamin E has proven better than the best drug for reducing symptoms in those with Alzheimer's.

Omega-3 fats, especially DHA found in oily fish, are helpful because of their anti-inflammatory properties. DHA also keeps the brain healthy by replenishing the fatty acids that make up brain cells. Try eating oily fish such as mackerel or wild or organic salmon three times a week, and supplementing 600mg of the omega-3 EPA and 400mg of DHA. The chemicals phosphatidyl choline and phosphatidyl serine aid mind and memory and are found in lecithin, so you can boost your levels by sprinkling a teaspoon of high phosphatidyl choline lecithin granules (known as Hi-PC lecithin) on your cereal in the morning. Otherwise, 'smart nutrients' such as glutamine (1,000mg), gingko biloba (150mg), pyroglutamate (250mg) and DMAE (100mg), found in many 'brain food' formulas, can help. And keep your mind and body active: exercise, and even just doing a daily crossword, can make a real difference.

Q *I've heard that Alzheimer's is caused by too much aluminium – what's your view?*

A While plenty of studies have shown increased accumulation of aluminium in the brains of people diagnosed with Alzheimer's disease, what isn't clear is whether this is a cause or a consequence of the disease. The likelihood is that it's a bit of both and is a significant contributor to memory problems. In a study in the 1980s of 647 Canadian gold miners who had routinely inhaled aluminium since the 1940s (once a common practice thought to prevent silica poisoning), all tested in the 'impaired' range for cognitive function, suggesting a clear link between aluminium and memory loss.

Aluminium is all around us – in aspirin, antacids, antidiarrhoeal drugs, cake mixes, self-raising flour, processed cheese, baking powder, drinking water, milk, talcum powder, tobacco smoke, drink cans, cooking utensils and pans, air pollution compounds and aluminium foil. It is poorly absorbed by the body unless you are zinc deficient, which half of the population are. It also becomes much more absorbable in acidic conditions. So if, for example, you boil tea (containing tannic acid) or rhubarb (containing oxalic acid), in an old aluminium pan, you can leach aluminium from the pan into the food or drink.

Your aluminium level is easily tested in a hair mineral analysis. If your level is high, it's important to identify the potential sources in your diet and lifestyle, and reduce them. I have often seen high levels in people who grill food directly on aluminium foil.

Q *Is there a link between mercury fillings and Alzheimer's?*

A I think the mercury in fillings is a serious cause for concern in relation to Alzheimer's and age-related memory loss. Autopsies of brains from Alzheimer's patients, compared to control patients of the same age, have shown raised levels of mercury. Researchers from the University of Basel in Switzerland have also found high blood mercury levels in Alzheimer's patients, more than double those of the control groups, with early-onset Alzheimer's patients having the highest mercury levels of all. Trace amounts of mercury can cause the type of damage to nerves that is characteristic of Alzheimer's, according to recent research at the University of Calgary Faculty of Medicine in Canada, strongly suggesting that the small amounts we are exposed to, for example from amalgam fillings, may be contributing to memory loss.

Although research on the links between mercury and Alzheimer's is in its infancy, it is certainly wise to reduce your exposure to this highly toxic metal. If you are experiencing significant decline in mental function, and have a mouth full of amalgam fillings, I'd recommend you seriously consider having them replaced. (See also 'Can Alzheimer's ever be reversed?', below.)

Q Can Alzheimer's ever be reversed?

A Yes, it can. The best case I know is that of Tom Warren. He was diagnosed with Alzheimer's disease in 1983 and was told by his doctor that he might have as long as seven years to live and there wasn't anything he could do. Brain scans confirmed that his brain was effectively shrinking. But today, Tom is completely cured of his dementia. His brain scans are normal and his mind is in tip-top condition. He has written two books about his experience (*Beating Alzheimer's* and *Reversing Chronic Disease*). His remarkable method involved getting all the mercury out of his mouth, dramatically improving his nutrition with diet and supplements, and eliminating all the substances he was allergic and chemically sensitive to.

I believe many people who are heading down the

path towards Alzheimer's are 'intoxicated' by environmental poisons – of which mercury from fillings is a prime candidate – and sub-optimally nourished. The brain, like any other organ, can't survive under these circumstances. I haven't heard of anyone reversing Alzheimer's with prescribed medication. However, it takes immense courage and determination to make all the changes to reverse such a condition. The important point is that it can be done, as Tom Warren's story shows.

Bipolar disorder/manic depression

Q *What causes manic depression, and what supplements can help to keep it under control?*

A People with manic depression experience swings from low moods to relatively normal or more or less manic periods. Quite a few people with the condition spend most of their time either in a normal mood or mildly depressed, although some people have severe, dramatic mood swings that can disrupt their lives and lead to breakdowns.

My first recommendation to someone with manic depression would be a full consultation with a nutritionist. They will be able to help you get to the root of your depression (the psychological angle aside) and give you a personally tailored nutritional strategy to help relieve your symptoms.

If mood changes are not owing to any drug intake (caffeine, alcohol or cocaine), the possibility of food allergy or hypoglycaemia should be carefully investigated. If your blood sugar levels are in serious imbalance, severe mood swings can result. Heavy stress may dissipate all the body's store of zinc and B6 so that the person becomes pyroluric, producing excessive amounts of chemicals called pyrroles, which can cause extreme mood swings, among a host of other symptoms ranging from nervous exhaustion to depression, seizures and confusion. Many patients with a diagnosis of manic depression who have weekly swings in mood are merely pyroluric, and are easily treated with adequate zinc and B6. A simple urine test can determine whether you have the condition. This test is available through nutritional therapists but sadly not through doctors. A hyperactive thyroid can induce mania, while an underactive thyroid can trigger depression, so thyroid function is well worth investigating.

Another possible factor in any type of depression is a lack of light. Some people suffer depression only in the winter and are diagnosed with seasonal affective disorder or SAD. Since light has a powerful effect on brain hormone balance, treatment via light boxes does produce beneficial results in some SAD patients (see Resources, page 483, for information on full spectrum lighting).

Lithium therapy is another possible treatment; numerous publications cite it as useful in treating chronic depression, alcoholism, premenstrual depression and hyperthyroidism. Under the guidance of a nutrition therapist it may be worth trying the amino acid tryptophan or 5-HTP in the normal phase and tyrosine in the depression phase. (See Resources, page 483, for a list of nutrition therapists.)

Concentration

Q **What foods improve your concentration?**

A The answer is eggs and fish. But they've got to be the right kind. Carnivorous, oily, fatty – whatever you call them, herring, wild or organic salmon, mackerel and trout contain the essential omega-3 fats that are proven to sharpen your mind. In fact, blood levels of omega-3s in newborn infants correlate with their IQ at the age of five. If you don't like eating fish, supplement an omega-3-rich fish oil every day. Oily fish, and especially sardines, also contain pyroglutamate, an amino acid that improves concentration.

Eggs, on the other hand, contain phospholipids that also help improve memory and concentration. But don't fry them, as this destroys the valuable nutrients, and always go for organic and/or free range. Columbus free-range eggs, available in your supermarket, are also rich in omega-3 fats because they feed their chickens a diet high in them.

Q **My daughter has exams coming up. What helps brain function?**

A There are lots of nutrients that can help brainpower and stress reduction in the run-up to exams. Some 20 per cent of the brain's dry weight is made up of the same kind of fats found in fish oils, which optimise the health of brain cells and the way they fire information to one another. Stress triggers the release of hormones that interfere with the way these fats are processed in the body, so taking supplements can bypass this interference. A recent study in Japan showed that students who took omega-3 fats in fish oils were calmer at exam time than those who took a dummy pill. Another group of nutrients important for helping the body cope with stress are the B vitamins, so your daughter could take a B complex daily, or a high-strength multivitamin. If she's particularly stressed, especially on the night before exams, give her 300mg of magnesium, which relaxes both mind and muscles.

Depression and anxiety

Q *I'm depressed and my doctor wants to put me on anti-depressants. Is there an alternative?*

 Emphatically, yes. Did you know that exercising more, keeping a diary and owning a cat are equally, if not more, effective than anti-depressant drugs? Simple things like going for walks in the countryside, or having someone to talk to, really do help put things into perspective. That said, many people, especially women, do suffer from low levels of the mood-boosting neurotransmitter serotonin. This is made directly from tryptophan, an amino acid found in dietary protein. Most weight-loss diets are low in tryptophan so, if you are on such a diet, or don't eat enough protein, you can end up going short. A form of tryptophan called 5-hydroxytryptophan (5-HTP) is the most easily used by the brain, and so is the best way to maintain normal serotonin levels and, through that, your moods. Beans are rich in 5-HTP, but I'd recommend supplementing it at 100mg, twice a day.

What you're eating and drinking may also be triggering negative feelings. I'd recommend avoiding all stimulants such as coffee, tea, cigarettes and sugar or sugary foods and drinks. These can cause anxiety as well as swings in mood, energy and concentration. Make sure you're eating plenty of fresh fruit and vegetables, wholegrains such as brown rice, and fibre such as beans and lentils, and keep up your intake of fish and chicken. A prime way of combating depression is to boost your levels of omega-3 essential fats, found in oily fish and flax seeds. These fats are abundant in the brain and essential for it to function, and there is increasing evidence that supplementing them can help many people prone to depression. In addition, I suggest you take a multivitamin high in B vitamins.

Finally, the herb St John's wort is becoming the top natural treatment for mild to moderate depression, with all the benefits of medication and none of the side effects. Take 300mg of the herb, standardised to contain 0.3 per cent hypericin, three times daily. I'd try 5-HTP first, and then St John's wort, each for two weeks. In the meantime take on all these suggestions – walking, a better diet, omega-3 fish oil supplementation, vitamins and cutting out stimulants and sugar – for a month before you decide to take anti-depressants.

Q **I'm often panicky, get mood swings and am always tired. Can nutrition help?**

A Sounds like you're adrenally exhausted. Your adrenal glands, which sit on top of the kidneys, produce hormones that help you cope with the ups and downs of life. However, if you overwork the adrenal glands they'll eventually underfunction. The classic signs are feeling tired on waking, unable to cope with stress, and experiencing sudden moods swings and general anxiety.

There are two ways to bring you back to balance. Firstly, stop stressing yourself out. The more sugar, coffee, nicotine and stress you consume or expose yourself to, the more adrenally exhausted you'll become. Secondly, you can support normal, healthy adrenal function with certain nutrients and herbs. Two amino acids, the constituents of protein, called tyrosine and dl-phenylalanine, are the building blocks of your stress hormones. Then there are the adaptogenic herbs Chinese ginseng, Siberian ginseng (eleutherococcus), rhodiola, ashwaganda and reishi. These help you to adapt to stress by supporting normal, healthy adrenal function. Alternatively, try supplementing 2g of tyrosine (see Resources, page 483).

Q *I'm prone to anxiety attacks. Which natural remedies can help?*

A If you are deficient in B vitamins or magnesium, this can leave your nervous system more hyped up. As a result, you can overreact to stress and find it harder to relax and to sleep. The easiest way to test this is to take a B complex supplement and 300mg of magnesium every day. Another possible factor is your blood sugar. If you crave sweet foods or stimulants such as tea, coffee, chocolate or cigarettes, you may have poor blood sugar control. Again, this can lead to overreactions to stressful situations. The solution here is to eat wholefoods and enough protein to balance out your carbohydrates, which will have a stabilising effect on your blood sugar levels. This means ensuring you have a handful of seeds with fruit, hummus with oatcakes, tofu or chicken with rice or potatoes and so on. Supplementing 200mcg of chromium can help, too.

With the recent ban on off-the-shelf kava kava, the most effective anti-anxiety herb, you need to look elsewhere for remedies. GABA is one. Anxiety arises when the body overproduces the stress hormone adrenalin. The body's own antidote to this is GABA, an amino acid. You can buy GABA in healthfood stores: take 500mg or 1,000mg when you are feeling anxious. However, don't overdo it – 5,000mg will make most people nauseated. Another amino acid, taurine, has a similar effect. The best available herbal remedies are hops, passion flower and valerian. Valerian is the strongest, although be aware that it also makes you sleepy. Combinations of these herbs and amino acids are most effective for relieving anxiety. (See Resources, page 483.)

It is vital to get to the root of what's making you anxious. A reputable counsellor or therapist can help. Or consider taking up yoga, t'ai chi or meditation to help you respond more calmly to life's inevitable stresses.

Q **What's your view on Prozac? I have just come off it after two years and am feeling very depressed, tearful and irritable.**

A Prozac belongs to the family of anti-depressants called serotonin reuptake inhibitors (SSRIs). These give serotonin, the brain's natural happy chemical, more 'miles per gallon'. Do they work? Yes, in roughly half of cases, but the side effects can be depressing in themselves. About a quarter of people on SSRIs experience a lowered libido, flattened moods, nausea, headaches and insomnia, to name just a few. What's more, the positive effects tend to wear off after six months to a year. Why? Probably because taking these anti-depressants does nothing to correct the underlying deficiency in serotonin.

The nutritional solution is to supplement the building blocks for serotonin, the amino acids trypto-phan or hydroxytryptophan, known as 5-HTP. Some supplements combine 5-HTP with niacin, folic acid, B6, and zinc, which all help the brain keep your neurotransmitters in balance. But there are plenty of other ways to raise serotonin levels: by meeting friends regularly or taking up a group activity such as dance, getting a hug from a partner, going for a brisk walk, increasing our exposure to daylight, reading an amusing book. Psychotherapy and counselling can help give you that extra boost you might need to get your life back on track.

Certain foods can also help you banish depression. Research is revealing that omega-3 fatty acids help with a number of mood disorders, so make sure you are eating cold-water fish such as salmon (go for wild or organically farmed) and mackerel three times a week, or sprinkle ground flax seeds on your cereal in the morning. I also recommend supplementing an omega-3-rich fish oil. Magnesium strengthens the nervous system, so eat plenty of magnesium-rich foods such as wheatgerm, cashew nuts, Brazil nuts, almonds, beans and peas, and include 200mg in your daily supplement programme. (See Resources, page 483, for supplement suppliers.)

Q *I'm on anti-depressant medication (Seroxat) and want to come off. How can I do this?*

A Any change in your medication *must* be agreed with your doctor, and should really be done under the guidance of a health care practitioner. Many people experience cessation effects when coming off such anti-depressants and the slower you do it, the better.

It's likely that cessation effects occur because anti-depressant drugs don't deal with the underlying cause of depression, which in many cases is serotonin deficiency. While the drugs do promote serotonin uptake as long as you're on them, once you're off them you're back to square one.

Supplementing the amino acid 5-HTP, together with tyrosine, B vitamins, TMG (trimethylglycine) and zinc, helps to restore normal serotonin levels. Some supplements contain these nutrients in combination (see Resources, page 483). Fish oils rich in the omega-3 fatty acids EPA and DHA are also very important for people who have been on anti-depressants, as shown in a recent study in the *American Journal of Psychiatry* (Nemets and others, March 2002). The recommended dose is 1,200mg of EPA/DHA; if you take fish oil supplements with 800mg of these fatty acids per capsule, that will mean taking two a day.

With the agreement of your doctor and under the supervision of a nutritional therapist, I would suggest gradually reducing the anti-depressant over three weeks and gradually increasing the supplemental levels of these nutrients.

Q *Since starting anti-depressants I've been getting angrier. Is this possible?*

A Yes, and it's not that uncommon. The serotonin reuptake inhibitors Prozac and Seroxat, two of the most frequently prescribed anti-depressants, have clearly been shown to cause agitation leading to potential aggressive and suicidal behaviour in as many as one in five patients, according to studies conducted by the drug companies themselves but only recently released in court. Last summer the family of a man who shot others and himself after taking anti-depressants won a court case against the makers, and were awarded $6.4 million. Dr David Healy of the North Wales Department of Psychological Medicine in Bangor, an expert witness in the case, reckons that these anti-depressants often cause aggressive reactions and both patients and doctors should be warned of this.

In my view, many people who are depressed are low in the brain chemical serotonin because they don't get enough of the nutrient tryptophan. By supplementing tryptophan, or 5-HTP, which is available in health-food stores, this deficiency symptom goes away, without all the side effects of anti-depressant drugs. Also effective, and safer, is the herb St John's wort and omega-3 fats (see 'I'm on anti-depressant medication', page 363, and 'I keep hearing mixed reports', below).

Q *I keep hearing mixed reports – is St John's wort really as good as anti-depressants?*

A The answer to that is pretty much a categorical yes for people with mild to moderate depression. There have been numerous studies backing this up, most recently one reported in the *British Medical Journal*. This found St John's wort to be more effective than the tricyclic anti-depressant imipramine. A group of 324 patients were given either St John's wort or an anti-depressant. Although both were equally effective in reducing the depression, St John's wort was better tolerated, in that the people had fewer side effects.

Remember that depression can have various causes, so for some people, St John's wort does not work. It may be a case of dealing with an issue, say with a therapist, or sorting out other slight chemical imbalances such as blood sugar levels or nutrient deficiencies that can be done with the help of a nutritionist. (For general dietary guidelines, see also 'I'm depressed', page 358.)

Q *I've been taking St John's wort and I'm on the Pill. Should I stop the St John's wort?*

A There isn't any direct research that shows taking St John's wort while you're on the Pill is dangerous, but I wouldn't recommend it. St John's wort accelerates certain biochemical pathways in the liver that can, in some cases, make certain medications less effective because they are processed more quickly by the liver and therefore effectively lowers their effect. More important, perhaps, is the fact that taking the Pill can actually trigger depression in the first place because it depletes certain nutrients. That doesn't necessarily mean you should stop taking the Pill; rather, that you would do well to increase your vitamin C (1g a day) and B vitamin intake, especially B6 (50mg a day) plus zinc and magnesium by taking a high-strength multivitamin. Deficiencies in these important nutrients can contribute to low moods. Take 1g of vitamin C and 50mg of B6 daily.

Q *What's your view on valerian?*

A Used by the ancient Greeks as a sedative, valerian is the most popular natural remedy for insomnia. It's no mystery: it really does work. Many studies have shown that valerian root makes you go to sleep faster and keeps you there longer. Valerian is also useful as a sedative at times of stress and anxiety, and as a painkiller. It appears to bind to the same brain receptors as Valium and other tranquilliser drugs. In trials comparing valerian with such drugs, it appears to have a similar sedative effect but not the same side effects, such as daytime drowsiness.

It comes either as a dried root or as a standardised powdered extract. For a standardised extract (usually 0.8 per cent valeric acid) you need 300mg half an hour before bed, as compared to 1,000mg or 2,000mg of the dried root. (See Resources, page 483.)

Q *I suffer from seasonal affective disorder (SAD) in the winter. What can I do?*

A You're not alone. Three million people in Britain officially suffer from SAD, and the real figure is

probably double. SAD is caused by low levels of serotonin, the 'happy' brain chemical, brought on by the
lack of light during the winter months.

Apart from emigrating, there are two things you
can do. The first is to get more light. You could start
by doing this simple exercise. Place an anglepoise
lamp containing a 60-watt opaque (not clear) bulb,
preferably with no writing on it, about a metre away
and directly in line with your line of vision. Make
sure you can turn the light on and off without moving your head. Turn the light on and look directly at
the bulb for *one* minute, no longer. After one minute,
turn the light off, close your eyes (put on a blindfold
if the room is not completely dark) and focus on the
after-image, the phosphene, without moving your
head, until it completely vanishes. This usually takes
three to four minutes.

The second vital task is to get to grips with your
nutritional needs. Balance your energy by eating a
wholefood diet rich in oily fish, nuts, seeds and
wholegrains, and lots of fresh fruit and vegetables,
while limiting the sugary foods and refined carbohydrates that can play havoc with your blood sugar
levels and moods. Supplement-wise, take a good
multivitamin and mineral supplement, plus the
amino acids phenylalanine or tyrosine (2g of either
or 1g of both), and 1.5g of tryptophan or 150mg of
5-HTP (the chemical from which the brain makes
serotonin), or 200mg of SAMe or 600mg of TMG
(trimethylglycine). SAMe is an amino acid that has
been well proven to boost mood by helping the

brain make serotonin. SAMe is, however, very expensive and unstable, so you might choose to take the amino acid TMG from which it is made. You need three times as much of TMG, but it is both cheaper and more stable. Some supplements provide all these nutrients in combination. (See Resources, page 483.)

Eating disorders

Q *I've heard zinc can help anorexia. Is this true?*

A Quite simply, yes. Although anorexia nervosa has deep-seated psychological aspects, ensuring a good supply of the mineral zinc has been shown to help speed recovery. One study showed that anorexics gained weight twice as quickly when they took zinc.

There are various reasons why zinc supplementation may be useful. One is that it is involved in appetite control and taste – so both would go if you were low in zinc. Studies have shown more than half of anorexics have zinc deficiencies. Since zinc is needed by the body to digest and use protein, an anorexic would need extra zinc once they started to eat and gain weight. Studies have also shown that taking zinc supplements help improve mood and reduce anxiety – which can help anorexics deal with the psychological aspects of their condition. So I recommend supplementing 30mg of zinc daily in addition to any other help they are getting.

Q *My daughter's recovering from bulimia. Is there anything I can do nutritionally to help?*

A First of all, many people who binge are drawn to wheat, sugar or milk-based foods. Wheat and milk both contains exorphins, substances that make you feel good, much like chocolate. The more you eat, the more you want to eat. I have had great success asking people to binge on anything, if they have to, but not on wheat or milk-based foods. Of course, some people binge on sugar. Here, the trick is to regulate your blood sugar. If the level of glucose in the blood goes too low, any of us can end up craving something sweet; so keep blood sugar up to a healthy level by snacking on fruit, preferably with a small handful of seeds and/or nuts, as soon as you start getting hungry, grouchy or tired.

The mineral zinc, which controls normal appetite reflexes, is another deficiency in those with anorexia and bulimia. Make sure your daughter supplements 10 to 15mg of zinc. Most good multis will give you 10mg.

Memory (see also Alzheimer's)

Q *What can I do to improve my memory?*

A The main 'memory molecule' in the brain is acetyl-choline. If the brain makes enough of it, your memory and concentration will be sharp. Many drugs designed to treat Alzheimer's try to promote this effect. Acetylcholine is made directly from phosphatidyl choline, which is found in eggs and organ meats such as liver. A precursor of phosphatidyl choline, called DMAE, is abundant in sardines. Also vital is phosphatidyl serine, which improves the brain's receptivity for acetylcholine. Phosphatidyl serine is the first nutrient the US Food and Drug Administration have allowed claims for, stating that it may reduce risk of dementia in the elderly. These three nutrients certainly help to support normal memory. Another brain-friendly nutrient is the omega-3 family of fats, found in fatty fish and fish oil supplements as well as flax seeds.

I believe memory need not decline as you get older, provided you are optimally nourished. Try supplementing 300mg of phosphatidyl serine a day, or adding a tablespoon of lecithin, which is rich in phosphatidyl choline, on your cereal. Also supplement an omega-3-rich fish oil capsule – about 1,000mg of EPA/DHA a day is effective. And finally, keep your brain active. Read, write, think, create, paint, play or compose music, even do the crosswords: whatever it is, use it or you really will lose it.

Q *I suffered a head injury 25 years ago and was in a coma for a month. I still have learning, memory and attention problems. What do you suggest?*

A For all these conditions, I recommend a combination of amino acids and herbs to stimulate memory and sharpen the mind; phospholipids, which are abundant in lecithin granules (sprinkle a tablespoon on your morning cereal each day); and omega-3 fish oil (aim to get 1,000mg of EPA/DHA, so take about three to four capsules a day, depending on the amount each capsule contains). In addition, a good antioxidant will help to protect the brain from oxidation – the damage caused by pollution and internal biochemical processes. The best brain food formulas provide phospholipids such as phosphatidyl serine and choline, plus DMAE and pyroglutamate, as well as gingko biloba. (See Resources, page 483.)

Q *I've heard ginkgo biloba is good for the memory – is that true?*

A Ginkgo biloba is a herbal remedy that has been used for memory enhancement in the East for thousands of years. It comes from one of the oldest species of tree known. Research has shown that it improves short-term and age-related memory loss, slow thinking, depression, circulation and blood flow to the brain. It has also been seen to have positive effects on Parkinson's and Alzheimer's diseases. Not all studies, however, have proven positive. It tends to be most effective as a mild brain enhancer for older people.

Gingko usually comes in capsule form and you should look for a brand that shows the flavonoid concentration, which determines strength. The recommended flavonoid concentration is 24 per cent; take 120 to 160mg of these supplements in two to three divided doses. I recommend that you try gingko for three months before evaluating the results, as the effects aren't often immediate.

Schizophrenia

Q *My son has been diagnosed with schizophrenia. Can this be linked to poor nutrition?*

A There is a very strong link between nutrition and schizophrenia. Some people tend to make certain abnormal chemicals in the brain more easily; and when the person is also deficient in certain nutrients, these brain chemicals can trigger the symptoms of schizophrenia, such as abnormal fears, hearing or seeing things, blank mind, compulsive behaviour, mood swings and depression. Supplementing large amounts of vitamin B3, B6, B12, folic acid and zinc have all been shown to help and sometimes cure schizophrenia.

In fact, one of Canada's former research directors for mental illness, the psychiatrist Dr Abram Hoffer, has treated 5,000 patients in this way and claims a very high success rate using nutritional approaches.

I strongly recommend you take your son to see a clinical nutritionist trained in this area. There are many avenues for them to explore. For instance, Dr Iain Glen of Aberdeen University's mental health department has found that 80 per cent of schizophrenics are deficient in the essential fatty acids found in oily fish, nuts and seeds. A lack of the antioxidant vitamins A, C and E could be a factor, as could allergies, blood sugar imbalances or high levels of histamine, a body chemical released during allergic reactions that is high in some people with schizophrenia.

Q *I am a schizophrenic and vegan, and am concerned that I am unable to convert EPA from flax seeds. What dosage would you recommend?*

A Many schizophrenics have been found to be deficient in the omega-3 fats DHA and EPA, which are essential for optimal brain function. These fats are found in oily fish and the oils extracted from them, but strict vegans would not regard that as an option. Your best option is therefore flax seeds, which contain the omega-3 fat alpha-linolenic acid (ALA) that can be converted by the body into EPA and DHA. However, as you've indicated, there can be a catch: quite a few people have a lazy enzyme that cannot convert ALA into DHA and EPA so easily. Now, you can take a vegan algae supplement to get the DHA, but it is the EPA that has proven helpful for some people with schizophrenia. It's up to you: either eat a heaped tablespoon of flax seeds a day in the hope that it will do the job, or break the rules and take a fish oil supplement.

And that's not the whole story. Further research has shown that the majority of people diagnosed with schizophrenia have an over-active enzyme, called phospholipase A2, that strips fat from the brain, hence increasing their need for both omega-3 and omega-6 fats. That means that supplementing with *both* omega-3s and omega-6s – EPA, DHA and GLA, the most important omega-6 fat – is the best choice. With that in mind, and given that not all schizophrenics respond well to essential fatty acid supplementation anyway, I'd recommend you see a nutritional therapist to sort out the best route for you (see Resources, page 483).

DIG DEEPER: For more on nutrition and mental health, covering a range of conditions from autism to schizophrenia, see my book *Optimum Nutrition for the Mind* (Piatkus, 2003) and visit www.mentalhealthproject.com.

SEX

Profoundly relaxing yet invigorating, sex adds a vital dimension to our lives, and is a wonderful antidote to the crazed pace of our century. But when we're sub-optimally nourished, it's not just our skin, hair or moods that can suffer – it's our sex lives, too. Optimum nutrition can bring the zing back to sexual performance and enjoyment; and supplementing with certain important nutrients can also sort out a number of sexual problems, as these questions show.

Q *I get depressed when my girlfriend and I have sex a lot. Why?*

A Although most people walk around on cloud nine when they're getting lots of loving, there is a very good reason why you are down in the dumps. Sperm is loaded with zinc and a man loses about 3mg of zinc with each ejaculation. Thus you could easily end up low in this important nutrient. Depression is just one symptom of a deficiency in zinc; another is impotence, so you're right to be concerned.

If you have made a definite link between lots of

sex and your moods, then increase your intake of zinc-rich foods – that means eating more oysters, meats, nuts, eggs and wholegrains. Also take a multi-vitamin that contains at least 15mg of zinc.

Q *I heard about supplements that can give your libido a boost. Which are the best?*

A There are several natural substances around that enhance sex drive, all of which claim to make bed-time (or perhaps any time) more alluring. B vitamins are needed for testosterone production – and a defi-ciency in testosterone causes low sex drive in both men and women – as well as adrenal support, energy production and healthy nerves. So you could take a high-strength multivitamin or B complex. On the herb front, there's ginseng, Muira puama and maca as well as damiana. If taking damiana alone, try 400 to 800mg twice daily. Ginseng is widely regarded as a sexual rejuvenator, and animal studies have shown ginseng to increase testosterone levels, help the body adapt to stress and boost energy. You need about 1g a day of either *Panax ginseng* (standardised to 10 per cent ginsenosides) or Siberian ginseng (standardised to 1 per cent eleutherosides). Muira pauma, native to the Brazilian Amazon, is traditionally used to allevi-ate menstrual cramps and the discomforts of the menopause – that is, it tones up the female sex organs. Try 1g a day. Maca (*Lepidium meyenii*) is native to Peru's central highlands, where it has been used in traditional Andean culture to awaken healthy passion. Try 3 to 5g ground up. These amounts are for the individual herbs, so I'd try one or two at a time – otherwise you might be up all night!

Q **Are oysters really an aphrodisiac?**

A One oyster contains about 15mg of zinc – so you're certainly charging yourself up by eating half a dozen for dinner. Why? The mineral zinc is crucial for healthy sperm and for the healthy growth of a baby. Not only is zinc vital for male fertility, it is vital for women's too. Research has found that men low in zinc were found to be low in testosterone, have a low sex drive and a low sperm count. So, given that the average man only takes in 7.6mg of zinc a day from his diet, a plate of oysters on the half shell is probably a very good idea on a romantic evening.

Q **I rarely have orgasms. Have you got any suggestions?**

A You are not alone. One survey in the US found that as many as one in three women rarely achieved orgasms with sex. Apart from technique, and there are many books now that explain how to maximise stimulation, there are some biochemical imbalances that can lower your odds of having an orgasm.

If you have a hormonal imbalance resulting in too

little testosterone, you may have difficulty attaining orgasm. Testosterone is made from progesterone and many women have low levels. A nutritional therapist can measure your progesterone and testosterone levels in saliva and advise you on what to do. Studies have shown that giving women testosterone implants raises their sex drive – with significant improvements in sexual desire, fantasy and response and a decrease in painful sex due to lack of excitement and lubrication.

I suspect that our ever-increasing exposure to oestrogen-like compounds found in pesticides, some plastics, household cleaning products, industrial pollutants and pharmaceutical drugs may be messing up the normal hormone production and messaging that contributes to a healthy sexual system. When men are exposed to high amounts of such so-called xeno-oestrogens, they can develop female characteristics such as breast growth. At the same time, these chemicals affect sex drive and other particularly male characteristics such as muscular strength and development.

Q *When I'm working hard or stressed my sex drive nose-dives. Why is this?*

A Stress is unquestionably a major cause of declining libido. Although the body needs its stress response to deal with everyday life, if stress is prolonged or extreme, the response can have negative effects on many aspects of health – including hormone balance.

Testosterone is a steroid hormone, derived from

cholesterol. Another important steroid hormone is cortisol, which is secreted as part of the body's response to stress. Both testosterone and cortisol are derived from progesterone. At times of stress, progesterone may make cortisol in preference to testosterone to help you cope with the strain, and this can leave you short on testosterone – and hence sex drive. Although in more serious cases, testosterone medication (on prescription only) may help, it is not getting to the root cause of the deficiency.

The real answer is to chill out, take some time off and give your sex drive breathing space.

Q *Is it bad to have too much sex?*

A From a nutritional point of view, it becomes bad for a man to have too much sex because it usually results in a depletion of zinc, among other nutrients, through ejaculation. Sperm is incredibly rich in nutrients and, in a sense, too many ejaculations rob you of these. Of course, provided you replace the zinc and other minerals, vitamins and essential fats, there should be no problem.

Interestingly, the net result of long-term zinc depletion would be growth problems and poor eyesight. So the old wives' tale about masturbation may be true after all! In the 18th century it was said that masturbation could make you mentally ill. Now we also know that zinc deficiency can cause depression, so, if you find yourself feeling low the day after a lot of sex, now you know why. There is another view of depletion via sex, concerning your vital energy, known as *chi* or *ki* in East Asian traditions. As you'd expect, there's a lot of *chi* in sperm, and it's lost in the process of orgasm. It's possible that women may also experience a loss of vital energy this way.

But let's not forget the massive plus side: sex is a great way to feel connected, and a fantastic relaxant. You'll just need to monitor how you feel the next day – more tired or more energised. My verdict is everything in moderation, including moderation.

SLEEP

One nutrient that is absolutely essential for our well-being is sleep. There's nothing that will help us more to get through the day bright-eyed, alert and calm as seven hours of deep, undisturbed sleep. It's the best tonic, and a huge boost to the body's own self-repair systems. And there's more. Research has shown that through dreaming, sleep 'knits up the ravelled sleeve of care', helping the brain lay anxieties quite literally to rest – and so leaving it, and us, ready for the next day's fray. But the sad truth is that many of us are failing to get enough sleep, and having difficulty getting to sleep and staying asleep. If you're concerned about your sleep patterns and feel tired and run down as a result, this section is for you.

Q **I don't sleep well so I'm often tired. Can nutrition help?**

A Nutrition can be a great way of enhancing sleep, alongside general relaxation and exercise. If you are highly stressed throughout the day, it is likely to interfere with a good night's sleep. So take a B complex supplement, 1,000mg of vitamin C and 300mg of magnesium daily to help your body balance energy levels. Another important factor is your blood sugar – fluctuating levels can disturb sleep. If you crave sweet foods or stimulants such as tea, coffee, chocolate or cigarettes, you may have poor blood sugar control. The solution is to eat wholefoods and fruit that have a stabilising effect on your blood sugar levels, and supplement 200mcg of chromium.

The herb valerian also promotes a good night's sleep. You need about 500 to 1,000mg taken one hour before going to sleep. A brisk walk before bedtime can also help to clear the mind and get you ready for a good night's snooze.

Q *I find it really hard to get to sleep and don't want to take sleeping pills. Any suggestions?*

A Your brain and nervous system may be too hyped up. I'd definitely recommend avoiding any stimulant drinks like tea or coffee for at least four hours before bedtime. The minerals calcium and magnesium have both been shown to calm down the nervous system and aid restful sleeping. You can buy powders of calcium and magnesium that dissolve in water. Try this before bed. See Supplements in Resources. The herb valerian also helps to induce sleep. You need about 500 to 1,000mg taken one hour before going to sleep. A brisk walk before bedtime can also help to clear the mind and get you ready for a good night's snooze.

Q **Can nutrition help me remember my dreams?**

A You should be able to remember your dreams with a little nutritional intervention. Your nervous system is dependent on B vitamins, which are present in many foods but removed by processing and refining (of grains, for example), and are depleted in the body by stress and alcohol. So many people today are not getting enough.

At the Institute for Optimum Nutrition, we found that the specific B vitamin related to dream recall is B6, but B vitamins do work together so it's best to take a complex plus extra B6. I'd recommend 50mg B complex with breakfast and dinner (either as a B complex or in a multi), plus 50mg B6 at breakfast, lunch and dinner (totalling 250mg of B6), and 15 mg zinc with breakfast. If this doesn't work, take an additional 50mg B6 before bed. Also reduce your alcohol intake and stress levels, and eat vitamin B-rich foods (wholegrains, brewer's yeast, lentils, most vegetables). One last thing . . . many people are reporting better dream recall with a supplement called Connect. (See Resources, page 483.)

Q **It takes me ages to wake up in the morning. Can you help?**

A There are two reasons. First, you may not be getting as good a quality of sleep as you think. The dream cycle in sleep is important for regenerating your mind and ironing out the difficulties of the preceding day, but many people have patchy sleep patterns and may wake up during the night, or don't sleep well enough for optimum dream activity. This can leave them exhausted in the morning. The amino acid GABA, and the herbs valerian, hops and passion flower, can all help. GABA is made in the body from glutamine, another amino acid. Combinations of these relaxing herbs and amino acids can help you sleep and wake up refreshed (see Resources, page 483).

The second reason is that you may be waking up with a low blood sugar level. If so, you need to review your diet and intake of sugar and stimulants, especially caffeinated drinks such as tea and coffee. Cut these right out, along with chocolate, and go for a diet high in vegetables and fruits, high-quality protein such as lean free-range chicken and tofu, and wholegrains such as rye and quinoa. Be sure to drink 1.5 litres of water a day, too.

Q **My boyfriend wakes me up with his snoring. Any suggestions?**

A What makes the snoring noise is air struggling to get through the throat when the uvula (the little hanging 'bell' of tissue) blocks it and the skin vibrates. (Vibrating mucus can also cause it, but that's not usually behind long-term snoring.) So one of the keys to stopping it is to unblock the throat and reduce that vibration.

One supplement that claims to reduce the noise level of snoring is Snor Away. A highly researched blend of olive, sunflower, almond, sesame and peppermint oils with vitamins, it comes in a spray that coats the back of the mouth and throat, effectively unblocking the uvula. Just two squirts will last six to eight hours because of the special time-release formula. Another similar product is Neversnore. They are both worth a try. (See Resources, page 483.)

Q **I grind my teeth in my sleep – are there any supplements I can take to stop this?**

A You're stressed. The first thing to do, before even considering supplements, is to reduce the sources of stress in your life. If that's difficult – say, you're in a highly demanding job and can't or don't want to quit right now – you can learn to manage your stress though regular exercise, yoga, massage, relaxing baths, enjoyable hobbies, down time just for you, meditation and relaxation techniques. These are all very much worth trying.

Having said all that, supplements *can* help. The nutrient most helpful for teeth grinding is vitamin B5. In addition to your multi or (100mg) B-complex supplement, take 100mg of B5 twice daily. B vitamins are generally good for your nervous system and can help improve your stress tolerance, as can vitamin C (1 to 2g twice daily) and Siberian ginseng (200 to 400mg daily). Finally, teeth grinding can often result from tension in the jaw, and this can be reduced by supplementing 200 to 400mg of magnesium – which relaxes the muscles – before bed.

SMOKING, DRINKING AND STIMULANTS

There's an old saying that 'if you don't drink and you don't smoke, you don't actually live longer – it just feels like it!' But if you've given up smoking and drinking or never taken them up in the first place, you'll know that the truth is quite other: there's actually nothing better than the clear, sharp energy you have when your brain and body are firing on all cylinders. Far too many of us, however, are dependent on caffeine to stay awake and alcohol or cigarettes to calm down. All of these substances are 'anti-nutrients' that leach nutrients from the body and, in the case of alcohol and cigarettes at least, lay us open to serious diseases. These answers explain their effects and how best to quit.

Smoking

Q *I'm finding it really hard to quit smoking. Can supplements help?*

A Cigarettes are carefully and insidiously designed to be addictive. Nicotine is just one of the chemicals in cigarettes which act as powerful stimulants that mess up your blood sugar balance. Each time your blood sugar levels fall, you get a craving.

But help is at hand. One of the most effective nutrients at helping to stabilise blood sugar and reduce cravings is the mineral chromium, so supplementing 200mcg chromium each day helps. Vitamin C helps protect you from the cancer-causing toxins in cigarettes: supplementing just 2g of vitamin C a day cuts your risk of cancer by a third if you smoke, and helps detoxify your body while you quit. While you are quitting, and for one month afterwards, supplementing 50mg of niacin (vitamin B3) a day also helps reduce cravings. Niacin dilates blood vessels and helps get toxins out of cells. (As a consequence, you may harmlessly blush for up to 30 minutes after taking it.)

Q *Why do I feel almost like I have a hangover the next day after being at a smoky party?*

A Even if you're not a smoker, a night at a smoky bar or party can easily leave you groggy from passive smoking. If you really feel terrible, though, it probably means that your body's detoxification processes aren't working too efficiently, so you'd do well to support your liver. Follow a sensible, wholefood diet rich in fruit and vegetables, with a measured amount of high-quality protein and grains like quinoa; and drink 1.5 litres of pure water a day. Vitamin C and other antioxidants are important for good liver detoxification – so especially after a night out, before you go to bed take a high-quality antioxidant and 1g of vitamin C (see Resources, page 483). The vitamin A in the antioxidant blend is also good for your lungs. Finally, check out the herb milk thistle, which offers excellent support for your liver.

Q **Why do smokers look older?**

A Every mouthful of cigarette smoke contains a trillion oxidants. Oxidants (otherwise known as free radicals) are bad news when it comes to keeping you looking young. Basically, early ageing – both inside and out – is inevitable if you smoke. The link between smoking and lung cancer is clear because of the damage it causes to the surface of your lungs, but oxidants damage every cell of your body – and that includes the skin, which they leave looking saggy, wrinkly and less elastic. Why? Your skin stays elastic via its collagen content, which the body needs vitamin C, a powerful antioxidant, to make. Yet with each cigarette you smoke you use up 35mg of vitamin C. You get the picture: so it's not surprising that research has shown that smokers actually have thinner skin than non-smokers.

Q *Why do smokers snore?*

A The oxidants in each toxic puff of that cigarette not only wreck your lungs and age your skin, but also damage the internal 'skin' of the throat. This makes the throat lose its elasticity – giving you in effect an internal turkey neck which wobbles as you breathe, making the snoring sound. The other reason for all that snoring is the mucus that coats the throat and nose. Smokers are, in effect, allergic to cigarette smoke, so the body does its best to protect itself from the damage by producing a layer of mucus. This then vibrates as the smoker sleeps, causing more of the snoring sound.

Clearly, the answer for snorers who smoke is to give up smoking. In the meantime, take a strong antioxidant supplement containing vitamins A, C, E and beta-carotene, plus zinc, selenium, glutathione and cysteine. You could also try the two anti-snore sprays Snor Away and Neversnore (see Resources, page 483).

Drinking

Q *Which is better for you – beer or wine?*

A Some questions in nutrition have no clear-cut answer, and this is one of them. While alcohol is a poison in the body, small amounts of red wine have been shown to reduce cardiovascular risk, albeit probably because of the anthocyanidins found in the grapes, not the alcohol. Women who drink alcohol every day, however, have an increased risk of breast cancer.

One of the best measures of health is a person's level of the amino acid homocysteine. The higher your homocysteine score, the greater the risk of disease. Both beer and wine in moderation has been shown to very slightly lower homocysteine. Both are fermented drinks and it is thought that it's the B vitamins in the yeast and to some extent the grapes that have this beneficial effect.

Overall, I'd vote for organic red wine in moderation, meaning four glasses a week maximum, especially for women. Women with low folic acid intake are more susceptible to the negative effects of alcohol as regards the breast cancer risk. Therefore, if you do drink wine on a regular basis, make sure you eat plenty of green vegetables or take a multivitamin or ideally both.

Q *Are some alcoholic drinks better for you than others?*

A Yes, because there's a lot more in most alcoholic drinks than just alcohol. Beers and, to a lesser extent, wines contain yeast which some people find they react to (champagne, though, is effectively yeast-free). Most wines contain sulphites, other preservatives and additives, which can cause headaches in some people. Red wine contains powerful antioxidants called anthocyanidins, so it's better for you than white. Nowadays there's a wide selection of great-tasting organic, chemical-free wines, champagnes and beers.

Of the spirits, vodka tends to be the purest. Stouts like Guinness contain B vitamins due to their yeast content – although I don't recommend beer for its vitamins, as alcohol destroys nutrients in the body. All alcohol dehydrates the body, too, so have plenty of water before, during and after drinking alcohol. Most importantly, don't drink too much. More than one drink a day is linked to an increased risk of cancer, diabetes and heart disease, no matter how pure the tipple.

Q *I get a rash when I drink wine or beer, but spirits and alcopops don't affect me that way. Is this an allergy?*

A You may have a sensitivity to yeast. Wine and beer both contain yeasts, while spirits, most alcopops and champagne do not. You may find that you also react to other yeast-containing foods such as bread, mushrooms or marmite, and fermented foods like soy sauce, sauerkraut or miso. I see many people with this problem, and a common sign, though not present in everyone, is patches of dry skin around the bridge of the nose, cheeks and/or eyebrows.

Visit a nutritional therapist for an IgG food intolerance test to confirm your sensitivity to yeast. Also have them check to see if you have an overgrowth of the fungus *Candida albicans* in your digestive system, which may be the reason for your sensitivity to yeast. Signs of this include sugar cravings, a white-coated tongue, digestive problems, general fatigue and sometimes joint stiffness or pain.

Q *Any tips for preventing hangovers?*

A Glutamine. Before you head out for that party, definitely up your intake of glutathione or N-acetyl cysteine. These help the liver to detoxify alcohol. I'd supplement 2g of the latter, or two good all-round antioxidant supplement, plus 2g of vitamin C, before going out; and take the same in the morning. In addition, try 5g (1 heaped teaspoon) of glutamine powder before going to bed after drinking, or, if you forget, the next morning. Depending on nutritional status, different things will work for different people. Most of all, drink as much water as alcohol, and if you forget at the party, drink a few glasses of water when you get home. I'm sure you'll find your magic formula somewhere in there.

Q *What's your cure for a hangover?*

A The symptoms of excess alcohol are half dehydration and half intoxication. Once the liver's ability to detoxify is exceeded, the body produces toxins from alcohol that trigger a headache. If you wake up with a thumping hangover, ensure you have a litre or two of pure water to hand – and drink it throughout the day. Have 5g (1 heaped teaspoon) of glutamine powder and supplement 1g of vitamin C every two hours, and take a high-potency multivitamin and an antioxidant complex. Also, drink cat's claw tea along with fruit or vegetable juices. Try a combination of carrot and apple – this will definitely speed up liver detoxification.

Q *I often feel paranoid and edgy the day after drinking alcohol. Why is this?*

A It's all to do with GABA, the brain's peacemaker. When you first drink alcohol it promotes relaxation and de-stresses by promoting GABA. But the next-day effects of alcohol are to suppress GABA, so you are more likely to feel anxious, irritable, edgy and even paranoid. The best solution is not to drink, but if you have, supplementing 1g of GABA in the morning can help calm down your brain. Unfortunately, GABA isn't available as a supplement in the UK, but is in the US. The next best thing is glutamine, from which the body can make GABA. This amino acid comes as a powder. I recommend 5g or one heaped teaspoon, taken with water on an empty stomach right before bed. As well as helping the liver, glutamine helps to repair the digestive tract, which gets damaged by alcohol.

Q *How can I get the natural high that I experience after drinking champagne?*

A Drinking alcohol releases dopamine, which stimulates you, followed by endorphins, which make you feel high, and then GABA, which makes you relax. The alcohol also gives your blood sugar a boost. Champagne makes you even higher because the bubbles get the alcohol into your bloodstream faster. But the euphoria can wear off after an hour or so, leaving you irritable, fuzzy and, for quite a few people, with a hangover the next day. My favourite 'natural high' is a combination of TMG, 5-HTP and sceletium, a herb from South Africa. These, together with B vitamins, give a very pleasant sense of being connected, without any of the down sides associated with alcohol. (See Resources, page 483.)

DIG DEEPER: If you'd like to find out more about natural highs, read my book *Natural Highs* (Piatkus, 2001), coauthored with Dr Hyla Cass.

Q *My boyfriend has an alcohol problem. Are there any nutritional remedies that can help him come off the booze?*

A The main thing is to reduce his cravings. There's a Chinese herb called kudzu root that appears to reduce dependency on alcohol – its Chinese nickname translates as 'drunkenness dispeller'. In a seven-week trial, 64 per cent of participants taking the root claimed to be drinking less and having fewer cravings; they also said they had more energy and were more alert. Your boyfriend will also need to keep his sugar levels balanced throughout the day, another excellent way of reducing cravings. That means eating little and often. A nutrient that is particularly useful, both for stabilising blood sugar and healing the gut, which gets damaged by alcohol, is glutamine, which provides the brain with fuel. Have your boyfriend take 3g three times a day. Since alcohol depletes just about every known nutrient, it's well worth suggesting he go on a comprehensive daily supplement programme, including a high strength multivitamin, an antioxidant complex, 2g of vitamin C and some essential omega-3 and 6 oils. (See Resources, page 483.)

Q *I'm a recovering alcoholic, but I smoke and crave chocolate and sugar. Can nutrition help?*

A Although you've stopped drinking (well done!), it's highly likely that you still have an underlying blood sugar problem – a condition shared by many alcoholics. And, as alcohol boosts production of the neurotransmitter dopamine, which has a stimulating or motivating effect, giving it up means you're left with a craving for stimulants. Smoking, chocolate and sugar give you that stimulative kick – but inevitably exacerbate your blood sugar problems and leave you stuck in another unhealthy cycle of highs and lows.

I recommend you strictly follow my diet for stabilising blood sugar. Eat little and often: always have breakfast, lunch and dinner and two snacks in between, choosing specific foods that keep your blood sugar level even. For example, oats, brown basmati rice, pears and apples are in, while cornflakes, raisins and bananas are out. Eating good-quality protein helps, such as organic chicken or fish. Always combine protein with carbohydrates – for instance, eat hummus with a couple of rice cakes, lentils with rice or a piece of roast chicken with a baked potato. Eat plenty of organic vegetables. Ensure you drink 1.5 litres of pure water a day, and cut out stimulating drinks such as coffee, tea and colas entirely.

Also supplement two things: 200mcg of chromium twice a day to help stabilise your blood sugar levels, and 1,000mg of tyrosine twice a day on an empty stomach. Tyrosine, an amino acid, helps to up your levels of dopamine and thereby reduces cravings. These, plus a high-strength multivitamin and 2g of vitamin C, will help your brain and body return to balance.

DIG DEEPER: See my book, *The 30 Day Fat Burner Diet* (Piatkus, 1999), for more information on eating to keep your blood sugar on an even keel.

Coffee and other stimulants

Q **Is it true that coffee improves your concentration?**

A There's no denying the lift and the buzz you get from a cup of good coffee. Scientists have backed this up with research that showed two cups of coffee give you maximum alertness and concentration – but this is only short term, as over time you need more and more to get the same effect. In other words, you're addicted. Another study concludes that the benefits of coffee are at best meagre when you consider the negative effects of caffeine withdrawal, and that overall drinking coffee causes a decline in performance and health. Research on 1,500 psychology students showed that those who drank more coffee had higher levels of anxiety, depression and stress-related medical problems, and lower academic performance. So, all in all, I would say that the short-lived up from a cup of coffee is not worth the down side as far as your health and mental wellbeing are concerned.

Q **I've heard that decaf coffee is no better than regular. What's your view?**

A I'm not a great fan of decaf coffee. While there's no doubt about the harmful and energy-depleting effects of regular caffeine use, decaf still contains two of the three stimulants in regular coffee – theobromine and theophylline. (Theobromine is the addictive stuff in chocolate.) Both regular and decaf coffee also contain chlorogenic acid, which raises both cholesterol and homocysteine, both of which are associated with an increased risk of heart attack.

A recent trial tested whether decaffeinated coffee would stimulate the nervous system the way regular coffee does, thereby raising blood pressure and heart attack risk. It was found that even without the caffeine, a triple decaf espresso still managed to trigger this undesirable effect. However, my real concern with decaf coffee is that, if you are trying to cut back on caffeine, drinking decaf does little to stop your behavioural craving for the stuff. I'd suggest drinking something else entirely. Rooibosch tea is a great alternative, as are the many delicious herbal teas on offer these days (they're very different from the dusty, rather tasteless blends of yore). See 'Can you recommend a good coffee substitute?', below, for more ideas.

Q *Can you recommend a good coffee substitute?*

A There's a wonderful array. My favourites are the barley/chicory blends such as Yannoh, Caro Extra and Barleycup, and dandelion root 'coffee' – these make rich, tasty drinks and are great substitutes for anyone cutting out coffee entirely. You could also try rooibosch tea, a South African tea that comes closest to normal tea in taste and is good with milk, unlike most herbal varieties. Yogi Tea, available from healthfood shops and some supermarkets, has some great blends. Also look out for Teechino, a delicious variety that's widely available in the US, but hard to find in the UK.

Q **I can't get going in the morning without a couple of strong cups of coffee. What's the remedy?**

A The chances are you are caught up in an all-too-common vicious cycle of stress, stimulants and fatigue. In the morning, when your blood sugar is at its lowest, you've got used to kickstarting your system, and no doubt propping it up throughout the day, with stress, sugar and stimulants – say, through overwork, 'elevenses' such as biscuits and plenty of coffee. In time the effects become blunted, so you'll need even more stimulation. In short, it's an addiction.

The cure is to stabilise your blood sugar with the right diet and supplements. For breakfast, try Get Up & Go, a powdered wholefood drink that you blend with milk (or soya milk) and a banana. (See Resources, page 483.) Supplement a high-strength multivitamin, one 1g vitamin C tablets in the morning and one in the afternoon, and 200mcg of the mineral chromium ... and stay off coffee! Instead, try Caro Extra, the best-tasting alternative. Follow a sensible diet rich in organic vegetables and good-quality proteins, cut out sugary snacks and drink plenty of pure water. You'll feel the difference within days as your blood sugar and your energy levels start to even out.

Q *Why do drinks such as tea, coffee and alcohol dehydrate us?*

A The reason for this is that caffeine and tannins in coffee and tea bind to the minerals that boost water excretion via the kidneys, including sodium, potassium, magnesium and calcium, therefore making the cells dehydrated. Alcohol is processed by a similar mechanism. All these drinks not only use up water during metabolism, but also act as diuretics, increasing the amount of water excreted so that you end up with a deficit.

Q *What's your view on green tea?*

A Contrary to popular belief, green tea is from the same plant as normal black tea, and it does contain caffeine. The difference is that green tea is made from only the leaf bud and the top two leaves of each branch on the bush. And while black tea is fermented, green tea is only lightly steamed, which leaves the potent antioxidant family of polyphenols in that part of the plant intact.

These substances have been investigated for their cancer-protective effects, which have been found to be even more powerful than those in vitamins C and E. It's believed that green tea consumption in Japan, which averages about three cups a day, is partly responsible for the low levels of cancer found in that country. If you are looking for a particularly high intake of antioxidants for cancer protection, or therapeutically for a disease such as an eye disorder, you may want to take green tea supplements. Take a daily dose of 300 to 400mg and choose ones standardised to contain 80 per cent polyphenol and 55 per cent epigallocatechin gallate.

Tea also has a blood-thinning effect, similar to that of aspirin. As it turns out, black tea also contains polyphenols and catechins, but with proportionately more caffeine along with them. Green tea contains only 20 to 30mg of caffeine per cup, as compared to 50mg in a regular cup of tea, and is consequently less stimulating – for many people, it's actually relaxing. In fact, East Asian monks have traditionally used green tea to stay alert, yet calm, during meditation. So all in all, you can count green tea in moderation (meaning two cups a day) as an acceptable natural stimulant.

Q *What's your view on guarana?*

A The name 'guarana' conjures up exotic images of tribal people in the Amazonian rainforests, living in harmony with nature. And if it's 'natural', it must be good for you. Right? Well, not exactly.

The seeds and leaves of the guarana plant, a climbing shrub native to Brazil and Uruguay, are high in caffeine, theobromine and theophylline, just like coffee. But there are mitigating factors. The plant itself contains saponins, compounds also found in ginseng that have tonic or balancing properties with a mild and long-lasting effect. These are less irritating to the gastrointestinal tract than coffee – probably because of the presence of fats and oils in the seeds, which prolong absorption. Guarana also reduces fluid retention and appetite, relieves tension headaches and period pains, and gives your energy a boost.

The problems with guarana lie in the processing. With many commercially prepared guarana products, the caffeine is absorbed and used up in the body as quickly as with a cup of coffee. So in this form guarana is over-stimulating, much like tea and coffee, and has the same ill effect on you. Like all stimulants it raises your blood sugar level, giving you a short-term lift in energy followed by a drop. I'd suggest going for a diluted, milder form of guarana, and only as an occasional pick-me-up. Supplements come in 500mg strengths, with a recommended intake of 1,000mg, which provides 35mg of caffeine – roughly that found in a cup of tea or a weak cup of coffee.

SPORTS NUTRITION

Whether you go for a daily walk, visit the gym three times a week, play Sunday football with friends or indulge in the occasional bout of extreme sports, finding the right nutrition for your energy needs is vital. The harder you drive your body, the more it needs in the way of nutrients. Athletes not only find they need improved nutrition to avoid burnout, but that optimum nutrition is a key factor in maximising their performance in any sport. Here I answer the most frequently asked questions about sports nutrition.

Q *What do you recommend to improve performance at sport?*

A Apart from lots of practice, the two key requirements in sport are energy and focus. Both of these are affected by how well your blood sugar is balanced. Poor blood sugar balance is very common and causes fatigue, as well as poor concentration, memory and mood, and cravings for carbohydrates. The condition results from nutrient deficiencies, a diet high in refined carbohydrates and low in wholefoods, and excessive use of stimulants such as colas, coffee and tea.

To keep energy and focus high, concentrate on fruits, vegetables, wholegrains and high-quality proteins such as lean free-range chicken and tofu. Always have a good breakfast, lunch and dinner plus two snacks a day (say, a handful of seeds or nuts and a piece of fruit, or a rice cake with hummus), balance carbohydrates and proteins 2:1, avoid sugar and drink plenty of water. On the day, have a good breakfast, eat a fruit/nut/seed snack before and during the event, and drink plenty of water instead of sugary drinks.

Q *My husband is training hard. What are the best carb/protein meal replacements to take, and what are your views on creatine?*

A Creatine is a substance in the body made of three amino acids – arginine, methionine and glycine. Not surprisingly, meat is naturally rich in it. Creatine is also sold as a supplement, and it's a top seller among sports people because it promotes muscle regeneration and recovery after exercise, as well as improving energy during intensive exercise.

Normally, muscle cells derive energy by breaking down adenosine triphosphate or ATP to ADP. When supplies of ATP are exhausted, for example during a sprint, creatine can quickly replace the phosphate needed to 'reload' the cell. Because muscles can work harder with extra creatine, and also increase their water concentration, the extra activity also results in more muscle growth as well as increased muscle size. So here's a caution. If your husband takes creatine, it is vital that he drinks plenty of water, as some people experience high blood pressure if they don't. Others also get diarrhoea. While there is good evidence that creatine gives you the edge, it is ideally suited for sports where every second counts. Your husband would need 2 to 5g a day, although some recommend 'loading up' for five days before an event with 20g.

In terms of carb/protein meal replacements, ideally your husband should just eat more of what he normally does, with a focus on white meat and fish, limited red meat, lots of fresh organic vegetables and fruit and wholegrains (brown rice, wholemeal pasta, quinoa and so on).

Q *What is the optimum food/drink intake, if any, before exercise to maximise fat burning?*

A To burn fat, you'll need to increase the amount of protein you eat and reduce carbohydrates, going only for wholegrain carbs such as raw oats, brown rice, wholemeal pasta, quinoa or sweet potatoes. Aim for the same size in portions of protein and carb on your plate.

So for breakfast, choose either skimmed or soya milk, a boiled free-range egg (limiting eggs to five a week) or yoghurt for protein, and team it with either a cup of raw oats topped with sliced apple, a banana, or two slices of wholegrain rye bread for carbohydrates. Add a dessertspoon of flax or pumpkin seeds for essential fats (which don't impede fat burning). For lunch and dinner, team carbs like brown rice, sweetcorn, broad beans or couscous with proteins like tofu or other soya products, cottage cheese, fish or lentils – then have double the quantity of non-starchy vegetables such as broccoli, runner beans, kale or tomatoes. This way you don't flood your blood with glucose (the breakdown product of carbohydrate that our bodies use as fuel and convert to fat if there's an excess), and that helps to burn fat and balance energy levels. Eat nothing for at least an hour, preferably two, before you exercise, but drink plenty of water to stop you from becoming dehydrated. And avoid all coffee, tea, colas – even diet – as stimulants can play merry hell with blood sugar too.

Q **Is an isotonic sports drink the best way to fuel a day's walking?**

A It's a bit of a buzzword, isotonic. What you are looking to do is replace minerals lost through excessive perspiration – sodium, potassium, magnesium and chloride. Also, muscles use up calcium and magnesium during prolonged exertion. And your blood sugar dips, so you need a relatively fast-releasing sugar, at least when you are climbing a mountain.

You can make your own mineral-rich energy cocktail to carry with you: coconut water is particularly good for the minerals, grape juice for fast-releasing sugars and apple juice for more sustaining energy. I recommend eating apples for walking and bananas for climbing. Most so-called isotonic drinks are just glucose and water, with a few added minerals. Quite acceptable, and welcome, if you've just climbed a mountain, but otherwise (or anyway) I'd stick to these other natural 'isotonic' foods and drinks.

Q *I'm training for the London marathon. What should I eat?*

A Complex carbohydrates are the best fuels for the body, so eat plenty of fruit, vegetables, wholegrains and baked potatoes. Avoid sugar and refined carbohydrates – they may give you a rush but then leave you more tired than you were before. Make sure you have a good breakfast every day – oats are best so go for muesli or porridge – and eat small regular meals throughout the day to keep your blood sugar levels even. Ensure you eat enough protein to repair fatigued muscles. That means at least half as much protein as carbohydrates at each meal and snack, so have fruit with nuts or seeds, rice with fish or lentils, baked potatoes with bean or tuna salad, oatcakes with hummus, and so on. Remember too that a demanding exercise regime generates more oxidants, so eat plenty of antioxidant-rich foods – orange, red and blue fruit and vegetables are best, especially berries. Don't forget to drink plenty of water – dehydration is a leading cause of fatigue. I'd also recommend supplementing a high-strength multivitamin, 2g of extra vitamin C every day, and 5g of glutamine powder before bed to aid muscle recovery. Good luck!

Q *What will help my muscles grow on a weight-training programme? Should I be buying protein drinks?*

A The notion held by many bodybuilders that you need to consume tons of protein to build muscle is a myth. A dozen eggs and a steak for breakfast are likely to give you a heart attack rather than a muscled body. With extremely hard training, the maximum amount of muscle you can put on in a year is 8lb (3.6kg), no matter how much protein you eat. That represents a gain of 2.5oz (71g) each week, or 0.3oz (9.5g) a day. Muscle is only 22 per cent protein, so an increased consumption of less than a tenth of an ounce, or 2.8g a day – equivalent to a quarter of a teaspoonful – is all you need to gain the maximum bulk of muscles!

So, instead of cramming in unnecessary protein, which taxes the body more than it helps it, follow the rules of moderation to make proper use of the protein in your diet. Eat fish as well as good-quality meat, and make sure some of your protein comes from vegetable sources such as beans, lentils, the protein-rich grain quinoa and soya. As the actual formation of muscle depends on amino acids, zinc and B6, ensure your supplement programme contains 15mg of zinc, 50mg of B6 and a free-form amino acid complex. There is also some evidence that the amino acids arginine and ornithine stimulate muscle growth. These are available as supplements and in powdered supplements that can be made into a drink.

Q **What can you recommend for eating and drinking during ultra distance endurance sports and during training sessions?**

A When you're depleting your body's resources through extreme exercise, you need something that will instantly replenish lost glucose, water and minerals to keep you going. PowerBars are excellent for a carbohydrate fix (they also have a good ratio of protein to slow down energy release), or try Multipower protein and energy bars. Zone bars are not bad either, apparently. These are available from most healthfood shops.

Two hours before events, you can also boost your glucose stores by eating lots of complex carbohydrates such as fruit, vegetables, wholegrains like wholemeal pasta or rye bread, and baked potatoes. But avoid sugar and refined carbohydrates – they may give you a rush but they will leave you more tired than you were before. Ensure you eat enough protein to repair muscles – at least half as much protein as carbohydrates at each meal and snack. So have nuts or seeds with fresh or dried fruit, rice with fish, tofu or lentils, and so on (the combinations are legion). Remember too that a demanding exercise regime generates more oxidants, so eat plenty of anti-oxidant-rich foods – go for fruit and vegetables in the orange, red and blue range, especially berries. Drink 1.5 to 2 litres of water at least, and supplement a high-strength multivitamin, 2g of extra vitamin C every day, and 5g of glutamine powder before bed to aid muscle recovery.

Q *When I exercise I have more energy. Why?*

A Probably because exercise increases the body's metabolic rate – which is, in essence, its ability to turn food into energy. One session of exercise can do this for up to 48 hours. So exercising three times a week keeps your inner 'fire' burning, which you experience as energy. Aerobic exercise (such as running, dancing or swimming, but not working with weights) also makes you breathe more deeply which, provided you don't overdo it, oxygenates the body. Some forms of exercise also loosen up the body to allow 'vital energy', also known as *chi* or *ki* in the Far East and *prana* in India, to flow more freely. This further increases your available energy. The best forms of exercise for this are yoga and t'ai chi.

DIG DEEPER: The best book I know of on sports nutrition is *Optimum Sports Nutrition* by Michael Colgan (Advanced Research Press, 1993). This is out of print, so if you cannot pin down a copy, try his *Sports Nutrition Guide* (Apple Publishing, 2002).

SUPPLEMENTS

Eating well and exercising will take you a long way towards good health, but for superhealth – a tuned-up immune system, high energy, emotional balance and a sharp mind – you'll need to take supplements. The question is, which are right for you? If you're a newcomer to supplementing, healthfood stores can seem bewildering – the sheer number of vitamins, minerals, phytonutrients, amino acids and other supplements on offer these days is huge. More, people's nutrient needs can differ profoundly, so you'll need to tailor what you take to your own. The answers below should make choosing the supplements you need a breeze.

Starting out

Q *How do I know what vitamins I need?*

A Taking vitamins is a sure way to optimise your health, but remember that supplements are just that – an adjunct to a good diet.

The basis of any supplement programme is a good high-strength multivitamin/mineral plus 1g of vitamin C. A good multi should contain all the vitamins and minerals, with between 25 and 50mg of each of the B vitamins and 10mg of zinc. I also take an antioxidant formula giving extra beta-carotene, C and E, with extras such as anthocyanidins because they protect from pollution and slow down ageing.

Since everyone is unique, the best way to find out exactly what you need is to have a personal assessment by a nutritional therapist. They take your diet, your lifestyle and your current health signs and symptoms into account. If necessary they can also run tests to find what you are lacking and what you need to be super-healthy. Most nutritionists charge from £45 to £60 for such an assessment, and will spend an enlightening hour with you. Alternatively, especially if you don't have any major health issues, you can have an on-line 'mynutrition' assessment. (See Resources, page 483.)

Q *How do you identify a good-quality vitamin supplement?*

A As with most things, you pay for quality, so, within reason, price is a place to start. The cheapest supplements are usually so for a reason – cheaper forms of nutrients, or lower amounts, are used. For example, iron sulphate is less absorbable than iron amino acid chelate; and natural vitamin E (called d-alpha tocopherol) is more potent than synthetic. So look for supplements that use natural forms of nutrients, absorbable forms of minerals (citrate, ascorbates or amino acid chelates) and the right kind of dosage. A couple of yardsticks for a good quality multivitamin are that it should contain at least 25mg of each of the B vitamins and 10mg of zinc. Capsules are no better absorbed than tablets, but with these you are not getting added extras like colourings or sugar coating. A reputable company will also list all ingredients and state that the product is free from colourings and undesirable additives – so always check the small print.

Q *I take my supplements during breakfast. Can tea interfere with their absorption?*

A Tea does interfere with the absorption of supplements because it contains methylxanthines and tannins – both of which will render minerals less absorbable. So as you take your supplements with breakfast, have your tea at least half an hour before. Or, even better, try rooibusch tea from South Africa, which tastes a lot like regular tea but doesn't contain any of the compounds that interfere with absorption.

It is best to take vitamin, mineral or essential fatty acid supplements while food is in your digestive tract, so this can mean 15 minutes before or up to 30 minutes after eating. However, individual amino acids are best taken on an empty stomach, although some compete for absorption better than others. Tryptophan, for example, competes poorly and is best absorbed when taken alone and eaten with carbohydrate, such as a banana. But lysine competes far better so it's less important to take it separately. As a general rule, take supplements with food.

Q *I've heard that most vitamin supplements can't be assimilated unless bound to other nutrients. Is this true?*

A There are a lot of myths about vitamin and mineral absorption, usually from companies trying to claim their products are much better than everybody else's. Vitamins are not difficult for the body to absorb. Minerals, on the other hand, do need to be bound to something else to be absorbed. The best forms of minerals are ascorbates (bound to vitamin C), citrates (bound to citric acid) and amino acid chelates (bound to amino acids). If you look closely at the label of a multivitamin, for example, you'll see 'selenomethionine' – selenium bound to the amino acid methionine, or perhaps zinc oxide or zinc citrate. In this case, zinc citrate is the better form. These binding agents – citrates, amino acid chelates or ascorbates – help to carry the mineral through the gut wall into the blood. Most forms of minerals in food are bound in similar ways.

Q *Can you take too many supplements and are there certain combinations to avoid?*

A If you're pregnant, don't supplement more than 3,000mcg of retinol, the animal form of vitamin A.

Theoretically, you can supplement too much vitamin B6 (1,000mg a day is potentially harmful) and vitamin D (above 3,000mcg can be toxic), but these are massive amounts, 10 times higher than what you find in most megadose supplements.

You have to be more careful with minerals. As little as 3,000mg of ferrous sulphate can cause death in an infant. Some prescribed iron supplements provide 300mg. Therefore, supplements containing a significant amount of iron should be kept in a childproof container away from children. Since iron competes with zinc for absorption, don't take extra iron without taking extra zinc. Zinc also competes with copper. You need 10 times more zinc than copper. That's why you are much better off starting by taking an all-round multivitamin/mineral supplement, then adding individual minerals as you need them.

Q *Are megadoses of vitamins harmful for you?*

A This is one of the longest-running myths in nutrition today. The truth is there has never been a single death attributed to a vitamin supplement. The most commonly reported scares are that vitamin C can give you kidney stones and increase your risk of heart disease and that vitamin B6 can damage your nerves. Both of these statements have been proven untrue, even at doses 10 times above the highest you'll find in supplements. While it is true that massively high doses of vitamins A, D and B6 can harm you, in reality these levels are very hard to achieve. The Institute for Optimum Nutrition has monitored over 50,000 people taking supplements and has never seen a case of vitamin overdose.

Having said this, when a person takes a large amount of an individual nutrient, without any others, this can have less desirable effects. That's why I always say the starting point is a high-strength multivitamin. Beta-carotene is a case in point. Hundreds of studies show that beta-carotene in food protects against cancer. Other studies show that beta-carotene, if supplemented with vitamin C and E, reduces cancer risk. But a couple of studies have suggested that beta-carotene, on its own, may modestly increase risk in smokers. So the way is clear – go for a good multi at the start.

Q **When you take all these high-dose supplements don't you just excrete them?**

A Water is the body's most essential nutrient. Yet, once it has done its job it is simply excreted. Does that mean you shouldn't drink water? The same is true for many nutrients. Supplementing vitamin C, for example, raises vitamin C levels in the blood for a few hours, then it's excreted. During that time, however, it protects cells from damage and makes it hard for any invading bacteria or viruses to survive. Nutrients come and go. In between they do their work.

Q *When I take a multivitamin my urine turns yellow. Does this mean I'm taking too much?*

A It is vitamin B2 (riboflavin) that makes your urine yellow. Once the body has used it, or if there is any excess, it is simply eliminated. But don't look at it as a wasteful excess, as it only stays in your body for about four hours, so you're unlikely to use all of it. It also just so happens that people are rarely deficient in vitamin B2, unlike some other B vitamins, so keep on taking the multivitamin to make sure you're getting a full range of nutrients. If your urine is particularly yellow, you may need to increase your intake of pure water – be sure to have at least 1.5 litres a day.

Q *What is your opinion on food-form supplements?*

A Given that we have evolved over millions of years to use the nutrients available to us in foods, it certainly makes good sense to provide nutrients in supplements in a form as close as possible to that found in nature. And that's what food-state supplements are – nutrients incorporated into a food matrix, similar to what you find in food itself.

Researchers at the University of Scranton in Pennsylvania in the US, headed by professor of chemistry Joe Vinson, have put these 'food-form' vitamins to the test. From their findings, it looks as if the complex way food incorporates nutrients, which is what the food-form process mimics, allows the nutrients to be more easily released, transported and used. So the laboratory research is looking good. However, it isn't as simple as that. While nutrients in food often perform better than isolated nutrients they don't always. For example, folic acid in supplements is much more effective, mg for mg, than folic acid in food. We don't yet know why.

What we also don't yet have is evidence that these food-form supplements result in better clinical outcomes compared to equivalent amounts of non-food-form supplements. Until we have the evidence that food-form nutrients are more effective in clinical applications, I will sit on the fence on this one.

Problems with supplements

Q *Since starting to take supplements I feel worse, not better, and have developed spots and headaches! Why?*

A To check if you're reacting adversely to the supplements or to something in them, the obvious thing to do would be to stop taking them and see if you feel better and your new symptoms clear. However, what may be going on (and this is very common) is that your body is detoxifying. Any changes to your diet or nutrient levels can trigger the body to begin to clear out toxins that have been hindering your overall health for some time. In the short term this can cause spots, headaches and general malaise, but these should pass within a couple of weeks.

You can aid your body in its efforts to detoxify by drinking plenty of water, eating a 'clean' diet (cutting out or reducing your consumption of meat, dairy, fats, fried foods, stimulants like coffee and so on), plenty of fibre (to aid elimination via the bowels), and perhaps the herb milk thistle to support your liver.

Q *What's your advice for someone who has trouble swallowing supplements?*

A Swallowing is a skill, and an inability to swallow is a lack of this skill, or can be psychological. As the throat naturally opens for food or drinks, small supplements can be swallowed between or with gulps of a fruit smoothie. Think positively about all the beneficial nutrients you are swallowing as you do it. Multis and other supplements tend to be large, but there's no problem with crushing tablets and emptying capsules. Another option is something like Get Up & Go, a powdered multinutrient supplement, or Optio's vitamin enriched drinks. (See Resources, page 483, for details.)

Q *My multi is low in calcium but contains 200 per cent RDA of vitamin D. I want to supplement more calcium as I do not eat dairy, but all the calcium tablets I see have lots of vitamin D as well. Will I be overdosing on vitamin D if I take both?*

A While dairy products are of course a rich source of calcium, it's quite possible to get enough from other food sources – after all, we evolved over millions of years only having milk as babies. So I suggest you eat plenty of green leafy vegetables, almonds, pumpkin seeds, prunes and bone-in fish – all great sources of calcium. And if you still want to supplement, it's quite OK to take more than the RDA, which is the amount that's calculated to stop you from getting deficiency diseases, rather than the amount you need to be in optimum health. You can take up to 1,200mg of calcium and 20mcg of vitamin D, which is four times the RDA, quite safely. Be aware, though, that for calcium to be absorbed, you also need a good intake of magnesium, boron and vitamin K – so you may be best off taking a multivitamin and mineral complex. (See Resources, page 483.)

Vitamin and mineral supplements A-Z

Q *What exactly are antioxidants?*

A Antioxidants are special nutrients that protect us from harmful toxins called oxidants or free radicals, which damage cells, accelerate ageing and cause disease. These by-products of oxygen are like the 'sparks' that emanate from anything that's burnt, including cigarettes, petrol and fried or barbecued food. Even the process we use to 'burn' food for energy inside our body cells ends up making a bucketful of oxidants every year.

Antioxidants are like fireproof gloves, catching the sparks and protecting us. Each antioxidant becomes 'hot' and passes the oxidant to another until there is no more danger – so they work cooperatively.

The key players are vitamin E (seeds, nuts and fish); vitamin C (fruits and vegetables); vitamin A and beta-carotene (orange or red foods); glutathione (onions and garlic); and anthocyanidins (berries and beet-root). You can top these up with an all-round antioxidant supplement that contains each of the above.

Q **What's your view on vitamin B6?**

A Vitamin B6 (pyridoxine) is an essential nutrient and has proven helpful in a variety of conditions, from PMS to cardiovascular disease. In the US, supplementing vitamin B6 is considered essential for minimising the risk of a heart attack.

For the body to make use of protein, you need B6 and, together with zinc, it is needed to make the enzymes that digest food – the process essential for turning food into energy. B6 also boosts brainpower as well as immunity. It helps make the brain chemical serotonin, a deficiency in which can cause depression. One study showed that about a fifth of depressed people are deficient in pyridoxine. It can become toxic above 1,000mg a day. The ideal amount to supplement is 50 to 100mg a day. Good multivitamins provide around 50mg.

Q **What is the best source of vitamin C?**

A An ideal daily intake of vitamin C is between 400 and 1,500mg. You can get 400mg of vitamin C by having five servings of fresh fruit and vegetables a day, so achieving more than this means taking supplements. These come in three forms – ascorbic acid, which is the least expensive; ascorbate, also known as 'buffered' C; and 'ester C', which is a more absorbable form of the vitamin. With ester C you may not need to supplement as much, so it's probably the best option.

The best easily available food sources of vitamin C are broccoli and peppers; a serving of broccoli gives twice as much vitamin C as an orange. Next best are kiwi fruits, followed by lemons, strawberries and oranges. Watercress, cabbage and cauliflower are also good sources.

Q *Isn't it dangerous to take large amounts of vitamin C?*

A Countless studies have demonstrated the positive effects of taking vitamin C. However, one research trial at the University of Leicester caught the headlines by stating that vitamin C could have a pro-cancer effect. After much criticism of their conclusions, the researchers retracted their statement and said that vitamin C had a profoundly protective effect. Another myth is that large doses of vitamin C can cause kidney stones. True, some studies have shown that massive doses of vitamin C injected into the bloodstream can increase the risk, but supplementation has not been shown to do this. If you do take excess vitamin C, the only likely reaction is that you'd get loose bowels – and for most people this only happens if they take more than 5g a day.

Q *What's your view on chromium?*

A If your get up and go has got up and gone, you may be low in chromium. This mineral helps to give your energy a boost by keeping your blood sugar level even. The trouble is that refining food to make white bread, rice or sugar destroys 90 per cent of the chromium in food. Supplementing 200mcg of chromium a day can help stabilise your blood sugar and give you consistent energy, stable moods and more resistance to stress. Numerous research studies have shown that chromium helps lessen the symptoms of diabetes and may also help you lose weight by improving the body's ability to burn fat.

Classic symptoms of deficiency include fatigue, dizziness if you don't eat, craving sweet foods, sweating a lot and a need for frequent meals. If this sounds like you, or if you're under a lot of stress, take 200mcg of either chromium picolinate or chromium polynicotinate in the morning with food. Chromium is only toxic in very large amounts, unachievable by supplementation.

Q *What exactly are colloidal minerals?*

A Colloidal minerals are insoluble mineral particles which are small enough to remain suspended in liquid, such as water, and are reputed to have health-giving properties. Colloidal silver, for example, has been used since the 1940s as an antibiotic. The colloidal method of supplying minerals is worthy of research, but a number of claims for them – such as that they have 98 per cent absorption – are unfounded. Also, complexes that claim to contain 70 or more minerals may include toxic ones such as aluminium and mercury. Another critical issue is dose. No colloidal blends I've come across contain anything like enough of Britain's two most commonly deficient minerals – at least 15mg of zinc and 300mg of magnesium. Most contain only 1 or 2mg of zinc, and even if you absorb 100 per cent of that, it's still only a tenth of what you need.

Q *What are your views on vitamin E?*

A Vitamin E is undoubtedly a star among nutrients. One of the most essential antioxidants, it helps the body use oxygen properly and so provides great protection from pollution and against cancer, as well as slowing down the ageing process. It also helps reduce the likelihood of blood clots and thrombosis. Studies have shown that vitamin E reduces the risk of heart attacks, colon cancer, Alzheimer's and cataracts. Vitamin E is essential for a healthy immune system. As a fat-soluble antioxidant, it works particularly well in tandem with vitamin C, which is water-soluble. This is because the body's tissues and fluids are either water or fat-based, so vitamins E and C act as a dynamic duo.

You can get vitamin E from nuts, seeds and their oils, unrefined corn oil and wheatgerm. For optimum health, make sure your multivitamin contains at least 100mg (150iu) of vitamin E. If you are at risk of heart disease or want extra protection, take 400mg (600iu).

Q *What's your view on niacin?*

A Niacin, otherwise known as vitamin B3, has many remarkable properties. It improves cholesterol levels, can stop a migraine in its tracks, and gives energy a boost. It is also a great detoxifier because it acts as a vasodilator, widening the blood vessels and helping to remove toxins and deliver nutrients into your body cells. During this process you blush for 20 to 30 minutes, and may get a little hot and itchy as your circulation improves. If you want to detoxify your body, try taking niacin every day for a week, as well as eating healthy foods. Take 100mg of niacin on an empty stomach in a restful environment (don't do this at work – the blushing effect, although quite safe, is pronounced in some people and might look a bit alarming!). When the blushing starts have a relaxing bath and then lie down. You'll find it relaxes your body and mind and leaves you feeling thoroughly detoxified.

Q *What's your view on selenium?*

A Selenium is the vital constituent of the antioxidant enzyme glutathione peroxidase, and like all antioxidants wards off the effects of oxides or free radicals in the body. The need for it first came to light in connection with Keshan disease, a heart condition common in a region of China where the soil is low in selenium. Selenium deficiency has since been associated with a form of arthritis found in certain parts of Russia.

But perhaps the most significant finding in relation to selenium is its protective effects against certain kinds of cancer. It has been found that a tenfold increase in dietary selenium causes a doubling of glutathione peroxidase, which disarms oxides, in the body. Since many oxides, for example from smoking or deep-fried food, are cancer-producing, and since cancer cells destroy other cells by releasing oxides, it is likely to be selenium's role in promoting glutathione peroxidase that gives it its protective properties against cancer. Selenium may also be essential for the working of the thyroid gland, which controls the body's rate of metabolism.

I recommend supplementing 30mcg of selenium a day, minimum. There is a good case, however, for supplementing 100mcg and even double this amount if you are at risk of cancer or fighting an infectious disease. Selenium is found predominantly in wholefoods, seafoods, seeds (especially sesame seeds) and nuts, but food sources, which should provide up to 50mcg a day, are unreliable.

Q *What's your view on zinc?*

A Zinc is one of the most important minerals for health, yet a large part of the population is at risk of being deficient – half of us eat less than 50 per cent of the RDA. Symptoms of deficiency are white marks on the nails, a poor appetite or lack of appetite control, pallor, infertility, lack of resistance to infection, poor growth (including hair growth), skin problems such as acne, dermatitis and stretch marks, and mental and emotional problems. Zinc deficiency plays a role in nearly every major disease including diabetes and cancer: it is needed to make insulin, to boost the immune system and make the antioxidant enzyme SOD. Zinc also plays a part in the body's manufacture of prostaglandins (hormone-like substances) from essential fatty acids, which help balance hormones, control inflammation and balance the stickiness of the blood. Sucking zinc lozenges can help to shorten the duration of a cold.

Meat is high in zinc, so you're more likely to be deficient if you're vegetarian. Stress, smoking and alcohol deplete zinc – as does frequent sex, at least in men, since semen has the highest concentration of zinc in the human body.

I recommend supplementing 10 to 15mg of zinc each day, in a more absorbable form such as zinc ascorbate, glycinate or citrate. Zinc is somewhat better absorbed on an empty stomach, but can be mildly irritating in large amounts. Good food sources of zinc include oysters, lamb, pecan nuts, Brazil nuts, oats, rye and egg yolks.

Other nutritional supplements A–Z

Q **What's your view on bioflavonoids?**

A These remarkable nutrients are found in plants, especially citrus fruits, berries, broccoli, cherries, red grapes, rosehips, papaya and tomatoes, as well as tea and red wine. Bioflavonoids do a number of vital jobs: act as powerful antioxidants; bind to toxic metals (such as lead) and escort them out of the body; support the body's use of vitamin C; prevent some bacteria from multiplying; and protect against cancer. In one study, footballers were shown to get fewer injuries and heal better when taking bioflavonoids. Bioflavonoids are particularly useful for dealing with problems related to fragile blood capillaries such as bleeding gums, varicose veins, haemorrhoids, thrombosis and bruises, as well as strains and sprains. If you are suffering from any of these, take a good bioflavonoid complex to give your capillaries maximum support.

Q **Does cod liver oil really oil the joints?**

A It's no coincidence that the most popular over-the-counter remedy for relieving joint aches is cod liver oil – it really does work. But this is not because it oils the joints. Cod liver oil is high in vitamin D, which is needed for healthy bones. This was one of the reasons for its original popularity in the 1930s, as it prevented rickets and other bone problems. It has since been found that cod liver oil is a rich source of omega-3 essential fats. These fats don't actually oil the joints as such by lubricating them, but they contain substances called prostaglandins that help reduce inflammation. Many studies have found that people with joint problems have found an improvement in pain, stiffness and swelling when they take fish oil supplements. Look for cod liver oil supplements labelled as high in omega-3 fats. You want one that gives around 400mg of EPA and DHA per capsule. Take two every day if you suffer from joint problems.

Q *What's your view on Co-Q10?*

A Coenzyme Q10 (CoQ10) is not classified as a vitamin because most of us can make it in the body. It's a vital antioxidant that protects cells from carcinogens and also helps in the recycling of vitamin E. But its magical properties lie in its ability to improve the cell's use of oxygen.

Here's how it works. In the final, and most significant part of catabolism – the body process to do with breaking down complex substances into simpler ones that happens with the release of energy – hydrogen is released to react with oxygen. The actual reaction, of course, occurs at atomic level. Electrons of these elements are passed from one atom to the next in what is called the electron transfer pathway. These tiny charged particles are highly reactive and need to be very carefully handled. They are like nuclear fuel – a very potent, but very dangerous, energy source. It is in this last, vital stage that CoQ10 gets in on the act, by controlling the flow of oxygen, making the production of energy most efficient, and preventing damage caused by dangerous oxides or free radicals.

There is evidence that CoQ10 levels are lower in people with cancer and that the need for CoQ10 increases when you have the disease. For this reason, researchers are now looking at supplementing with extra CoQ10 as a cancer treatment. It is also highly beneficial in the treatment of cardiovascular disease and essential to take if you're on statin medication, since this drug inhibits the body from making CoQ10.

No studies have reported toxicity of CoQ10 even at extremely high doses taken over many years. There is no reason to assume that continued supplementation with CoQ10, as is advised for many vitamins, should have anything but extremely positive results.

CoQ exists in many foods but not always in a form that we can use. There are many different types of CoQ, from CoQ1 up to CoQ10. Yeast, for example, contains CoQ6 and CoQ7. Only CoQ10 is found in human tissue, and this is the form that should be supplemented. However, we can utilise 'lower' forms of CoQ and convert them into CoQ10. This conversion process, which occurs in the liver, allows us to make use of CoQ found in almost all foods. Problems arise for some people, especially the elderly, whose ability to convert lower forms of CoQ into the active CoQ10 becomes impaired or non-existent. Exactly why and to what extent this occurs is not known. But for them, CoQ10 is effectively an essential nutrient – that is, they need to supplement it as their bodies cannot make it, which is probably why so many people are deficient.

Some foods contain relatively more CoQ10 – all meat and fish (especially sardines), eggs, spinach, broccoli, alfalfa, potatoes, soya beans and soya oil, wheat (especially wheatgerm), rice bran, buckwheat, millet, and most beans, nuts and seeds.

Many supplement companies produce CoQ10 products. The best dosage is probably between 10 and 90mg a day, and it's best taken in an oil-soluble form.

Q *What's your view on digestive enzymes?*

A If you often feel bloated, get indigestion after meals or suffer from excessive flatulence, you may not be making enough enzymes to digest your food properly. It's a vicious circle, because with fewer enzymes you absorb fewer nutrients, and with fewer nutrients you make fewer enzymes. If this is your problem, there's a simple solution: supplement a digestive enzyme tablet with each meal. The good ones contain lipase (for digesting fat), amylase (for digesting carbohydrate) and protease (for digesting protein). Some also contain papain (from papaya) or bromelain (from pineapple). These fruits also aid digestion. (See Resources, page 483.)

It's also a good idea to supplement a multivitamin and mineral containing 15mg of zinc, because zinc is needed to make stomach acid. If you eat a high-nutrient diet too, you may well find that, within a month, you can stop the digestive enzymes and stay well.

Q *I've heard that fish oil supplements aren't safe because they contain toxic PCBs. Is this true?*

A It all depends on the brand. If you buy the cheapest fish oil supplements, you are very likely to get the cheapest the producer could find, and it's more likely that the oil has not had the PCBs removed. These harmful industrial pollutants are found in most oceans, and hence in marine fish.

There are several good brands of fish oil that are free of such toxins. Two that have consistently come out the purest in independent tests are Seven Seas and Higher Nature (see Resources, page 483). They manage this by either initially sourcing their oils from minimally polluted waters, and/or using effective methods for removing any traces of toxins. With this in mind, it's completely safe to take fish oil supplements as long as you choose a reputable brand. If you're very concerned, you could ask the manufacturer whether they guarantee their supplements to be PCB-free.

Q *What's your view on flax seed oil?*

A Flax seed oil, also known as linseed oil, is by far the richest plant source of the essential omega-3 fats. Used by Native Americans for a wide variety of health problems, flax seed oil balances hormones and helps with PMS, menopausal problems and male infertility. It contains a fat called alpha linolenic acid, which is converted by the body into the fatty acids EPA and DHA. These two fatty acids are essential for the functioning of the brain, immune system, heart and arteries. Children who are deficient in these omega-3 fats are prone to learning difficulties, hyperactivity and poor coordination, and pregnant women need to pave the way for healthy brain development in the foetus by taking these fats, too. The richest sources are fish and flax seed oil; but while fish oil is a direct source, flax seed oil needs to go through a stage of processing in the body to create EPA and DHA.

If you're deficient, this may show up as dry skin. In most cases a daily tablespoon of flax seed oil, which is best either drunk with some orange juice, or added to salad dressings, soups or cereals, improves dry skin within a week. Alternatively, you can supplement capsules – four 1,000mg caps is an ideal daily amount. With omega-3-rich fish oils, however, limit your supplementation to a *total* of 1,000mg a day.

Q *I've read that glucosamine prevents and repairs joint damage. What's your view?*

A Glucosamine sulphate (GS) is an essential part of the building material for joints, and the cellular 'glue' that holds the entire body together – although joint cartilage contains the highest concentration of GS. GS appears to stop or reverse joint degeneration by providing the body with the materials needed to build and repair damaged cartilage – a process recently proved by a research team in Belgium. (Scientists had originally thought GS just helped reduce the pain of arthritis.) So if you do have any joint problems from injury or arthritis, glucosamine could well help you rebuild the damage. Glucosamine hydrocholoride is more bio-available than glucosamine sulphate, so look for that form. The usual dosage of GS is 500mg, three times daily.

Q *What's your view on melatonin?*

A Best known for beating jetlag, melatonin can also be a remarkably effective solution to other problems – from insomnia to depression and perhaps even ageing. The substance is produced by the pineal gland, at the base of the brain, and is depleted by stress and also decreases naturally as we age. Melatonin is released at night, when it's dark.

If the body's levels are low, supplementing melatonin can help you sleep better. Body levels are naturally higher at night, so it should be taken no more than two hours before bedtime. Melatonin boosts immunity, and is a very powerful antioxidant that can help protect against heart disease and cancer. At night, when it is highest, it helps to 'clean up' the body and brain, reducing cancer risk. Low melatonin levels are often found in people with brain, breast and prostate cancer. Low melatonin levels are believed to be the cause of seasonal affective disorder, or SAD – the winter blues.

Electromagnetic radiation has negative effects on melatonin. So, for example, if you have a cordless phone base station next to your bed, or even a radio clock, the radiation from these devices could be perceived as if they were light, consequently affecting your sleeping and dreaming, and lowering your production of melatonin. So, make sure you sleep in a dark room, without any sources of electromagnetic radiation close to you head.

Melatonin, which is a hormone, not a nutrient, is prescription-only in the UK, and is best taken under the guidance of a health professional. It is also available in the US, over the counter. Suppliers can easily be found on the Web.

Q **What's your view on NADH?**

A The main benefit of this supplement, which has a ridiculously long name (nicotinamide adenine dinucleotide-hydrogen) is, quite simply, energy. I hesitate to suggest that any one substance is a magic route to super-energy, but this comes about as close as you can get. NADH is an essential molecule in the body's production of energy from food, so the more each of your cells has, the more energy they can produce. It is also a powerful antioxidant substance that protects the body from the harmful effects of pollution, fried food and even its own waste products. But there's even more: it's involved in the immune defence system; it can stimulate the production of hormones that boost mood, alertness and sex drive; and it has even been shown to lower cholesterol levels and blood pressure. As an energy boost, try 5mg a day.

Q What's your view on phosphatidyl serine?

A Known as the 'memory molecule', phosphatidyl serine (PS) can genuinely boost your brain power. PS is a type of phospholipid that is essential for the health of the liver, immune system, nerves and brain. PS is especially rich in the brain and there is growing scientific evidence that supplementing 300mg a day improves memory, mood, stress, learning and concentration.

While the body can make its own PS, we rely on receiving some directly from what we eat, making PS a semi-essential nutrient. The trouble is, modern diets are deficient in PS unless you happen to eat a lot of organ meats, in which case you may take in 50mg a day. A vegetarian diet is unlikely to result in even 10mg a day.

The secret of the memory-boosting properties of PS is probably its ability to help brain cells communicate. It is particularly helpful for those with learning difficulties or age-related memory decline and, in one study, only 12 weeks on 300mg of PS significantly improved the ability of the people who were tested to match names to faces. With sixteen clinical trials proving that it works, phosphatidyl serine is a tried and tested nutritional support for memory. (See Resources, page 483.)

Q **What's your view on probiotics?**

A As we all know, our guts are teeming with beneficial bacteria. When we take antibiotics for an infection, or develop a stomach bug, these are wiped out, and our immune defences can become weak. Probiotics – supplements containing some of the same beneficial bacteria found in the gut – can be a good alternative to antibiotics, or at least should be taken along with them to ensure they don't kill off all the bacterial 'good guys'. Probiotics work by helping out existing gut bacteria, and reinforcing the body's immune defences. They can halve the recovery time from a bout of diarrhoea. Most good probiotics will contain *Lactobacillus acidophilus* and *Bifidobacterium bifidus*. Some yoghurts have these bacteria too (check the label), although supplements are a more direct way to boost your defences. (See Resources, page 483.)

Q ***What's your view on SAMe supplements?***

A SAMe, or s-adenosyl-methionine, is a body chemical that helps keep your brain and nervous system well tuned. In fact, as far as the chemistry of connection is concerned, SAMe is the master tuner.

Although the body can make it, many people find supplementing SAMe helpful. SAMe helps neurotransmitters – the nervous system's chemical messengers – deliver their messages to the receptor sites. It can also aid a good night's sleep and stimulate dreaming because it is one of the precursors of the sleep hormone melatonin. SAMe has been proven to be a good anti-depressant, and can generally enhance feelings of wellbeing and connection. It should be taken on an empty stomach, preferably one hour away from food. Start with a dosage of 200mg twice daily, but that can be increased to a maximum of 400mg four times daily, if needed. SAMe should also be taken with its cofactors, vitamins B6, B12 and folic acid.

You may find SAMe too expensive, however; and it is also relatively unstable as a supplement. A good alternative is to supplement TMG (trimethylglycine), the chemical from which the body makes SAMe, as it's cheaper and much more stable. You need three times as much TMG as SAMe, so start with 1,200mg. (See Resources, page 483.)

Q *What's your view on spirulina?*

A Spirulina is an alga, and one of nature's wonderful 'green' superfoods. Its green colour is all down to chlorophyll, which is very cleansing and nourishing and contains the important mineral magnesium. As a wholefood in itself, spirulina provides an easily absorbable spectrum of nutrients, helps detoxify the body, and can be a good all-round tonic. Not only does it contain most vitamins and minerals, from beta-carotene to B vitamins, but also essential fats, protein and phytonutrients – plant nutrients with health-promoting antioxidant properties.

Spirulina has been shown to boost immunity, nourish the skin and increase energy. It would, however, be a mistake to consider it a 'magic bullet' that will protect you from a poor diet or unhealthy lifestyle. It's available in capsules, tablets or powder: quality can vary greatly, so choose an organic variety.

Q *What's your view on 5-HTP?*

A The substance 5-hydroxytryptophan, or 5-HTP for short, is derived from an African plant called griffonia. In the body, 5-HTP is the substance from which serotonin, the 'happy' neurotransmitter, is made. Studies have proven that this nutrient is as effective as the best anti-depressants, but without the side effects. It also appears to control appetite and is sometimes taken as a support to a weight loss diet.

Compared to many people's experiences with the so-called serotonin reuptake inhibitors, which work by blocking the breakdown of serotonin, the action of 5-HTP seems relatively problem-free. If you're depressed, the recommended dosage is 100mg of 5-HTP, twice a day. Note that if it makes you feel sleepy, you probably don't need it. Don't, however, take it if you are on anti-depressant medication.

DIG DEEPER: For more on supplements, and building your own supplement programme, read my book *Supplements for Superhealth* (Piatkus, 2000).

WEIGHT
LOSS

If you're the right weight for your build, you're more likely to feel energised and balanced – and to live a long and healthy life, too. But for many of us, staying trim is an elusive goal. Perhaps this isn't so surprising. Myths about weight loss continue to proliferate along with the diets that publicise them, and finding the ideal method for getting and keeping weight off for life can feel like negotiating a labyrinth. Here I give you a number of threads to get you out of the maze, and into a sensible, practical and above all do-able way of painlessly losing extra pounds.

Q **What do you think of the Atkins diet?**

A If you stick to the low-carbohydrate Atkins diet, it will probably work in the short term – but it is neither the healthiest nor the most effective way to lose weight. The idea behind it is that by eating very few carbohydrates and lots of protein, mainly meat and fish, your blood sugar is stabilised and your body is forced to burn fat. I agree that stabilising your blood sugar is critical for weight loss because this, more than anything, halts food cravings – but the ban on fruit and the extremely high protein intake are another story.

The problem with these rules is twofold. First, although this is refuted in the book, some researchers have shown that high-protein diets can cause a loss in bone mass. Excessive protein creates an acidic environment in the whole body, and triggers an extraction of calcium from the bones to neutralise it, potentially leading to bone-density problems such as osteoporosis in the future. This was recently confirmed in a major article in *New Scientist* (15 December 2001, page 42).

Secondly, most people are desperately short in B vitamins and other nutrients – hence the big emphasis on eating five servings of fruit and vegetables a day. To compensate for this lack in his diet, Dr Atkins does recommend supplements. I'd say they are essential for anyone on a weight-loss diet, not least because the level of the amino acid homocysteine, which is a marker for heart disease, goes up when people on such diets fail to supplement B vitamins, which most do. And while the low-carbohydrate rule is nice and linear, the fact is that slow-releasing carbohydrates, such as oats or apples, don't cause big increases in blood sugar. The Atkins diet is certainly not a 'diet for life', so in the long term it isn't the best way to lose weight and maintain weight control. Instead, eat a well-balanced, largely organic diet with a big emphasis on fresh fruit and vegetables and no high-fat meat, cheese and fried food – a diet in which high-quality protein and carbohydrates such as brown rice and rye bread both have a place, such as my Fatburner Diet. But, which approach works better for losing weight?

Thanks to recent trials published in top medical journals we can make a comparison. To compare 'like with like' the studies featured here all involved people given the diets to follow, who say they follow them 'as best they can'.

So let's first look at Atkins-type diets versus conventional low-calorie, low-fat diets. Two trials carried out at the University of Pennsylvania Medical Center (Samaha and Foster et al.) showed that after six months, those on the Atkins or an Atkins-type diet had lost between 10 pounds and 12.7 pounds, versus 4 pounds to 4.5 pounds on a conventional low fat diet.

So over a six-month period, these studies show that:

Atkins dieters tend to lose, on average, 11.35 pounds after SIX months

while

Conventional, low fat dieters tend to lose, on average, 4.25 pounds.

However, after 12 months there was no significant difference in weight loss in either diet in either study.

But why do Atkins-type diets lead to short-term weight loss? A review of all studies to date on low carb diets (Bravata) concludes that 'weight loss was principally associated with decreased calorie intake'. So although the research in these studies implies that the Atkins Diet works, it finds the results aren't that spectacular and are probably due to eating less.

Nevertheless, Atkins tends to outperform conventional low-calorie low-fat diets in terms of weight loss. But does Atkins help you lose as much weight as my Fatburner Diet, that recommends only 'good' slow-releasing carbohydrates, less 'bad' saturated fat, more 'good' omega 3 fat foods (fish and seeds)?

A study in Ireland (Maconaghie) compared the Fatburner Diet with Unislim, a conventional low calorie, low-fat diet with support group meetings. The average weight loss after 3 months was 13.7 pounds on the Fatburner Diet, versus 2 pounds on the Unislim diet. Not only do Fatburner Dieters appear to lose *more* weight in half the time than the average Atkins dieter, but they also feel better and have none of the risks of bone or kidney stress associated with the Atkins diet, or the risk of dry skin and essential fat deficiency associated with low fat diets.

Q **CLA is touted as the new weight-loss miracle. What's your view?**

A It may not quite have miracle status, but CLA (conjugated linoleic acid) may well help with weight loss. CLA boosts the action of enzymes in the body that encourage the release of stored fat to be burned as fuel. It also appears to reduce the action of another enzyme that facilitates the storage of fat in fat cells. Studies on fat loss in people taking CLA have been mixed – some showing a significant effect and some not much. The richest food sources of CLA are lamb and other meats as well as dairy products, but it's best taken in supplement form. (See Resources, page 483.)

Q *Can you only get fat from eating too many calories?*

A There's much more to weight loss and indeed to food than calories, as shown by the fact that obesity is increasing while the overall intake of calories is generally reducing slightly, and the percentage from fat is decreasing. We are, however, eating proportionately more calories from sugar, consuming more stimulants such as coffee, experiencing more stress, both of which effect blood sugar control, and exercising less.

What is just as important as the quantity (calories) is the quality of the food (as even foods with the same calorific value have a completely different effect on weight. For example, essential fats (from fish or seeds), while having the same number of calories as saturated fats (from meat or dairy produce), can be put to good use in the brain, immune system, cardiovascular system and skin, leaving less to add to your unwanted fat stores. There is also some evidednce that omega 3 fats help utilise body fat as fuel, hence helping to burn fat. Saturated fats, on the other hand, can only be used to make energy, so an excess will affect weight.

Then there's the blood sugar phenomenon, which I think is the crux to most people's weight problems. Many overweight people have wildly fluctuating blood sugar levels due to excess sugar, stimulants and stress. When their blood sugar levels are too high and there's more than the body can use for energy, the excess is turned to fat. So weight loss involves far more than just calorie counting.

Q **Do slimming drinks like Calorad really work?**

A Calorad was recently exposed as a scam and the importer was found guilty of making false claims about the product. There's certainly nothing in it that offers instant weight loss. Although not all slimming drinks are such a con, most make unrealistic claims. They leave you craving food, and even if they do the trick in the short term, the weight usually piles right back on afterwards. A sensible (solid) diet is almost always best. As far as supplements are concerned, hydroxycitric acid (HCA), which is extracted from the tamarind plant, can help stop excess carbohydrates being stored as fat, as can 200mcg a day of the mineral chromium.

Q *Why do men seem to lose weight more easily than women?*

A Women have a higher percentage of body fat and are literally designed to store more fat. Why? Because fats are essential for foetal development, both for the infant's brain and also to ensure there are enough calories around to keep mother and baby nourished. This basic design also means that men, proportionately, have more lean body – or muscle – mass. Muscle tissue burns a lot more calories than fat tissue. So if a man decides to lose weight by cutting calories, he'll have more muscle to burn off unwanted fat. The genetic programming of a man also means that men build muscle quicker, and the more muscle you have the more you can burn off fat. That's one big reason why exercise, plus fewer calories, works as a weight-loss method. Of course, the same applies for women even if the results are a little slower.

Q *In the last two years I've become more 'pear shaped'. Why is this?*

A This kind of weight gain isn't just gravity. It's often caused by 'oestrogen dominance'. When you have an excess of oestrogen to progesterone, fat starts to accumulate on the bum, hips and thighs. You can actually test for this with an ingenious saliva test: ask your doctor for details, or visit a nutritionist.

If you find you do have oestrogen dominance,

there are a number of things you can do. First, cut right back on meat and dairy products and eat more fish and seeds instead. Meat and dairy are often high in hormones and hormone-like chemicals, as well as saturated fat, while fish and seeds provide highly beneficial essential fats – and one of the benefits is that they balance your hormones. Also cut out sugar and refined carbohydrates and eat more wholefoods, such as brown rice, lentils and beans. Beans are especially good because they help to lower the body's oestrogen overload. It's also worth going organic as much as possible. Many pesticides and herbicides act like oestrogen in the body. If your oestrogen level is very high, and your progesterone level very low, you may need to use some transdermal natural progesterone for a few months to bring your hormones back into balance. Any weight-loss diet based on the general advice for balancing your blood sugar will work.

That means cutting out all stimulants such as coffee, sugary snacks and drinks, and saturated fats; eating little and often; and choosing oats, brown basmati rice, pears, apples and other slow-release carbs, and good-quality protein such as organic chicken, tofu or fish. Always combine carbohydrates with protein. For instance, with brown rice, eat lentils, broccoli and tofu stir-fry, or a piece of roast chicken; with a piece of rye bread, eat bean salad; or with a piece of fruit, have a dessertspoon of pumpkin seeds or a few almonds. Go organic, ensure you drink 1.5 litres of pure water a day and take 200mcg of chromium a day.

> **DIG DEEPER:** For details on natural progesterone, contact the Natural Progesterone Information Service on 07000 784849.

Q *What's the best type of exercise to burn fat?*

A You might think that the best fat-burning exercise is whatever burns the most calories. However, the real trick to keeping slim is to have more muscle and less fat. Muscle cells require more calories (energy) to stay alive, so they burn fat around the clock, while fat cells require very few calories to stay alive. So, as you start to gain lean muscle you are becoming a fat burner rather than a fat storer. You will lose inches, but possibly not so many pounds in the first month. This is because lean muscle weighs more than fat. But who cares, as long as you look good and feel good?

So, what achieves this? Any active, strengthening exercise that you can stick to. My favourites are Astanga yoga, a very active form of yoga, and Psychocalisthenics, a brilliant 15-minute exercise that is like aerobic yoga –you learn it in a half-day's worth of training and can do it at home without any equipment (see Resources, page 483). I'd recommend Psychocalisthenics as a daily regime at home, plus two other exercise classes (good aerobic, step or circuit training), brisk walks, cycle rides or jogs a week.

Q *What supplements or foods can boost your body's metabolism?*

A A regular exercise regime is actually the only way to raise your basal metabolic rate. The effect lasts for about 15 hours after you stop exercising. And while nutrients cannot themselves change your metabolism, certain foods and supplements can enhance the way your body turns food to energy. The B vitamins are essential for this process, so take a B complex. Keeping an even blood sugar level also helps – so avoid refined foods, sugar and coffee and take 200mcg of the mineral chromium a day. A substance called hydroxycitric acid (HCA), an extract from the tamarind plant, has also been shown to enhance the body's use of fat for making energy, reduce the conversion of excess sugar to fat and lessen appetite. (See Resources, page 483.)

Q *Does food combining work for weight loss?*

A The answer is yes and no. People do tend to lose weight on food combining diets, but the reason is unclear. The food combining principles of Dr Hay, now described and amended in various books, extol the virtues of wholefoods, cutting out sugar, eating more fresh fruit and vegetables and less meat and processed foods – and all of this is good, sensible advice which in and of itself could easily help you lose weight.

But the keystone of food combining is to separate protein-rich foods from carbohydrate-rich foods. In order to test whether this method affected weight loss, some students of mine put two groups of people on a 'food combining diet', with all the healthy foods recommended; one group ate them in any combination, and the other ate proteins and carbohydrates separately. Both groups lost weight, but there was marginally more weight lost in the group that followed strict food combining principles. Whether this was due to the food combining itself, or the awkwardness of the process (it isn't easy to 'food combine' and eat out, so you can end up eating less) is unclear.

DIG DEEPER: For more on effective weight loss, see my book *The 30 Day Fatburner Diet* (Piatkus, 1999).

WOMEN'S HEALTH

In some very important ways, the last decade has been a brilliant one for women's health. A number of phytonutrients and herbal supplements have emerged as excellent alternatives to risk-laden hormone replacement therapy for treating symptoms of the menopause. More generally, optimum nutrition, including supplementing omega-3 oils, is emerging as a prime way of keeping hormones balanced and nurturing a healthy foetus. You'll find a range of information on women's health issues here, from menstruation through pregnancy and the menopause. (Advice on nutrition and breast cancer can be found on page 145.)

Contraception

Q *I've been on the Pill since I was 16. I'm worried about my fertility and the risk of cancer. What's your view?*

A You have reason to be concerned. Some contraceptive pills contain oestradiol, and taking this form of oestrogen is ill advised for young girls before their breasts are fully developed. It is well known that girls taking the Pill between the ages of 13 and 18 can increase their risk of getting breast cancer by as much as 60 per cent. This is because undeveloped breasts contain more stem cells, which are vulnerable to the known cancer-promoting effects of hormones in the Pill. Oestrogen-containing pills can encourage 'oestrogen dominance', which is a major cause of infertility. Progesterone is the female hormone that not only balances out oestrogen, but is also vital for maintaining a healthy pregnancy. In the body, oestrogen makes things grow, such as the lining of the womb, while progesterone's job is to keep these uterine cells healthy. I'd recommend waiting six months after coming off the Pill before trying to get pregnant. Your doctor can test your oestrogen and progesterone levels at this point to check that everything is OK. B vitamins such as vitamin B6, B12 and folic acid, together with magnesium and zinc, help to protect against the harmful effects of the Pill. (See Resources, page 483.)

Q **Can vitamin C stop the Pill from working?**

A There was a concern that vitamin C could make oestrogen more potent, though this has been thoroughly investigated and shown not to be the case. There is one other concern about vitamin C in relation to the Pill: it can cause loose stools if taken in excess, and diarrhoea, as you probably know, can stop the Pill from working. Again, I do not share this concern, as the problem with diarrhoea is that it usually involves an infection and/or reduced absorption (of food and the Pill), whereas the loose stools caused by excessive vitamin C do not involve a reduced nutrient absorption, and so should not affect the Pill's effectiveness. In other words, in my opinion, vitamin C is fine to take when you're on the Pill.

But you have to decide for yourself. The Pill isn't 100 per cent effective, so should it fail, you can't know whether it was because of the vitamin C or not. Therefore, most take a very cautionary line and recommend no more than 1g of C per day if you're on the Pill. I feel this is a reasonable position. If you need more vitamin C, consider another form of contraception.

Q **I have just started taking the Pill – what supplements should I take?**

A The Pill increases your need for vitamins B6, B12, folic acid and zinc. It is especially important to achieve optimum amounts of these, and you can do that easily with a good all-round multivitamin and mineral. (See Resources, page 483.) Zinc is important because copper levels tend to go up in Pill users, and zinc counteracts copper. You want a supplement that gives you at least ten times as much zinc as copper (if it has any copper at all). Drinking filtered water also helps because much of our water passes through copper pipes and can pick up some copper as a result. (This is particularly a problem in new houses and in soft water areas. The softer the water, the less the pipes get calcified, and the more acidic is the water, which means copper can pass more easiliy into the water. New houses have new copper pipes, with lots of rough edges in the bends.)

Fertility

Q *I'm having difficulty getting pregnant. What kind of diet and supplements should I be on?*

A No doubt you're aware of folic acid. However, folic acid is but one of several nutrients that maximise fertility and lower the risk of pregnancy problems. Folic acid is important because, along with vitamins B2, B6 and B12, it helps the body to methylate, a fundamental chemical process involved in building new cells. Women who have a high level of a protein in the blood called homocysteine are poor methylators, and are much less likely to conceive, and more likely to have miscarriages. For this reason I'd recommend having your homocysteine level checked (see Resources, page 483). If it's high, take more of these B vitamins, plus zinc. There are specific supplements designed to help maintain normal, healthy homocysteine levels.

Also vital are essential fats, especially the omega-3 fat DHA. This is found in wild salmon, herring, sardines and mackerel, and supports reproductive health in both men and women. It's also an essential nerve builder in the growing foetus.

Q *What can my husband and I do to increase our chances of conceiving?*

A Remember that you're aiming to create a new body from your own (and from healthy sperm, in the case of your husband). So for three months before you start trying to conceive, aim for a superhealthy lifestyle.

Give up smoking, minimise alcohol, cut out all recreational drugs and take as few medical drugs as possible. Start eating a diet rich in nutrients, focusing on organic foods, fresh fruit and vegetables, fish and wholegrains, and cutting out processed and junk foods. Take a good-quality multivitamin and mineral with at least 400mcg of folic acid and 15mg of zinc – or supplement extra. Essential fatty acids are crucial, as they support your monthly cycle and the health of your husband's sperm as well as the development of the nervous system (including the eyes and brain) and immunity in the growing foetus. So ensure you're getting enough of these beneficial fats by eating good-quality mackerel, wild or organic salmon and other oily fish three times a week, and pumpkin, sunflower and flax seeds as snacks or with your morning cereal – or supplement a high-quality, PCB-free fish oil capsule. (See Resources, page 483.) And finally, correct any underlying health issues such as ongoing fatigue, digestive problems or high blood pressure.

Q *I am having a fertility problem because my hormones are out of balance. What can I do?*

A While any long-term hormonal imbalance cannot be addressed overnight, there is plenty you can do to gently shift the situation. There are several herbs that are very useful in rebalancing hormones, particularly one called Vitex agnus castus or chasteberry. Others are false unicorn root, sarsasparilla, white peony, dong quai and black cohosh. A blend of Agnus castus and other nutrients is very helpful in supporting the pituitary gland, the master gland for directing hormone production. Your overall health has a knock-on effect on all parts of the body including hormone regulation, so eating a healthy diet is key: concentrate on fresh fruit and vegetables, fish, lean meat, wholegrains, beans and lentils, and impose a ban on coffee, tea, alcohol, sugar, and sugary and processed foods.

Q *I'm trying to have a baby but my partner's got a low sperm count. Any advice?*

A Given today's diets and lifestyles, it's not surprising that many men have low sperm counts. Assuming nothing mechanical is wrong, there's plenty your partner can do to help raise his fertility. Of all the nutrients known to affect male fertility, the mineral zinc is best researched. Not only does the body need zinc to release vitamin A (essential for making the male sex hormones) from the liver, but an adequate supply of zinc is needed for the formation of healthy sperm as it is found in high concentrations in the outer layer and tail of sperm. Beans, nuts and seeds are good, easily available sources of zinc as well as arginine, an amino acid particularly abundant in sperm. So in addition to avoiding 'anti-nutrients' such as smoking, and reducing alcohol and stress, get your partner to take a good multivitamin which contains at least 15mg of zinc, eat a moderate handful of nuts and seeds a day, and introduce more beans into his diet – easily done, as they're a tasty addition to soups, curries, stir-fries, stews and salads.

The Menopause

Q *What are the best natural remedies for menopausal symptoms?*

 You are very wise to be looking for natural alternatives, given that HRT increases your risk of breast cancer, and also that its bone-protecting benefits disappear as soon as you stop taking it. Several herbs such as dong quai and Mexican yam are age-old remedies, while nutrients such as vitamin E and magnesium have also been shown to help. There have been great results with extracts from soya and red clover, which contain active substances called isoflavones, in scientific tests. The herb St John's wort, famous as an anti-depressant, can also relieve other menopausal symptoms (see 'What are the best herbs for hot flushes?' below). So a blend of two or three of these could be highly effective in combating menopausal symptoms. (See Resources, page 483.)

Q **What are the best herbs for hot flushes?**

A There are three herbs that are coming up strong in recent research. Most promising are the results with the herb black cohosh which helps hot flushes, sweating, insomnia, and anxiety. Also encouraging is new research that shows that black cohosh doesn't have a down side – it doesn't increase cancer risk nor is it anti-oestrogenic. The usual recommended amount is 50mg, however much larger amounts, up to 500mg, are more effective. It also helps raise serotonin, relieving depression.

The combination of black cohosh and St John's wort (300mg a day) is particularly effective for women who experience depression, irritability and fatigue. St John's wort, reknowned for its anti-depressant effects, has been demonstrated to relieve other menopausal symptoms including headaches, palpitations, lack of concentration and decreased libido. A medical trial in Germany found that 80 per cent of women felt their symptoms had gone or substantially improved at the end of 12 weeks.

The other 'hot' herb for hot flushes is dong quai, officially called Angelica sinensis. One placebo-controlled experiment giving dong quai plus camomile to 55 postmenopausal women who complained of hot flushes and refused hormonal therapy found there was a big reduction, almost 80 per cent, in the number of hot flushes. These results became apparent after one month. Try 600mg a day. The best results are often achieved by a combination of herbs, in which case you can often use half the therapeutic amount of the herb. Whatever you try give it six weeks for a fair trial.

Q *I've stopped HRT because of the risks, but the hot flushes are back. What can I do?*

A Hot flushes happen when the ovaries stop producing enough oestrogen. The pituitary gland in the brain then overproduces certain hormones in an attempt to kickstart the ovaries into action. It is this over-production of pituitary hormones that triggers hot flushes. If you take oestrogen they tend to stop, but oestrogen HRT does have problems – not least of which is the increased risk of breast cancer. Recent research has shown that the hormone progesterone works just as well, if not better, at stopping hot flushes. The good news is that progesterone reverses breast cancer risk, and is therefore better than oestrogen HRT. However, do not confuse 'natural' progesterone, which comes as transdermal cream that's absorbed through the skin, with synthetic progestins used in HRT preparations. The latter are not the same thing at all and do have associated problems. A recent US study showed that menopausal symptoms in 83 per cent of women using natural progesterone cream were significantly better or disappeared. Natural progesterone is available on prescription from your doctor.

Vitamin E supplements (400mg/600iu) and the herb agnus castus are helpful, but isoflavones, plant oestrogens found in soya, red clover and chickpeas, have a more powerful effect. Supplementing isoflavones from red clover or from soya has been shown to reduce hot flushes quite significantly. The herb St John's wort, widely used as an anti-depressant, can also relieve menopausal symptoms such as headaches, palpitations and decreased libido. So a combination of these substances could be a highly effective alternative to HRT. (See Resources, page 483.)

DIG DEEPER: You can get more details on natural progesterone from the Natural Progesterone Information Service on 07000 784849, or send a first class stamp to NPIS, PO Box 24, Buxton SK17 9FB.

 I am on HRT but am losing my hair. What can I do?

A HRT has many side effects, of which hair loss is one. The main culprit behind this appears to be progesterone rather than oestrogen deficiency. When progesterone is low, the body compensates by making more androgens, and it's this that can lead to male-pattern baldness.

When you go though the menopause your body produces less oestrogen, but it doesn't necessarily mean you are deficient. Oestrogen is made in body fat and in sufficient quantities usually until around the age of 80. However, progesterone deficiency is far more common. Conventional HRT uses synthetic progestin, which the body cannot use as effectively. So women on HRT are likely to be more progesterone deficient.

HRT is frequently prescribed without first checking a woman's hormone levels – and even if this is done, the usual blood test only measures redundant hormones and not those in circulation. The most effective way to test is via a saliva test, which shows the level of active hormones (see Resources, page 483). In the unlikely event that oestrogen is deficient, appropriate levels need to be prescribed. Where progesterone is deficient, natural progesterone cream, available on prescription (see 'I've stopped HRT', page 483), helps to correct this. Then the excess androgens reduce and scalp hair returns to normal.

Also helpful for relieving menopausal symptoms are vitamin B6 and E, zinc and magnesium, and herbs such as dong quai and white peony, in addition to the essential fats found in evening primrose and borage oil. There are supplements that contain combinations of these nutrients and herbs.

Q *I am 43 years old and have not had a period for four months. Are there any nutritional guidelines for encouraging ovarian activity?*

A There are many factors that can cause periods to stop. These include stress, inadequate nutrition (from dieting, not eating enough or following a diet high in nutrient-deficient foods) or pregnancy! If your periods don't return within six months, you should visit your doctor for referral to a gynaecologist. But in the meantime, to help bring your body back into balance, follow the advice below:

- Check your weight – if you are significantly under- or overweight your periods can stop. Dieting can also have the same effect if you're losing a lot of weight very quickly and are starving your body of essential nutrients.
- Eat a wholefood diet rich in wholegrains such as brown rice, rye bread and oat cakes, fresh fruits and vegetables, lean meat, tofu, oily fish, nuts and seeds.
- Supplement your diet with a good multivitamin and mineral supplement with good levels of zinc (15 to 20mg) and magnesium (375 to 500mg).
- Also take a B-complex supplement. Choose one that contains good levels of all the B vitamins, including folic acid. Folic acid is absolutely crucial for your cells to multiply normally. When working on getting your periods back, it's important that your ovaries are able to produce eggs, and that the cells in those eggs are able to divide properly.

- The herb agnus castus is also useful for helping to bring hormones back into balance. It works on the pituitary gland by balancing the levels of FSH (follicle stimulating hormone) and LH (luteinising hormone), which then sends a message to the ovaries. The result is that progesterone levels go up and your cycle kicks back into action. This can take between three and six months. Try your local healthfood shop for this herb.

Pregnancy and birth

Q *Do you recommend an anti-candida regime during pregnancy?*

A Candida albicans is a kind of yeast that lives in the intestines and on the skin. Ordinarily, it's kept in check by friendly bacteria; but it can break out under the effects of hormonal disturbance and poor diet, and emerge as thrush, cystitis and a number of other complaints such as bloating and chronic fatigue. However uncomfortable the symptoms, it's best to avoid a targeted anti-candida regime using supplements during pregnancy. Instead, you can maintain a candida-unfriendly diet by cutting out sugar, yeast, all alcohol, fermented products, mushrooms and so on, and using a probiotic pessary (or live yoghurt) to ensure you do not get thrush around the time of birth. This is because thrush can be passed to the sterile gut of your baby.

If you're not yet pregnant and know you have candida, this is the best time to clear it. The main reason for doing it now is that an anti-candida regime, if successful, creates a 'healing crisis' where the body has even more toxins to deal with as a result of the die-off reaction. That would severely overload an already taxed body if you were pregnant. An anti-candida regime is best embarked upon under the guidance of a qualified nutritional therapist. See Resources, page 483, for a list of nutritional therapists.

Q **What should I supplement to stay healthy in pregnancy, and have a healthy baby?**

A Although the most famous baby supplement – folic acid – is important, there are many other nutrients that are needed for a healthy baby. Omega-3 fats, found in oily fish and flax seeds, are important for the formation of the baby's brain and nervous system. Recent research has also shown that taking choline during pregnancy can create a 'superbrain' in the baby. Although the study was on baby rats, I'd still recommend taking choline in the form of lecithin, derived from soya. Sprinkle a heaped teaspoon on your cereal in the morning. I'd also recommend a good multi so that you get not only your folic acid (400mcg), but also a spectrum of nutrients including zinc (15mg), which is crucial for the healthy development of your baby before it is born.

Q *Is it dangerous to supplement vitamin A in pregnancy?*

A Only in very large amounts in the animal form, known as retinol. Beta-carotene, which is the vegetable form of vitamin A, is not toxic because the more you take in, the less the body converts into retinol. Retinol is risky because it can store in the liver, and excessive amounts of it may increase risk of birth defects, although this has never been proven in humans, only animals. The concern was orginally raised because there have been cases of birth defects reported in women taking a synthetic relative of vitamin A, sold as the drug Roaccutane. In any case, it is probably wise not to supplement more than 3,000mcg (10,000ius) of vitamin A during pregnancy. Neither should you eat liver frequently, as it's a very concentrated source of retinol. However, it is a good idea to supplement a multivitamin containing vitamin A below this level, as well as folic acid, as multivitamin supplementation during pregnancy has been shown to reduce the risk of birth defects by 75 per cent, according to research published in the *Journal of the American Medical Association.*

Q *Is it safe to take a fish oil supplement during pregnancy? And is it safe to eat tuna?*

A Omega-3 oils are vital during pregnancy, both for your own wellbeing and for nerve and brain development in the growing foetus. But you need to pick and choose your oil carefully. Firstly, you want a pure oil, free from PCBs. Two brands that have consistently come out purest on independent tests are Higher Nature and Seven Seas.

Secondly, you don't want to supplement more than 3,000mcg (10,000ius) of vitamin A in the form of retinol during pregnancy (see 'Is it dangerous to supplement vitamin A in pregnancy?', opposite). Cod liver oil, which is an excellent source of omega-3, can be too high in retinol, so check the label. That said, most cod liver oil supplements rarely supply more than 800mcg (2,640ius) of vitamin A, so in practical terms this means that you are fine taking two or three of these high-strength caps. In terms of the omega-3 fatty acids DHA and EPA, you want about 1,000mg a day.

As for tuna, it has been found to be high in mercury, so you should eat other oily fish, preferably from waters that are as unpolluted as possible (for example, wild salmon from the Arctic), or organic fish.

Q *Which supplements can I take while pregnant and after the birth to avoid excessive weight gain without harming my baby's health?*

A During pregnancy, your main focus has to be keeping your body optimally nourished for the ongoing healthy development of your baby. It is best not to try to lose weight at this very important time in your life. In any case, 'eating for two' doesn't mean letting go and tearing into mountains of munchies, although various models and starlets have recently been in the news revelling in this brief opportunity to 'get fat'.

Really eating for two is following the very same healthy eating patterns that will keep you, yourself, optimally nourished, and that doesn't entail excessive weight gain. A well-balanced menu of high-quality proteins such as lean free-range chicken, tofu, lentils, beans and quinoa, teamed with plenty of organic fruit and vegetables and slow-release carbohydrates such as wholemeal pasta and rye bread, will leave you and baby in splendid shape. I suggest that in addition to following the principles of optimum nutrition you take a high strength multivitamin containing at least 10mg of zinc and a PCB-free omega-3 fish oil supplement to optimise your health and the growth of your baby.

Q **I've had early miscarriages. Is there anything I can do to prevent this happening again?**

A Overall, the better your nutrition, the better your chances, so I would certainly recommend you see a nutrition therapist to get yourself in the best possible condition. Deficiencies in zinc, for example, are linked to miscarriages. So too are high levels of the amino acid homocysteine. These can be tested for (see Resources, page 483) and, if present, specific dietary supplements can be recommended to get you into good health. These will contain the vitamins B6, B12, folic acid and an amino acid called trimethylglycine (TMG), all of which have been shown to lower levels of homocysteine.

Another extremely common cause of early miscarriage is progesterone deficiency. Progesterone is the hormone that the womb needs to stay healthy. Again, a nutritionist can test if you are low in this hormone. If you are, your doctor can prescribe natural progesterone, given as a transdermal skin cream. Supplement small amounts of progesterone in this way until you are three months pregnant, by which time the placenta takes over producing the hormones necessary to maintain a healthy pregnancy.

DIG DEEPER: You can get more details on natural progesterone from the Natural Progesterone Information Service on 07000 784849, or send a first class stamp to NPIS, PO Box 24, Buxton SK17 9FB.

Q *What can you recommend for morning sickness?*

A Morning sickness has been shown to respond well to 50mg of vitamin B6 twice a day and 200 to 500mg of magnesium once a day, plus sufficient B12 and folic acid (which you will get from a good multivitamin). Ginger may also help to relieve the sickness and settle your stomach – take either in capsules or as tea. To make the tea, chop or grate fresh ginger root into a cup and add boiling water. Steep for five minutes before drinking.

Q *Last time I was pregnant I got stretch marks. How can I prevent this?*

A Up your intake of vitamins A (to a maximum of 3,000mcg when pregnant), C, E and the mineral zinc, which are all key for skin health. A stretch mark is a tear in the collagen fibre of your skin, so while these nutrients can't necessarily repair it, they can help increase skin elasticity and tone, and prevent any further stretch marks developing. Applying vitamin E oil directly to your stomach and areas where any stretch marks appeared in your previous pregnancy will also help to condition your skin and reduce the appearance of existing marks. Just prick a vitamin E supplement capsule with a pin, and rub the contents directly into the skin. Alternatively, use a strong vitamin E cream. Also, make sure you have a good intake of essential fats, preferably by eating a tablespoon of ground seeds every day and supplementing 1,000mg of omega-3 fish oil containing EPA and DHA – essential in pregnancy for maximising brain development in the growing foetus.

Q *What is your view on vitamin K given to newborn babies?*

A Vitamin K is important for blood clotting and is manufactured by gut bacteria. It is given to all newborns either orally or as an injection because a very small number of babies get haemorrhagic disease in which they bleed uncontrollably. When they are first born, babies do not yet have sufficient gut bacteria to produce their own vitamin K, but can receive it via breast milk, provided the mother is not deficient. The mother may be deficient if she has an imbalance in her gut bacteria, does not eat cruciferous vegetables (which provide vitamin K), takes certain drugs or excessive vitamin A supplements, or has liver or gut disease. Breastfeeding encourages the growth of healthy gut bacteria in the baby, who can then make their own vitamin K within a few days. This process is obviously hindered by antibiotics.

So, if the mother has good digestive health, eats cruciferous vegetables, breastfeeds, and if the newborn is healthy enough to not require antibiotics in the first few weeks of life, there seems no need for vitamin K supplementation, though oral drops seem an unobtrusive intervention that can benefit a small number of infants. I doubt that there is anything to the suspected link between vitamin K injections and cancer, though an injection does seem an unnecessary trauma for the vast majority of newborns. I didn't opt for this at the birth of my children.

Q *If I'm unable to breastfeed, what would be the best alternative?*

A There are plenty of formulas on offer, but you need to be careful. Babies often become allergic to formula made from cow's milk, and sometimes also become sensitised to soya milk formula. This happens simply because their digestive tracts and immune systems are immature and designed for human milk. One of the best tolerated alternatives is a goat's milk formula called Nanny. It is made by Vitacare and their freephone helpline is 0800 328 5826. I'd go for this.

Q *Do children, and pregnant and breastfeeding women, need milk?*

A Yes – in that they need calcium, the main touting-ground for milk. But that does not mean they need *milk*. In fact, there are reasons why they would do well to avoid it. Firstly, dairy consumption by infants under three months old or their breastfeeding mothers is a risk factor for diabetes in children who are genetically susceptible to it. Secondly, milk is the most common food allergen for children and a common one in adults, and avoidance in early years reduces that risk. Thirdly, milk contains significant quantities of oestrogen-like chemicals from pesticides and pollutants that get stored in the fat of cows. These so-called xenoestrogens are increasingly associated with hormonal imbalances, reproductive problems and cancer risk in later life. Of course, organic milk is better in this respect. Luckily, there are many other great food sources for calcium (nuts, seeds, root vegetables and sardines) and for protein (fish, lentils and beans, free-range chicken and lean meat).

Q *Can you recommend anything for post-natal depression?*

A Serious post-natal depression is thought to affect up to 15 per cent of new mothers, and feeling weepy or down is even more common. Although there's a psychological component – from shouldering the huge responsibility of a baby – post-natal depression is usually triggered by hormonal and chemical changes, and these can be supported with good nutrition.

Before you give birth, you transfer a large supply of zinc to your baby, and if you didn't have a good supply yourself, the chances are you're now deficient, especially if your labour was long and difficult or you had a caesarean. Depression is a common side effect of zinc deficiency, as are white marks on more than two fingernails, a poor appetite, stretch marks and a weak immune system. So if you have any of these additional symptoms, up your supplementary zinc intake to 15mg twice a day until your mood improves. As zinc works with the B vitamin family, particularly B6, also take a B complex supplement.

The other common deficiency in post-natal depression is in essential fats. In a study of 11,721 British women, those who consumed fish two or three times a week were half as likely to suffer from depression as women with the lowest intakes. So eat more oily fish (organic salmon, sardines and mackerel, although go easy on fresh tuna, as it can contain mercury) and some fresh pumpkin and sunflower seeds each day to boost essential fats in your diet. Also take an all-round essential fat supplement containing 600mg of EPA, 400mg DHA and 200mg GLA.

Problems with periods

Q *My breasts become very tender a week before my period. Is there anything I can do?*

A There are several key nutrients that can help reduce the water retention that you get before a period, and that makes your breasts swollen and tender. First up are vitamin B6, magnesium and zinc. Magnesium is particularly helpful – supplement 300mg along with 100mg of vitamin B6 and 20mg of zinc. Some supplements contain a blend of these nutrients and herbs aimed at preventing premenstrual problems (see Resources, page 483). Another important one is gamma-linolenic acid, or GLA, which is found in evening primrose oil. The trouble is that most people don't take enough. You need about 250mg of GLA, *not* of the oil – and so should supplement five capsules. A much more cost effective way is to supplement a concentrated borage (starflower) oil capsule – you usually only need one of these a day. Also, in addition to a healthy diet free of stimulants and sugar, be sure to drink 1.5 litres of pure water a day, as this will help prevent water retention.

Q *I get desperately depressed before my period. What can I do?*

A Unconnected as it may seem, a key factor in balancing your premenstrual moods is to balance your blood sugar levels throughout the month. If your blood sugar levels are all over the place, your moods and energy are likely to follow. For this, cut your intake of tea, coffee, alcohol and sugar right down; eat 'little and often'; and have some good protein at each meal such as eggs, tofu, fish, lean meat or nuts. Taking 200mcg of the mineral chromium also helps regulate blood sugar levels. Many women who have premenstrual depression are deficient in the hormone progesterone – but natural progesterone is available in a cream.

DIG DEEPER: You can get more details on natural progesterone from the Natural Progesterone Information Service on 07000 784849, or send a first class stamp to NPIS, PO Box 24, Buxton SK17 9FB.

Q *Which supplements are best for PMS?*

A For years, the key nutrient for avoiding PMS has been vitamin B6. It was then discovered than B6 works better with zinc. Then research found that magnesium is especially helpful for women with breast tenderness. Many women also find relief with evening primrose oil, which is high in an essential fat called GLA. GLA is converted in the body into prostaglandins, which among other things help reduce PMS symptoms such as water retention, irritability and fatigue. And to tie it all together, scientists have now established that the conversion in the body of GLA to prostaglandins depends on adequate B6, magnesium and zinc. There are supplements that combine these three nutrients; and in addition, I recommend you supplement the equivalent of 250mg of GLA. So take one starflower oil (or borage oil) 1,000mg capsule, or five evening primrose oil 500mg capsules.

Keeping blood sugar levels even throughout the month helps minimise PMS. For this, eat regularly, have protein (fish, yoghurt, lean meat, soya) and fibre (vegetables, fruit, wholegrains) at each meal, cut out sugar, processed foods, coffee, tea and alcohol and take 200mcg of the mineral chromium each day.

Q *Can chocolate help alleviate PMS?*

A Yes – but don't start eyeing up the oversized bars in your local supermarket. Chocolate can in fact ease symptoms of PMS psychologically, and to a certain extent nutritionally. A good-quality plain chocolate does contain nutrients such as calcium and magnesium (which help to relieve muscle spasms), B6 (which helps to regulate hormone function) and the amino acid tryptophan (which boosts serotonin levels, so reducing anxiety and balancing mood). But unless it's got very high cocoa content (70 per cent plus), and you eat enough of it, it's unlikely that you'll get sufficient quantities of these nutrients to make any real impact. As chocolate also contains sugar and stimulants, eating more than a few squares at a time can affect blood sugar balance and unsettle your energy levels – which will both make PMS worse.

Q *I suffer from PMS and mood swings but since taking pregnenolone I feel great. Are there long-term side effects, though?*

A While pregnenolone is a naturally occurring hormone, that doesn't make it harmless. It can be used by the body to make adrenal and sex hormones, so it can have a powerful effect. Although pregnenelone levels normally decline as we age, supplementing it, or too much of it, means your body needs to work harder to get rid of any potential excess. (In this regard, hormones aren't like vitamins. The body is well designed to excrete excess vitamins. Hormonal levels are controlled more by reducing production than by promoting excretion.) So more is not necessarily better. Even though it does help those with adrenal exhaustion, blood sugar problems and hormonal imbalances, it really isn't advisable to take unless supervised by a qualified nutritional consultation.

Reproductive health

Q *I've been diagnosed with fibroids. What can I do?*

A These benign lumps affect as many as 30 per cent of women, usually in their late thirties and early forties. Symptoms are irregular, heavy and painful periods and sometimes stress incontinence. The usual treatment is surgical removal. Fibroids are, however, caused by 'unopposed' oestrogen, which means you have a relatively high level of oestrogen in relation to progesterone. So applying natural progesterone, which comes in transdermal skin cream, could help. Other things you can do to help are reduce your exposure to plastics that contain oestrogen-like chemicals, and eat organic foods naturally high in fibre (such as beans, fruit, vegetables and brown rice). Various herbs, including agnus castus, support hormonal balance.

DIG DEEPER: You can get more details on natural progesterone from the Natural Progesterone Information Service on 07000 784849, or send a first class stamp to NPIS, PO Box 24, Buxton SK17 9FB.

Q *I have polycystic ovarian syndrome (PCOS) and have now developed impaired glucose tolerance. What can I do?*

A PCOS is a complex problem, and not clearly understood. It has been linked to high insulin levels, as well as excessive testosterone. The latter is why many sufferers put on weight and develop excess hair. Other symptoms can mimic those of a sluggish thyroid, and you may have heavy periods and severe chocolate cravings. Luckily, there is much you can do nutritionally.

Much of the clinical research on PCOS has focused on poor insulin mechanisms. My main recommendations are to work hard on blood sugar balance and insulin sensitivity. Include protein-rich foods at every meal (such as fish, eggs, soya, pulses and beans), avoid refined foods (and that means no grains and bread subjected to over-processing or using refined flours, and no sugar) and eat wholegrains such as brown rice, quinoa and wholemeal pasta instead. Eat plenty of fruits and vegetables, but if you like to snack on fruit, have it with a handful of fresh, unsalted nuts or seeds, as the protein will prevent a sugar high and a subsequent nasty slump. Ensure you're taking in enough essential fatty acids, found in oily fish and seeds such as pumpkin and flax seeds. Taking 200mcg of chromium daily will also help, and a good B complex supplement or high-strength multivitamin.

Herbally, I find a blend including agnus castus helps regulate hormone balance, while some herbalists recommend taking saw palmetto to help lower the conversion of testosterone to its more potent form DHT; but it is worth checking this with a qualified herbalist.

DIG DEEPER: For more on women's health, read my books *Balancing Hormones Naturally* (Piatkus, 2003) coauthored with Kate Neil, and *Optimum Nutrition Before, During and After Pregnancy* (Piatkus, 2004), coathored with Susannah Lawson.

RESOURCES

Useful Contacts

Full-spectrum light bulbs
FSL supply a wide range of full-spectrum lighting including bulbs and tubes

FSL, Unit 1, Riverside Business Centre, Victoria Street, High Wycombe, Bucks HP11 2LT. Tel: 01494 448727.

Nutrition consultations
For a personal referral by Patrick Holford to a nutritional therapist in the UK in your area, visit www.patrick holford.com and select 'consultations' for an immediate online referral. This website also gives you details on who to see outside of the UK and how to get an online consultation if there's no one near you.

Nutritional therapy training
Institute for Optimum Nutrition (ION) offers a three-year foundation degree course in nutritional therapy that includes training in the optimum nutrition approach to mental health. There is a clinic, a list of nutrition practitioners across the UK, an information service and a quarterly journal – *Optimum Nutrition*. Contact ION at Avalon House, 72 Lower Mortlake Road, Richmond TW9 2JY.

Tel: +44 (0) 20 8877 9993 or visit www.ion.ac.uk. To find a nutritional therapist near you who we recommend, visit www.patrickholford.com and click on 'consultations'.

Psychocalisthenics

Psychocalisthenics is an excellent exercise system that takes less than twenty minutes a day, and develops strength, suppleness and stamina and generates vital energy. The best way to learn it is to do the Psychocalisthenics Training. See www.patrickholford.com (seminars) for details or call 020 8871 2949. Also available is the book *Master Level Exercise, Psychocalisthenics*, the Psychocalisthenics CD and DVD. For more information please see www.pcals.com

Water filters

There are many water filters on the market. One of the best is offered by the Fresh Water Filter Company who provide mains-attached water-filtering units.

Tel: 020 8597 3223. Website: www.freshwaterfilter.com

Tests

Homocysteine tests

YorkTest Laboratories produce a home test kit where you can take your own pinprick blood sample and return it to the lab for analysis. If your homocysteine level is high, full instructions are provided to help you reduce it. At the time of going to press, the test costs £75.

Tel: 0800 074 6185. Website: www.yorktest.com

Also see www.thehfactor.com for details of other labs, supplements and to order *The H Factor* (see Recommended Reading).

Food or chemical allergy and intolerance tests

YorkTest also sell a home test kit for food and chemical allergies that requires a pinprick blood sample. YorkTest laboratories will test you for sensitivity to all foods including gluten, gliadin, wheat and yeast. They send you a home test kit that enables you to take a pinprick of blood, so you don't have to go to your doctor.

Call them for a Food Sensitivity Test kit on freephone Tel: 0800 074 6185. Visit www.yorktest.com for more information and prices.

Hair mineral analysis

To determine the presence of any toxic metals, a hair analysis can be arranged via your local nutritional therapist (see www.patrickholford.com for a referral).

Parasite and digestive stool analysis

This helps to identify causes of digestive disorders. These tests can be arranged through your local nutritional therapist (see www.patrickholford.com for a referral).

Supplement, Remedy and Supplier Directory

Finding you own perfect supplement programme can be confusing, but my website, www.patrickholford.com, offers useful guidance.

The backbone of a good supplement programme is:

- A high-strength multivitamin
- Additional vitamin C
- An all-round antioxidant complex
- An essential fat supplement containing omega-3 and omega-6 oils.

In this section I list some of my favourite herbal, food and nutritional supplements. The addresses of the companies whose products I've referred to are given at the end.

Herbal, food and nutritional supplements

Adaptogenic herbs

These include ashwagandha, Asian and American ginseng (Panax), Siberian ginseng (Eleutherococcus), reishi, rhodiola and licorice. These herbs are available in supplements. The amino acids tyrosine and phenylalanine are also important as the building material for dopamine, adrenalin and noradrenalin. BioCare's Awake Food Formula contains tyrosine, ginseng, reishi and B vitamins. Liquorice provides adrenal support. Try Solgar's DGL Root Extract, morning only.

Aloe vera

This plant from the cactus family has many healing properties and supports healthy digestion, skin and immunity. As such it is a good all-round tonic. Aloe vera juices vary considerably in strength or dilution. What you should look for is the amount of MPS (mucopolysaccharide precipitating solids) per litre. You want more than 10,000 MPS for a high-quality product. My two favourites are Forever Living Products and BioCare's Aloe Vera capsules.

Antioxidants

A good all-round antioxidant complex should provide vitamin A (beta-carotene and/or retinol), vitamins C and E, zinc, selenium, glutathione or cysteine, anthocyanidins of berry extracts, lipoic acid and co-enzyme Q10. My favourite is BioCare's AGE Antioxidant followed by Solgar's Advanced Antioxidant Nutrients. Complexes of bioflavonoids, often found together with vitamin C, are available from both companies.

Bone health

Minerals such as calcium, magnesium, boron, zinc and silica plus vitamins C and D all help support bone health. My two favourite supplements are Solgar's Advanced Calcium Complex and BioCare's Osteoplex.

Brain support and phospholipid supplements

The brain needs essential fats (see page 490), phospholipids such as phosphatidyl choline and phosphatidyl serine, plus other key nutrients to function optimally. These include pyroglutamate and DMAE, from which the brain can make phosphatidyl choline. Biocare's Brain Food Formula contains all these, plus some ginkgo.

Phosphatidyl serine is available in 100mg capsules from Solgar and other companies. Phosphatidyl choline (PC) can be found in lecithin granules.

Calming nutrients and herbs

The contraction and relaxation of nerves and muscles is controlled by calcium and magnesium. BioCare's Chill Food contains a combination of amino acids, magnesium and herbs.

Hops, passion flower and valerian are traditionally classified as 'calming' herbs. Valerian, in fact, is more soporific. Try Solgar's Standardised Valerian Root Extract.

Colon cleansing and detox supplements

Various herbs and fibres help to cleanse the digestive tract and are a great support for a detox programme. BioCare's Psyllium Plus contains psyllium husk which helps clear the digestive tract and provides tremendous support for any detox programme.

Creams and balms

For stiff or injured muscles or joints I recommend the herb boswellia, as well as ginger, capsaicin and peppermint. For skin healing, ascorbyl palmitate (vitamin C) and aloe vera are excellent, as is MSM, a form of sulphur. BioCare's Joint Protection is excellent for stiff or injured joints.

Digestive enzymes and support

Any decent digestive enzyme needs to contain enzymes to digest protein (protease), carbohydrate (amylase) and fat (lipase). Some also contain amyloglucosidase, which digests glucosides founds in certain beans and vegetables noted for their flatulent effects. One of my favourites is Solgar's Vegan Digestive Enzymes. BioCare's Digest Pro is also excellent.

Some people have low levels of betaine hydrochloride (stomach acid). You can supplement this on its own and, if it helps digestion, then this may be your problem. Solgar's Digestive Aid supplement contains betaine HCL, plus other digestive enzymes. It is not vegetarian.

Essential fats and fish oil supplements

The most important omega-3 fats are DHA and EPA, the richest source being cod liver oil. The most important omega-6 fat is GLA, the richest source being borage (also known as starflower) oil. My favourite supplement is BioCare's Essential Omegas, which provides a highly concentrated mix of EPA, DHA and GLA. They also produce an Omega 3 Fish Oil supplement – good value, as is Seven Seas Extra High Strength Cod Liver Oil. Both these products have consistently proven the purest when tested for PCB residues, which are in almost all fish. Cod liver oil also contains vitamin A. BioCare's Mega GLA Complex and Solgar's One-A-Day GLA are good value if you only want omega-6 fats.

Eye support

Eyes need antioxidants and a good supply helps support healthy eyesight. Solgar's Bilberry, BioCare EyeCare Plus and Solgar's Bilberry Ginkgo Eyebright Complex also provides vitamin A and other antioxidants such as vitamin C, E and selenium, which also protect against radiation from computer screens. BioCare's EyeCare Plus also contains lutein, bilberry anthocyanidins and grapeseed extracts which are powerful eye-friendly antioxidants.

Get Up & Go!

This tasty breakfast shake that you blend with some milk or juice, plus a banana or other fruit, provides significant amounts of vitamins and minerals plus protein from a blend of rice, soya and quinoa, plus fibre from rice and oat bran, plus essential fatty acids from sesame, sunflower and pumpkin seeds. At less than 500 calories, this adds up to a substantial and sustaining healthy breakfast. Available from BioCare.

Hair and skin

Particularly for women who are losing their hair, Nature's Best NutriHair (mail order on 01892 552118), best taken three times a day, is excellent. My favourite skin formula is The Sher System Skin Support Formula, formulated by skin guru Helen Sher and sold by Higher Nature. MSM, the highly bioavailable form of sulphur, is also great for the skin. MSM 1,000mg tablets, 500mg vegetarian capsules, and powder, are also available from BioCare.

Hormone friendly supplements

There are many herbs, vitamins, minerals and phytonutrients, such as isoflavones, that influence hormonal health.

For the thyroid try BioCare's Thyro Complex. For women with periods try BioCare's Female Balance. For men, try BioCare's Muira Puama and Damiana and Saw Palmetto & Pygeum Bark.

Immune support and vitamin C supplements

Vitamin C is the nutrient most vital for keeping your immune system healthy. Also important are zinc, bioflavanoids and anthocyanidins which are found in berries, the best of which are elderberry and bilberry. Of the herbs, echinacea and cat's claw (*Uncaria tomentosa*) offer the best immune support. BioCare's ImmuneC® provides all the above, except echinacea. Grapefruit seed extract, known as citricidal, is also an important part of a natural immune protection programme. Citricidal is available through BioCare.

Multivitamin and mineral supplements

Supplementing the right multivitamin is the most important supplement decision you make. Most multis are based on RDA levels of nutrients, which are not the same as optimum nutrition levels. The best multivitamin, based on optimum nutrition levels, is BioCare's Advanced Optimum Nutrition Formula. The second best is Solgar's VM2000. Both of these recommend 2 tablets a day. Advanced Optimum Nutrition Formula has better mineral levels, especially for calcium and magnesium. Ideally, both should be taken with an extra 1g of vitamin C.

Probiotics

Probiotics are supplements of beneficial bacteria, the two main strains being *Lactobacillus acidophilus* and *Bifidobacterium bifidus*. There are various types of strain within these two, some more important in children, others in adults. There is quite some variability in amounts of bacteria (some labels say things like 'a billion viable organisms per capsule') and quality. I consider the following supplements to be high quality and well formulated: BioCare's Bifidoinfantis can be taken from birth to weaning; once weaned, babies and children can take BioCare's Banana or Strawberry Acidophilus powder, plain Bio-acidophilus capsules or Solgar's ABCDophilus. Adults can try BioCare's Bio-Acidophilus.

Supplements for snoring

I would recommend Snore Way (mail order on 01355 243091).

Weight loss support

There are three supplements worth considering to support proper metabolism while you are on a weight loss diet. These are 200 mcg of chromium, 750mg HCA (hydroxycitric acid) and 1,000mg CLA (conjugated linoleic acid). BioCare's Cinnachrome is the best, followed by Solgar's HCA and chromium supplements. Take chromium once a day in the morning, and HCA and CLA with each meal.

Supplement Company Directory

In the UK

The following companies produce good-quality supplements that are widely available in the UK.

BioCare Available in most healthfood shops. Tel: 0121 433 3727. Website: www.BioCare.co.uk

Seven Seas Specialise in cod liver oil, rich in omega-3 fats. Available in healthfood stores and pharmacies. Website: www.seven-seas.ltd.uk

Solgar Available in most healthfood shops. Contact Solgar on 01442 890355 for your nearest supplier. Website: www.solgar.co.uk

Health Products for Life It is the best 'e'-health food shop that stocks all the products I recommend, from supplements to water filters. But you can also order by phone on 020 8874 8038. Website: www.healthproductsforlife.com

In other regions

South Africa Bioharmony produce a wide range of products in South Africa and other African countries. For details of your nearest supplier contact 0860 888 339 or visit www.bioharmony.co.za

Australia Solgar supplements are available in Australia. Contact Solgar on 1800 029 871 (free call) for your nearest supplier. Website: www.solgar.com.au. Another good brand is Blackmores.

New Zealand BioCare products are available in New Zealand. Contact Aurora Natural Therapies, 4 La Trobe Track, KareKare, Waitakere City, Auckland 1232, New Zealand. www.Aurora.org.nz

Singapore BioCare and Solgar products are available in Singapore. Contact Essential Living on 6276 1380 for your nearest supplier or visit www.essliv.com

INDEX

Index

Index

fractures 77, 229–30
frankinscence 187
free radicals 15–16, 206–7, 334, 422, 432
fried foods 61, 80, 141, 216, 217, 264, 428
frozen vegetables 90
fructose 106, 107
fruit 82–92
  for acid reflux 180
  and acne 25
  as alkali-forming food 74
  for Alzheimer's prevention 351
  anti-inflammatory effects 255
  and cancer 142, 146
  citrus 12–13, 27, 30, 48, 86, 302
  for constipation 32
  daily requirements 65
  for detox programmes 60, 62, 149, 291
  dried 61, 106
  for eye conditions 195–6
  for flying support 318–19
  for glandular fever 201
  for pollution support 207
  as snack 69
  for weaning 26
fruit juice 42, 60, 85–6, 106, 201
frying 72–3

GABA 287, 361, 385, 394, 395
galactosides 179
gallbladder flush 199, 200
gallbladder problems 198–200
gallstones 198–200
  calcified stones 199–200
  fat deposits 199–200
garlic 34, 86–7, 142, 176, 213, 223–4, 262, 294, 302
  anti-cancer effects 146
  blood-thinning properties 324
  as insect bite deterrent 316
  for sinus infections 322
  topical 28

gastrointestinal reflux 35–6, 180–1
genetically modified (GM) food 115–17
genistein 100, 144, 151
genital herpes 200–1
germ 113
Giardia 176, 183
ginger 3, 137, 139, 165, 187, 211, 236, 328–9, 471
gingko biloba 194, 196, 211, 213, 257–8, 324, 352, 372–3
ginseng 173, 288, 301, 324, 343, 377, 403
  American 329
  Asian 189, 194
  Chinese/Korean 329–30, 343, 360, 377
  Siberian 189, 194, 227, 329, 343, 360, 377, 386
GLA (gamma-linolenic acid)
  for asthma 29–30
  for menstrual problems 476, 478
  for the nerves 241
  and pain 252
  for pregnancy 476
  for schizophrenia 375
  for the skin 35, 186, 273, 277
glandular fever 201–2
glaucoma 84
Glen, Iain 373
gliadin 111, 192, 232
glucosamine 137, 223–4, 436
glucose 73, 105
  see also blood sugar levels
  impaired tolerance 480–1
glucosides 83
glucosinolates 59, 85, 91, 190
glutamine 4, 20–1, 33, 48, 61, 62–3, 166, 167, 176, 229, 262, 287, 385, 396
  for Alzheimer's prevention 352
  for chemotherapy 155
  for hangovers 393, 394

for physical exercise 409, 411
for stomach ulcers 299
for travellers' diarrhoea 319
glutathione 188, 308, 393, 423
  for Alzheimer's prevention 351
  anti-ageing effects 16, 17
  for detox programmes 59
  for fatigue 236
  for hay fever 5
  for the nerves 240
  for paracetamol toxicity 253
  for smoking 390
glutathione peroxidase 428
gluten (wheat protein)
  allergies 8–9, 12–13, 32, 45, 47–8, 49, 110–11, 136–7, 167, 180, 185, 191–2, 232, 258, 302
  and candida 293–4
  and Graves' disease 203, 204
  and systemic lupus erythamatosis 292
  and thyroid function 297
gluten-free products 32
glycaemic indices 73–4
glycaemic load 74
glycine 20–1, 405
Goddard, Frank 28
goldenseal 176
gout 202–3
grains 60, 95, 119, 127
  see also specific grains; wholegrains
grapefruit seed extract 34, 140, 183–4, 186, 294, 319, 330
grapes 86, 408
grasses 5
Graves' disease 203–4
green tea 401–2
griffonia 441
growing pains 36
guarana 402–3
gums, bleeding 244, 430

haemorrhagic disease 472–3
haemorrhoids 204–5, 430

Index

Index

multiple sclerosis (MS)
240–1
multivitamins and minerals
34, 65, 66, 135, 262,
339, 377, 391, 413–14,
417, 422, 423, 434,
465, 486
absorption 416
for alcohol problems 396,
397
for children 40, 45, 50,
54–5
for diabetes 170
for dizziness 185
for eczema 186
for fatigue 236
for fertility 460
for fibromyalgia 198
for flatulence/bloating
179
for glandular fever 201,
202
for hair and scalp 282,
283, 285
for hangovers 394
and headaches 208
for nails 285, 286
for the nerves 241
for osteoporosis 246
for physical exercises 409,
411
for pregnancy 467, 468
for restless leg syndrome
259
for seasonal affective
disorder 368
for skin 266, 270
for stress support 288
for superbugs 289
suppliers 492
for systemic lupus
erythamatosis 292
for tiredness 190
for vegans/vegetarians
126, 128
and yellow urine 419
muscles
problems 229–30, 237–9
relaxants 102, 212, 216
and weight loss 449, 451
and weight training
409–10
mushrooms 334–5
shitake 142, 334–5

mustard 325
myelin sheath 239, 240, 241

N-acetyl cysteine (NAC)
226, 351, 393
N-acetyl glucosamine
(NAG) 138
nails 285–6
nasal sprays, saline solution
321
naturopaths 200, 225
nausea/vomiting 328, 329
of morning sickness 471
of motion sickness 236–7
support for during cancer
therapy 155, 156
travel-related 183–4
necks, painful 238
nervous system conditions
239–41
neutral foods 75
*New England Journal of
Medicine* 153–4
New Scientist (journal)
444
newborns, vitamin K for
472–3
niacinamide 212–13
nicotinamide adenine
dinucleotide-hydrogen
(NADH) 437–8
nicotine 388
night blindness 49, 84
nightshade family of plants
48
nitric oxide 343
non-steroidal anti-
inflammatory drugs
(NSAIDs) 61
nonylphenol 311
noradrenalin 256
nosebleeds 242
nutrition *see* diet and
nutrition
nutritional therapists 33,
61, 70–1, 150, 166,
177, 179, 200, 203,
212, 240, 259, 279,
301, 356, 379, 393,
467, 483
training 483
nuts 96–102, 125–6, 127,
275, 290
for bones 251

for detox programmes
61
roasted 99
Nystatin 51, 294, 348

oats 3–4, 111, 232–3
oesophageal sphincter 35
oestradiol 454–5
oestrogen 227, 333, 462,
464
see also phyto-oestrogens
deficiency 264–5
dominance 147, 158,
225–6, 249, 346,
449–50, 455
in tap water 130
testing levels 248
unopposed 480
oestrogen-mimicking
chemicals (xeno-
oestrogens) 130,
145–6, 305–6, 311,
346, 379, 450, 474,
480
oils
see also specific oils
for detox programmes 61
oleic acid 99
olive leaf extract 183–4
olive oil 80, 141, 200
omega-3 essential fatty acids
6, 79, 81, 169, 309,
314, 454, 486
see also ALA; DHA; EPA
and alcohol problems 396
for Alzheimer's
prevention 351
anti-cancer effects 146,
150
anti-inflammatory effects
166, 167, 253, 254,
297, 299
for arthritis 137–8, 139
for asthma 29
for autism 47
blood-thinning qualities
262
for the brain 92, 93, 357,
358, 359, 360, 371,
372
for children 29, 47, 53,
54, 55–6
in eggs 76
for emphysema 188

Index

Index

Index

vitamin B5 (pantothenic
acid) – *contd*
deficiency signs 252
for hair 283, 284, 285
for hay fever 5
for lowering
homocysteine 351
sources 252
for teeth grinding 386
vitamin B6 (pyridoxine)
356, 362, 440
for acne 265
anti-inflammatory effects
255
for autism 47
for cancer treatment
support 155, 156
defining 423
for diabetes 170, 171
for fatigue 236
for glandular fever 201
for gout 202, 203
for Graves' disease 204
and heart health 215,
217–19
for homocysteine levels
350, 351
for kidney stones 234
for the menopause 464
for menstrual problems
476, 477, 478
as mood enhancer 366–7
for muscles 410
for oral/dental problems
242–3
for Parkinson's disease
256
for Pill support 455, 456
and pregnancy 470–1
for pregnancy 457, 475
for schizophrenia 373
as sleep aid 384
for superbugs 289
taking too much 417–18
for water retention 303
vitamin B12 155, 440
for anaemia 128, 135
anti-ageing effects 17, 18
anti-inflammatory effects
255
for diabetes 171
for fatigue 236
for glandular fever 201
for Graves' disease 204

for hair 18, 284
and heart health 215,
217–19
for homocysteine levels
350, 351
for Parkinson's disease 256
for Pill support 455, 456
and pregnancy 457,
470–1, 471
for schizophrenia 373
vegan/vegetarian sources
126, 128
vitamin B complex 78, 208,
227, 291, 310, 395,
465
for acne rosacea 268
and alcohol 392
for anaemia 135
anti-ageing effects 17, 18,
19, 21
anti-inflammatory effects
255
and the Atkins diet 444
for bones 230
for the brain 358, 359,
361
for children 40
for the circulation 258
detoxifying properties
260
for diabetes 171
for dizziness 184, 185
for exhaustion 192–3
for food allergies 7
general requirements 414,
415
and hair 18
and heart health 216–17
for heavy perspiration
148
for HIV/AIDS 226
for homocysteine levels
350
for irritable bowel
syndrome 233
and methylation 15
for nails 285–6
for the nerves 241
for oral/dental problems
243
and osteoporosis 246
for Pill support 455
for polycystic ovary
syndrome 481

for restless leg syndrome
259
for the sex drive 377
for shock 230
as sleep aid 382–3, 384
sources 109, 113
for teeth grinding 386
for thinning blood 213
and urine colour 133
and vision 84
for weight loss 452
vitamin C 83–4, 208, 227,
291, 308, 310, 348,
423, 430, 486
and alcohol problems 396
for allergies 316
for Alzheimer's
prevention 351
anti-ageing effects 15, 16,
22
anti-cancer effects 146,
149, 151, 152, 157
as antihistamine 324
ascorbate/buffered C 424
ascorbic acid 424
for asthma 29, 139
for autism 47
for bleeding gums 244
for bones 230
for children 55
for cholesterol levels 80
for circulation 278
for colds 159–60, 163,
165
for detoxification 59, 62,
260, 262, 339, 389
for diabetes 169, 172
for emphysema 188
ester C 424
excretion 418
for exhaustion 192
for eye conditions 194,
195, 197
for fatigue 236
for flying 318–19
for food allergies 7
forms 424
for general anaesthetic
support 262
general requirements 414
for genital herpes 201
for glandular fever 201,
202
for gout 203